EMBRACE PLEASURE

"In a world where pleasure is pathologized, *Embrace Pleasure* is a breath of fresh air. This is the book the world needs to begin to heal its sexuality and move from trauma to joy. Reading it helped me understand my journey and has given me a clear path to support others in healing. Full of fascinating information, this is essential reading for anyone seeking deeper self-awareness and more pleasure in life."

TAMMY NELSON PHD, TEDX SPEAKER, HOST OF THE PODCAST
THE TROUBLE WITH SEX, AND AUTHOR OF *OPEN MONOGAMY*

"Under the guidance of a master clinician and fellow traveler, *Embrace Pleasure* is a groundbreaking book that integrates sexuality, psychedelics, and profound personal growth. Suited for experienced practitioners, newbies, and curious observers, it provides an overview of the use of psychedelics that has until this point been woefully inattentive to the impact of individual and collective trauma on intimacy, connection, and pleasure. Goldpaugh takes direct aim at the personal, cultural, and professional narratives that have hindered expansive experiences of sexuality and healing. The personal stories of transformation are the heart of this book and include a wide variety of storytellers interviewed by Goldpaugh with moving skill and sensitivity. At a time of such great uncertainty and trauma, this book is urgently needed. Run, don't walk, to your nearest bookseller!"

SUZANNE IASENZA, PHD, AUTHOR OF *TRANSFORMING SEXUAL NARRATIVES* AND COFOUNDER OF THE SEX THERAPY PROGRAM AT THE INSTITUTE FOR CONTEMPORARY PSYCHOTHERAPY

"Finally, a healing resource that combines the ancient power of sex with the wisdom and medicinal nourishment of psychedelics. Now more than ever, we need to embrace pleasure where we can find it, and this book is the warm hug we need to navigate tumultuous times—both inside and out. A must-read healing guide for weary hearts and hungry souls seeking to create meaningful sex and satisfying relationships."

CYNDI DARNELL, SEX AND RELATIONSHIPS THERAPIST AND AUTHOR OF *SEX WHEN YOU DON'T FEEL LIKE IT*

"There's no better author for this much-needed book on healthy eroticism. It is helpful, practical, and long overdue. Goldpaugh reminds us that the war on drugs has always been a war on pleasure and that 'being present with pleasure, sensation, and deep joy even for a moment is a radical act.'"

JULIE HOLLAND, MD, EDITOR OF *THE POT BOOK* AND AUTHOR OF *GOOD CHEMISTRY*

"Creative and erudite, Dee Dee Goldpaugh's *Embrace Pleasure* offers a highly readable and entertaining narrative style that is also deeply informed by scientific research and anthropological perspectives. Once you've read it, your perspectives on sexual trauma, psychedelic therapy, and the healing power of pleasure will be transformed."

JEFFREY GUSS, MD, PSYCHIATRIST, PSYCHOANALYST, AND CLINICAL ASSISTANT PROFESSOR OF PSYCHIATRY AT NEW YORK UNIVERSITY

"With a pleasurable rush, Dee Dee Goldpaugh's *Embrace Pleasure* fills the vacuum created by hundreds of grimly serious books about psychedelics. Imagine acquiring practical, well-researched knowledge that you can use to transmute your emotional pain by skillfully embracing pleasure! I wholeheartedly recommend it."

CHARLES WININGER, LP, LMHC, AUTHOR OF *LISTENING TO ECSTASY*

EMBRACE PLEASURE

HOW PSYCHEDELICS CAN HEAL OUR SEXUALITY

DEE DEE GOLDPAUGH

Park Street Press
Rochester, Vermont

Park Street Press
One Park Street
Rochester, Vermont 05767
www.ParkStPress.com

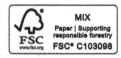

Park Street Press is a division of Inner Traditions International

Copyright © 2025 by Dee Dee Goldpaugh

All rights reserved. No part of this book may be reproduced or utilized in any form or by any means, electronic or mechanical, including photocopying, recording, or any information storage and retrieval system, without permission in writing from the publisher. No part of this book may be used or reproduced to train artificial intelligence technologies or systems.

Cataloging-in-Publication Data for this title is available from the Library of Congress

ISBN 979-8-88850-058-3 (print)
ISBN 979-8-88850-059-0 (ebook)

Printed and bound in the United States by Lake Book Manufacturing, LLC

10 9 8 7 6 5 4 3 2 1

Text design and layout by Virginia Scott Bowman
This book was typeset in Garamond Premier Pro with Oskar Inline used as the display typeface

To send correspondence to the author of this book, mail a first-class letter to the author c/o Inner Traditions • Bear & Company, One Park Street, Rochester, VT 05767, and we will forward the communication, or contact the author directly at **deedeegoldpaugh.com.**

Scan the QR code and save 25% at InnerTraditions.com. Browse over 2,000 titles on spirituality, the occult, ancient mysteries, new science, holistic health, and natural medicine.

Contents

Foreword by Alex Belser, PhD   vii

Acknowledgments   xi

INTRODUCTION
Things to Know Before You Begin Reading   1

1 Healing in Bliss   6
Psychedelics, Sexuality, and the War on Pleasure

2 Psychedelic Sexuality   39
Turn On, Tune In, and Connect

3 Sexual Healing   84
A Psychedelic Approach to Understanding Sexual Violence and Sexual Dysfunction

4 Psychedelic Preparation and Integration for Sexual Healing and Expanded Pleasure   123
Living Ritual

5 High Impact   160
Recovered Memories, Sexual Abuse, and Power Dynamics in Psychedelic Healing

6 In the Garden of Earthly Delights   194
Psychedelic Medicines for Sexual Healing

7 Stories of Transformation   248
Personal Narratives of Psychedelic Sexual Flourishing

8 Big Love   285
A Psychedelic Philosophy of the Heart

Glossary of Psychedelic Terms   297

Notes   304

Bibliography   316

Index   331

Foreword

Alex Belser, PhD

Dear reader,

"Pleasure" is the longest four letter word in the English language.

I'm considering this knotty thought while under a mosquito net in the sweltering heat of the Peruvian Amazon. I'm on an intercultural exchange trip with the Shipibo-Konibo people outside of Pucallpa, staying in a little hut in the rainforest.

For a New Yorker like me, it may seem there is not much pleasure to be had here—the brutal heat sticks to everything, the mosquitos are our constant companions, there is no Wi-Fi. But there are pleasures here too: the sweet savor of maduro at breakfast, a deep sense of relaxation in my bones after a week of rest, and the profound feelings of the psychedelic experience.

There is also the dear pleasure of reading this very book you are now holding.

When Dee Dee Goldpaugh invited me to pen a foreword for their book, I was delighted. Dee Dee is such a beloved figure in the psychedelic world. They are brilliant but not brash, grounded clinically with an abiding heart, and they are able to tackle tough issues with a sense of humor. They aren't afraid to critique the often invisible structures of oppression girding our practices—structures that leave us feeling disconnected from ourselves, estranged from one another, and separate from the cosmos.

Embrace Pleasure: How Psychedelics Can Heal Our Sexuality is part of a broader project to reclaim what has been lost and expand the scope of what may be gained. Dee Dee explores the intricate dynamics of trauma, consent, healing, love, erotic vitality, sexually diverse relationships structures, sexuality with self and others, with a clear-eyed view on how psychedelics can serve as catalysts for healing, growth, and connection.

Dee Dee, with their clear and empathic voice, articulates a vision for a psychedelic philosophy of sexuality, intimacy, and pleasure. In a culture where psychedelics are illegal and pleasure is often seen as naughty, it's quite a feat to bridge the two into a coherent discourse that challenges prevailing societal norms. Dee Dee's book emerges at a crucial time, as our society grapples with the ongoing aftermath of fifty years of the War on Drugs and a prevailing sex-negative attitude that infuses much of our culture, including much of the contemporary psychedelic world. They navigate the historical contexts of psychedelics with great subtlety, from their use in psychotherapy and couples' work to their controversial ban and reemergence as powerful medicines for hard to treat psychiatric conditions. They advocate for the rightful place of psychedelics as a legitimate form of practice for personal and collective healing. They confront the taboo of seeking pleasure as part of a healing path, especially in the "drug" context of psychedelics. In a world where pleasure is an epithet, when we embrace pleasure, it is not only a means of healing trauma, but it's also a revolutionary act.

As you delve into the pages of this book, you are invited to reconsider your own beliefs about pleasure, trauma, and healing. It is likely to be a deeply personal read for you; it was for me. I was able to reconnect to my own body—my knees and joints and muscle and tendons and all the workings of the human organism, and to experience the sensations arising as forms of pleasure to be enjoyed—not as a problem to be solved, but as a reality to be experienced.

Goldpaugh offers not just a theoretical framework, but a practical guide to integrating these insights into your life, fostering a "love bubble" with yourself and your loved ones. Their narrative is a testament to the power of psychedelics to transform our experience of sexuality and intimacy. They urge us towards a future where pleasure is reclaimed as our birthright. As they write, "The question is, are we ready to receive a love that big?"

In our personal conversations on this topic, Dee Dee shared insights that cut to the core of our society's deeply medicalized narratives as they relate to mental health and wellness. Their vision moves beyond the traditional objectification of patients and the so-called delivery of treatment within the health care system, envisioning a shift towards a community-centric, intersubjective approach to healing that values personal connections over impersonal treatments.

They confront the risks of boundary violations and ethical breaches that may accompany psychedelic sexual healing. Dee Dee does not shy away from sexual trauma and offers compassionate guidance. They underscore the critical need for explicit conversations about erotic transference and countertransference in supervisory contexts and in peer-led, community-based support for psychedelic practitioners. Without these discussions, practitioners are left without the tools to appropriately navigate and hold the erotic power that may arise in psychedelic work.

The therapeutic framework needs to be large enough to make sense of the psychedelic phenomena. The attempt to shoehorn complex psychedelic experiences into prescriptive and contained therapeutic modalities such as Cognitive Behavioral Therapy serves to disavow powerful erotic undercurrents that are often present in highly charged treatment settings. This is a significant limitation in current practices for training practitioners in psychedelic therapy.

Dee Dee's critique of the misuse of psychedelics and the dangers of spiritual bypassing is both necessary and timely, as is the call for a sex-positive approach to psychedelic therapy. They speak passionately about including pleasure and the erotic as celebratory aspects of our existence, rather than sources of fear or shame to be pathologized.

In reading, I came to untangle some of my own knots of anxiety and self-doubt and came to face my own fears and longstanding inhibitions. Dee Dee shows us it's possible to write from a place of "safety, embodiment, pleasure, and joy." Lying under that mosquito net, I listened to my body's wisdom. I began to see my doubts as disconnections from deeper truths about pleasure, sexuality, and psychedelics that Dee Dee seeks to heal.

In the same way that "pleasure," our longest four-letter word, encompasses an expanse of experiences and emotions, this book stretches beyond the conventional boundaries of understanding and feeling.

Embrace Pleasure is more than a book. It is a lively manifesto of healing, understanding, and, ultimately, how to feel truly good in our bodies and our hearts. Dee Dee Goldpaugh has crafted a love letter to the world that stands as a testament to the healing power of psychedelics and the revolutionary act of claiming our pleasure. I encourage you to approach the book with an open mind, ready to heal your own sexuality, reclaim pleasure, reconnect with our collective self, and maybe even rediscover the joy of feeling good.

ALEX BELSER, PHD

ALEX BELSER, PHD, is a clinical scientist, author, and licensed psychologist exploring psychedelic therapies. A cofounder of early psychedelic organizations, he researches the potential of psilocybin, DMT, ketamine, and MDMA therapies to improve human health and well-being. He is a coinvestigator at Yale University on a clinical trial to treat obsessive-compulsive disorder (OCD). He served as chief clinical officer at Cybin where he led their clinical programs in the United States and Europe. He is the coeditor of *Queering Psychedelics: From Oppression to Liberation in Psychedelic Medicine* (Synergetic Press). His latest book, *EMBARK Psychedelic Therapy: A New Approach for the Whole Person* (Oxford University Press) offers a clinical guide to working with psychedelic medicines.

Acknowledgments

THANK YOU TO MY PARTNER IN LIFE, Korneel, for walking this path with me and allowing me to share the story of our love. I'm so lucky to have you on this journey. For all that we've shared together and the experiences we are yet to have. I love you.

Thank you to the entire Inner Traditions team, especially my editor, Emilia Cataldo, for believing in this project and bringing this book to life.

Thank you to all of the experts who volunteered their time to share their thoughts with me in interviews and conversations that molded this book. To Alex Belser, who contributed the foreword to this book and who has been a great source of wisdom and perspective. To Justin Natoli, Laura Mae Northrup, Jeffrey Guss, Bill Brennan, Anne Wagner, Adele Lafrance, and Tommaso Barba for sharing their friendship, knowledge, and experience.

To my friends Daniel Grauer, Steve Schwartzberg, Don Shewey, Matthias Von Reusner and Rose Von Reusner and so many others who actually thought a book about psychedelic pleasure was a great idea and tirelessly cheered me on every step of the way and offered feedback on the project. A very special thank you to Charley Wininger, who guided me toward the perfect publisher and for being a ceaseless champion of psychedelic pleasure. Thank you to Lex Pelger for research support. Thank you to Thunder Bear who has been my friend, mentor, and a wise elder in my life who taught me so much about healing, love, and medicine during all of these years of friendship. And to Brett Greene, who once wordlessly handed me a crumpled piece of paper in the forest that contained the message that shaped the underlying philosophy of this book. It said, "Give love to people. Give hell to ideas."

Last, a very special thank you to the survivors, lovers, and psychonauts who shared the stories of their love, healing, and triumphs with psychedelics in chapter seven of this book. May the brave telling of your stories touch every reader.

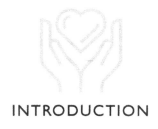

INTRODUCTION

Things to Know before You Begin Reading

THIS BOOK IS THE CULMINATION of a personal healing journey of over twenty years from trauma to transcendence; from isolation to connection; from numbness to being in touch with true pleasure. Western psychotherapy, spiritual practice, and loving relationships all had a role to play in my healing from sexual and relational abuse in childhood and sexual assault as an adult. But nothing has ever been capable of helping me feel, express, move through, and ultimately reconnect to pleasure in the way psychedelic medicines have. I believe this level of healing should be accessible to everyone who wants it. This book is a deeply personal expression because it is a reflection of the most profound healing I've experienced that I hope to share with others. Likewise, these ideas are also drawn from over seventeen years of professional experience as a psychotherapist supporting the healing of my clients. My training background is in somatically oriented trauma therapies including Internal Family Systems (IFS), Eye Movement Desensitization and Reprocessing (EMDR), sex therapy, and also in psychodynamic psychotherapy and relational therapies. I am also a ketamine-assisted psychotherapist and an expert in psychedelic integration psychotherapy, having developed and published specific techniques for sexual trauma survivors.

This book is born into a moment that is a turning point in the history of psychedelic medicines, and the messages contained within have no easy place in the corporate world of medicalized psychedelics which is becoming the dominant paradigm in the West. Readers interested in healing their sexuality, connecting more deeply to pleasure, experiencing more satisfaction in their lives, and who are interested in what role psychedelics might play in that process are the audience for whom I'm writing. However, it's important to know this book is written with the assumption the reader may have some experience with or preexisting knowledge of psychedelics. If you are just starting your exploration of these medicines, or are new to learning about emerging mainstream psychedelic science and the contexts in which it occurs, you may want to first pause and read the glossary of this book, where key concepts in psychedelic research and theory are defined. There are also many wonderful books and websites for learning the very basics about psychedelic medicines and healing. This book is not an attempt to replicate existing foundational texts in this field. My aim in writing this book is to contribute to a psychedelic philosophy of pleasure, as well as offer a critical analysis of, and insights into all that is emerging in the field of psychedelic science. I hope that it will provoke thought, as well as provide useful tools and perspectives for your own healing journey.

This book is not medical advice. It's intended to be information for all people seeking a deeper relationship with pleasure, survivors of sexual and relational trauma, and therapists who wish to offer support to their clients, more holistically empowering them to become active agents of their own healing. In the same spirit, this book is not a how-to on healing your trauma with psychedelics *without* clinical support. The support of highly trained therapists is often needed to heal severe sexual and relational trauma. The case vignettes that appear in this book are all composites from multiple people. No vignette represents a single individual (with the exception of the first-person accounts, all printed with full informed consent of all contributors that appear in chapter seven). The work that happens in the context of therapeutic confidentiality is sacred. The truth is, no one client ever has a story that is not mirrored in others as well. To protect the identities and stories of the people I've worked with, each vignette is a work of fiction inspired by, but removed from, real life.

I am a white, non-binary, queer, trauma survivor who grew up in an environment of financial disadvantage and have now attained education and stable income. As a white person living in the West, I will have blind spots in my perspective and analysis. I want to be clear that I do not presume to speak for the experience of marginalized individuals from communities to which I do not belong, and, while I offer thoughts and commentary on the experience of marginalized individuals from communities to which I *do* belong, no group is a monolith; the complex, intersecting dynamics of power, privilege, discrimination, and other social/cultural forces makes it impossible for me to speak on behalf of all individuals who happen to share a group identity.

It is important to acknowledge however the erasure of certain groups of people (such as BIPOC, disabled or queer people, for example) from contemporary psychedelic research. Many research studies often do not even ask questions that would help differentiate responses to psychedelics in these groups of people, so we really don't know if there are indeed differences that can be illuminated through study. In any discussion of healing from trauma, it is important to acknowledge the discrimination, violence, and increased risk of trauma that members of these and other traditionally marginalized communities have faced and continue to face, which adds to the challenges some people have in feeling safe. Believing we can "cure" depression and anxiety with psychedelics while neglecting to address systemic injustices stemming from the forces of racism, unbridled capitalism, patriarchy, misogyny, colonization, homophobia, transphobia, fatphobia, a Western model of science and medicine characterized by materialist reductionism, and extremist movements such as white supremacy and religious extremism (the list goes on and on) will leave us traumatized and isolated, and are doomed to fail. While I have touched on some of these forces throughout the book, it is impossible to incorporate a full discussion into the complexities surrounding each. It is my hope therefore that diverse future writers continue with this discourse and help it to evolve.

All that being said, while I advocate for a more holistic approach to use of psychedelics, I write from within the cultural context I am situated. While I have made efforts to highlight the research and perspectives of people from traditionally marginalized groups, it is important to note that because the history of Western psychedelic science and research has largely been shaped by white, Western men, I have necessarily relied on the work of many of them to support my endeavor in writing this book. As I say in chapter six: "You can't put toothpaste back in the tube. Here we are. We can only do everything in our power to act ethically given the current circumstances."

It is also important to note that when I use the term "psychedelic science" I am referring to the contemporary Western endeavor of intense research into the use of psychedelics for healing here in the West. While some psychedelics are Western inventions (usually lab-created), plant medicines have a long history of use by Indigenous people, and as such, their use deserves special consideration. While cultural appropriation is a topic worthy of consideration, and while it is difficult to define what avoiding it looks like in practical terms, I believe it is incumbent upon non-indigenous users to consider how they might engage with these medicines in a way that is equitable and enhancing to the community and lineage holders of the medicine, ask questions about whether the work is carried out in a sacred and respectful way, and make an effort to minimize harm to the environment and surrounding communities. Evgenia Fotiou says it best when she says: "Indigenous peoples are not a-historical others but historical agents here and now. Superficial representations of Indigenous peoples and their knowledge systems only cause further trauma. When using plants that have been previously used by Indigenous peoples, at the very least they should be consulted about respectful ways of using them."[1]

Whenever you see me referring to an individual using the pronouns "they/them," it is because the individuals I am referring to have specified that they prefer use of these pronouns when referring to them in the third person. Also, throughout the book the term "man" or "male" and/or "woman" or "female" includes all male-identified and female-identified people respectively.

As I write, all life forms on our planet are experiencing the hottest temperatures ever recorded. Extreme weather has marked the past few months around the globe. We caused this, and it will take massive, extreme collective action not just on the part of individuals, but of corporations and governments to slow down the death rattle of our home planet. She is dying before our eyes. If you've ever attended to the bed of a dying person, a wonderful and mysterious thing can happen. The edges soften. Family members who could not get along find their deeper purpose and put strife aside. Tones are hushed and arguments cease. We understand that we are in the presence of a great transition when someone we love is dying. Grief holds the power to garner perspective and to open our hearts to the present moment. That is the energy I wish to carry into this book. As I sit writing on this dying Earth, I let my heart be softened, filled with compassion. I feel a renewed call to explore pleasure and healing, not just for its own sake, but because connection with our bodies, with our loved ones, our hearts, and the Earth herself is what this moment requires of us. I hope this book and the medicines that this great Earth has offered us, both through science and through plants and animals, can be used to support a shift toward pleasure, healing, and toward love.

1
Healing in Bliss

Psychedelics, Sexuality, and the War on Pleasure

Birds flying high, you know how I feel
Sun in the sky, you know how I feel
Breeze driftin' on by, you know how I feel
It's a new dawn, a new day, a new life for me
And I'm feeling good . . .

"Feeling Good" as sung by Nina Simone

BEHOLD THE MUSHROOM. If we happen to be walking in the forest on a lush, damp day and come upon some fungi punctuating the landscape, what we are actually seeing is its fruiting body, the meaty, sensual, often interesting, sometimes alien-looking part that manifests into the world to which we assign use: culinary, visionary, or environmental. But the part of the mushroom that we don't see, the mycelium, is far more vast and profound than what can easily witnessed above ground. Mycelia can stretch for miles, consisting of a filigree of hyphae that soaks up nourishment for the fruiting body to manifest in its worldly habitat. Not only that, but the mycelia create a vast underground communication network that delivers necessary nutrients to the other plants around it, creating a symbiotic relationship deep beneath the forest floor. So powerful, mycelium can even break down toxic waste created by humans.

As you visualize this mushroom (perhaps it even looks like the famed *Amanita Muscaria*, the red-capped, white-dotted mushroom that has been ubiquitous to artistic renderings of all things psychedelic) the picture that most likely comes to mind is the fruiting body. The flashy, fleshy part of the mushroom. But if we seek to understand what's really going on, if we dare to inspect the scene more closely, we come to understand that the mushroom is being fueled by the expansive and unseen power grid of the mycelium. This is a perfect metaphor for the entheogenic inflection point into which this book has been born, some call a Psychedelic Renaissance. We are witnessing a massive cultural shift around the use and perception of psychedelics. Informed largely by the proliferation of psychedelic research into their therapeutic use in clinical settings, these substances are increasingly shirking their reputation as dangerous drugs of abuse, in favor of a new status as transformative medicines. But this new public perception, fueled by a plethora of mass media articles touting them as miracle cures, actually represents only a part of what psychedelics have to offer, and offers only a narrow view of how they are used. Their secret power, the attributes you won't read about in research studies or popular articles about the healing of depression or smoking cessation, is that the psychedelic experience can also be joyful, sensuous, erotic, ecstatic, and, dare I say, pleasurable.

This book is about a topic that has been overlooked, ignored, and even reviled in the current medicalized psychedelic landscape: the healing power of pleasure. The new psychedelic frontier is populated by psychedelic start-ups racing to design treatments for every type of disorder imaginable in the hopes of banking a massive profit, while wellness gurus, researchers, and expensive retreats centers pitch the promise of miracle transformation. But, in the midst of all the frenzied empire-building, I believe the most powerful healing attribute of psychedelic medicines is being neglected, which is the power of psychedelics to help us connect with deep feelings of pleasure and bliss, connect to ourselves and our bodies, support us in living joyfully, connect to the divine, and embrace love. My intention for this book is to explore a psychedelic philosophy of sexuality, intimacy, and pleasure. Sexuality and psychedelics is a topic interesting in its own right, but my deepest motivation is to shine light on the most neglected and hidden places within ourselves where we carry the most painful wounds that prevent us from fully being fully alive inside our own bodies and connected to profound expressions of love. Healing our sexuality means healing our creativity, healing our wounded inner children, and restoring our life force to balance. Ultimately, a cause far, far beyond merely optimizing erotic pleasure or sexual novelty. All the research, all of the clinical trials, mean nothing if we don't allow these medicines to wake us up to love.

This book is for the curious. That is the only essential ingredient to healing. Can we be curious enough to imagine the life that's possible if we were able to have a relationship to pleasure unmitigated by the stories, striving, and belief systems that conspire to keep us from it? Psychedelic medicines are not a panacea. They are helpers, elders, archangels, delivering to us the message that we are allowed, by virtue of being born in a body, to enjoy our body and the full expanse of our minds, free from shame and outside regulation. Pleasure is our birthright. In this book I aim to describe crucial aspects of how psychedelics can help us to heal our sexuality, deepen sexual satisfaction, connect with pleasure, and come to a renewed relationship with ourselves and deeper relationships with partners. To make this argument convincingly, we must explore what pleasure truly is and what prevents us from accessing it. I will present a perspective on psychedelics and sexuality including a frank discussion of the harms and risks associated with the use of psychedelics. I will also expand upon a definition of one of the primary reasons erotic pleasure eludes us: sexual and relational violence and trauma, and briefly touch upon some of harms perpetrated in psychedelic spaces. Later chapters of this book offer a look at a number of widely used psychedelic medicines and tells a different story, the story you won't hear in popular media, about each centered in their capacity to heal our sexuality and restore embodiment and pleasure.

IT'S THE END OF THE (PSYCHEDELIC) WORLD AS WE KNOW IT (AND I FEEL FINE)

Psychedelics have emerged from the shadow of stigma laid thick by decades of misinformation and prohibition and are now basking in the sun of mainstream attention and acceptance. Around the country, some of the efforts to decriminalize psychedelics are succeeding. Companies providing psychedelic education are training the first generation of clinicians in decades who will provide psychedelic treatments in medical contexts. Research studies on novel substances and proprietary molecules close to, but distinct from, ancestral sacred plant medicines are being pitched as a rapid cure for all manner of mental health disorders. We've now seen ourselves through the trend of microdosing—taking a small, sub-perceptual dose of a psychedelic to improve mental health and optimize performance—and are on to the development of psychedelics that aren't psychedelic at all. In other words, biotech companies, keen to maximize efficiency in the mental health arena, are working assiduously to remove the apparently nasty side effect of actually *tripping* from psychedelic substances.[1]

I entered the entheogenic world when psychedelic conferences meant a few hundred weirdos on folding chairs in a church basement applauding people doing the very limited research at the time and hearing personal stories of healing. Now, I'm lost in a sea of tech bros and investors, pitching pills and transformative retreats, trying to find their way to the business track auditorium of the conference, many of whom have never had any substantial personal experience themselves with these medicines. Once, psychedelics were a world of outlaws and cosmic mind pirates. Now, you can just as easily walk into a conversation about how someone's LSD microdosing schedule has improved their output at work, or a parent discussing how taking mushrooms improves their capacity to be present with their kids. It's a new world.

At the same time, Indigenous peoples and cultures from whom many of these medicines originate are being regarded with increasing respect. Traditionally underrepresented peoples are holding more prominent roles in the Western psychedelic establishment and their voices and contributions are being valued. People who never would have considered psychedelic medicines as something "for them" are becoming curious and engaged in their healing potential. State governments are coming to realize that people should not be prosecuted for accessing healing medicines and are enacting laws to reflect this new stance. It is essential that we consider the potential consequences of an attempt to fold psychedelics into a medical model absent meaningful reform of the health care system this model resides in. Similarly, decriminalizing plant medicines without equal vigor for protecting the environment (the same one these plants originate from) is an exercise in futility, one that may leave us with access to sacred plants, but relegate all of us to life on a dying Earth.

All that being said, some of the contemporary research into psychedelic medicines has truly been thrilling. We have increasing scientific evidence from credible studies that support psychedelic use not only as a powerfully effective method of addressing symptoms of depression and anxiety[2], trauma[3], but also utility in improving creativity,[4] life satisfaction,[5] and mindfulness.[6] These achievements of science sit as jewels atop a hard-won crown. Western scientific and anthropological interest in psychedelics began in the early twentieth century with the discovery of mescaline from the peyote cactus.[7]* But the story of psychedelics in Western science made a quantum leap in 1943 when Swiss chemist Albert Hofmann discovered his "problem child," LSD, a discovery that fueled both a cultural and scientific revolution in the United States.[8] During the 1950s, over 500 scientific articles were published on LSD, not in terms of addiction or social menace, but rather its potential role in psychiatry.[9]

Many of us know some version of what happens next. Psilocybin mushrooms and LSD (and decades later in the 1980s the synthetic entactogen MDMA), all meet the same fate. They all start as tools in the hands of therapists and psychiatrists with tremendous promise to help addiction, depression, and even as adjuncts to couple's therapy. But when people started using these very same substances as vehicles

---

*Indigenous use dates back thousands of years prior to this date.[10]

for personal spiritual growth, sexual enhancement, pleasure, and even political revolution—that is, in a manner not condoned by (and well outside of the bounds of) the medical establishment—they were recast by the authorities as threats to the public good, culminating in the passage of the Controlled Substances Act of 1970, which halted all research and banned the use of all known psychedelics. Not only were people interested in exploring their own consciousness suddenly criminals, but promising research that held the potential to save many lives ended abruptly. Although the reasons why are a book in and of itself, I posit that fear of interracial sex, shifting expectations of gender, the dismantling of sexual mores, and a general cultural prohibition on pleasure have all always been part of the secret impetus for banning psychedelics and other substances under the banner of "public safety."

It wasn't until the 1990s that a new cohort of intrepid psychedelic researchers gained enough institutional legitimacy to support the launch of small clinical studies of psychedelics, as well as the private or academic funding necessary to do so. But psychedelic research had another problem, a respectability problem. If you want to be sure you won't be perceived as a dangerous disruptor of the status quo which led to the demise of the first great wave of psychedelic research during in the 1950s and '60s (something I will explore more later), you better button up your shirt and make sure psychedelics are seen as serious business. A few decades and several thousand peer-reviewed articles later, psychedelics are now a revenant washed clean from the stink of the "Free Love" movement and repackaged as a viable treatment for woes that ail respectable citizens. But what have we sacrificed to arrive in this place? In forging this shiny new facade for psychedelic medicines, many have forgotten that psychedelics have more to offer us than medical science would have us believe. It is important for those of us who live in the West to remember that today's "cutting edge" research stands on the shoulders of Indigenous people who pioneered and refined the use of plant medicines, often over the course of generations, for purposes of healing, community cohesion, and spiritual and visionary practices that continue on to this day.[11] Not to mention the use of psychedelics by legions of "underground" users—largely anonymous psychonaut pioneers, all working outside the bounds of the medical or scientific establishment who—through the sharing of first-hand knowledge with others (first orally, later via the internet)—anonymously contributed to an informal, decentralized collection of "best practices" that long-time underground users have relied on for years to inform their own journeys.

While the Controlled Substances Act of 1970 may have rendered psychedelic research impossible and gave rise to the failed War on Drugs, it did not stop these generations of seekers from continuing to explore their own minds even at great peril of arrest or other dangers. Certain therapists also quietly continued to offer psychedelic treatments to their clients, finding it unconscionable to withhold the very medicines that have the power to heal us on the deepest levels.[12] When psychedelics were made illegal in the United States, they did not disappear: they simply went underground. And like the mycelium of the sacred mushroom, have flourished in darkness providing spiritual nourishment for those curious and intrepid enough to seek them out. But their reputation "above ground" continued to be mired in misinformation and scare tactics fueling the ongoing federal prohibition of these medicines. It is taboo to associate psychedelics with pleasure, especially sexual pleasure. Today's psychedelic research world has been so committed to resurrecting psychedelics and restoring them to legitimacy, that they have overlooked and sometimes vehemently rejected the very reason the vast majority of people drawn to psychedelics used them in the first place. Because they feel good! Because they bring us home to ourselves. Bring us home to the Earth. Bring us home to pleasure; interpersonal, sexual, and sensual. It is my thesis that the restoration of pleasure is the deepest level of healing we can achieve.

The clinical psychedelic literature is sparse on the topic of pleasure. There is abundant research that *points* to pleasure, but only indirectly. Increased mindfulness, openness, qualities of increased creativity and non-judgment, all of which I discuss in depth later in this book, are pleasure-enhancing, yet seem to be beside the point when it comes to contemporary psychedelic research. A notable exception is a paper by

Frederik Bøhling which endeavors to an "affective understanding of the joys of tripping." Bøhling examined 100 "trip reports" of users of psilocybin mushrooms and LSD published in online forums. The author puzzles as to why pleasure has been omitted from the clinical discourse explaining that ignoring pleasure limits our scientific understanding of why people use psychedelics and what happens when they do. After all, pleasure is by far the most common reason people seek to alter their consciousness with substances. Bøhling notes, "One important dimension of the psychedelic experience that the scientific literature does not tell us much about, for example, is that tripping can be extremely *fun*." He describes laughter, engagement with physical activities such as dance, and connection to other people and nature as common tropes in the experience of naturalistic psychedelic use. Bøhling's parting remark? "Using psychedelic drugs for pleasure is purposeless, if we look at it from the prevailing instrumental, neo-liberal, and medical paradigms of contemporary society, but . . . so are all the things that make life worth living."[13]

THE PRINCIPLE OF PLEASURE

Pleasure is a word that conjures strong emotional responses. I've seen this time and time again on the faces of my clients when I ask about pleasure in their lives, or on those of my colleagues when I talk about my work. For some, it evokes a quality of naughtiness, for some shame, for others fear. And for others, exhilaration and curiosity. We all know what pleasure is, we know it when we feel it. But because the cascade of human emotions around the notion of pleasure can be so fraught and so personal, I'd like to present a working definition for our exploration of psychedelics and pleasure. This definition is necessary given that we are molded by both the historical and contemporary rejection of pleasure stemming from Puritanism to modern day Christian extremism that conflates pleasure with sin, idleness, being lost in feeling, and unable to resist excess.

Just this morning I was having my coffee (probably the most pervasively used mind-altering substance in America today) and reading a

New York Times opinion piece about masculinity in American culture. The article quoted a book by a conservative Republican senator who states men are called to "confront evil, embrace servanthood, privilege duty over pleasure, discipline their bodies and order their souls."[14] This view, centered on moral righteousness and the attributes of a well-ordered society, is nothing new. In fact, we are well served to remember that America was colonized by Puritans, people too uptight and pious for England. This conservative perspective pits pleasure against morality and specifically links the denial of pleasure to an elevated form of being. If we are expected to believe that pleasure signifies reckless abandon and social decay, and if survivors of sexual relational traumas associate pleasure with overwhelming sensations that lead to or signal danger, what is an approach to pleasure that supports a hypothesis that pleasure heals?

Being present with pleasure, sensation, and deep joy even for a moment is a radical act. I would not argue that everything we may think of as pleasurable heals us. For example, we can eat ice cream or engage in sex, both activities we often associate with pleasure, and simply be going through the motions. Likewise, we can overdo it, steeping ourselves in so much (so-called) pleasure, whether from alcohol, relentlessly scrolling through social media, or watching pornography, that we end up trapped in a state of suspended animation, not present or alive at all. It is not the act of merely engaging in the activity itself, but rather the savoring; the curious, mindful, sensual unfolding of a moment . . . that's the kind of pleasure I'm talking about. *Pleasure is an act of present moment awareness with a sensation or experience that brings good feeling, positive emotion, and has a quality of savoring the sensual.* True pleasure does not numb us out or disconnect us from life, nor does it necessarily lead us down any morally problematic path. Pleasure is an explosion of authentic presence, an access point to peak living. I hope to convince you that psychedelics hold tremendous promise in their ability to help us connect to this quality of experience during an entheogenic experience, as well as help us expand our window of access to pleasure in post-medicine integration, to support our ability to maintain ongoing life enhancement.

In what I assume to be a bid to "redeem" itself from the bygone era of psychedelic sexual liberation, the current psychedelic ecosystem—firmly entrenched in the same medicalized approach characteristic of nearly all healing modalities in the West—is likely one of the major reasons why pleasure is omitted from the current discourse on these medicines. But why might we as *people* be so resistant to experiencing real pleasure? In my observation, the answer to this question is as systemic as it is personal. First, experiencing pleasure requires safety. Overwhelming stress can be a barrier to feeling safe and a reason people may struggle to feel pleasure. Our current societal condition, characterized by gross economic inequality, in which all adult members in a household may be working a full-time job, beholden to the fast-paced, highly competitive economic system—many struggling simply to meet their basic material needs—are all factors that can contribute to stress. Systemic issues like poverty, relational violence, and barriers to access (to capital, education, and adequate medical care, to name a few), along with the discrimination and violence members of traditionally oppressed communities face, also add to the difficulty of achieving the sense of safety required to experience true pleasure. All of these factors must be part of our foundational awareness as we explore pleasure, else we risk labeling individuals as deficient, responsible for their own suffering, inadequate at reaching for those old bootstraps, when they are simply trying to survive the stressors around them.

Individual survivors of interpersonal or relational traumas, including sexual trauma, have an additional obstacle to achieving the sense of safety necessary to experience true pleasure: the protective nature of the human nervous system. Trauma theorist Bessel van der Kolk shifted the perspective of trauma for many with his widely-read book *The Body Keeps the Score: Brain, Mind, and Body in The Healing of Trauma*.[15] Van der Kolk illustrates how trauma is less about the terrible event that happens to us, and more about how that event is stored in our body and adaptive nervous systems, grooming us to adopt a state of hyper-attunement to any stimulus in our environment that may signal danger. Survivors of sexual trauma, particularly in childhood, often experience even more severe psychological fragmentation leading to a lived experience that is constantly mediating between a safe present and a dangerous past.[16] How can we help our bodies to be present with the pleasure of the present moment if only some parts of us are actually *in* the present moment?

Life in a culture held captive by unbridled capitalism—which rewards profit, competition and material wealth above all else—is another reason we struggle to experience meaningful and enduring pleasure. Prioritizing pleasure might require loosening our grip on unrestrained ambition and productivity, both powerful social influences. As psychologist Stella Resnick puts it, "The fact that in our society people are more interested in peak performance than peak experience says something very significant about our popular values and why it can be hard for people to hold onto their happiness."[17]

Our culture awards achievement and self-control. We are socialized with the legacy of Puritanism that extols work as salvation and pleasure as a path to danger and social disenfranchisement (and perhaps even Hell). Not only might we be toggling between traumas of the past and the present, we are also confronting a toxic culture that values financial dominance over community stability, exertion over joy, and self-control over exaltation. Resnick continues, "While we now have a substantial body of evidence showing that feeling good is good for us, the grand irony is that most people, to varying degrees, hold themselves back from feeling as good as they can."[18] Why might we do that? Because—as mentioned earlier—the body cannot sustain a connection to pleasure unless it feels safe. The ability to take pleasure from situations of simulated danger or intensity (such as those commonly enacted in BDSM and kink play for example) is predicated upon knowledge of actual safety and enthusiastic consent that allows the experience to be pleasurable. We are able to enjoy experiences of high stimulation and exhilaration, sexual and otherwise, when we are fairly sure we won't be harmed.

When we imagine the role psychedelics might play in supporting our access to pleasure, it is essential to consider not just the healing potential of individual psychedelic experiences, but also how to create containers for healing that are truly safe. An effective container is characterized by safety from interpersonal harm, complete removal from (or given the reality of legal restrictions, partial mitigation of) legal risk, safe facilitation, and, in order to limit inherent risks associated with the ingestion of *any* medicine, only using substances known to be free from harmful adulterants in recommended doses. Psychedelic pleasure is not only about destigmatizing fun, it is also about equitable medical access for those who want it, decriminalization, culturally competent psychedelic training, and healing spaces hosted by the communities for whom they are created.

Learning how to reorient our relationship to pleasure plays an important role in healing our sexuality. Sexual pleasure can be any act of stimulation intended to elicit a sexual response, including erotic self-touch, partnered sexual connection, the reading of erotica . . . the menu of delights is limitless. But whether due to sexual abuse, poor sex education, a strict religious upbringing, or simply the struggle to navigate daily life in the modern world, for many of the clients with whom I've worked, the thought of any of these overtly sexual activities is panic-inducing.

Healing our sexuality can also stem from *sensual* pleasures and connection with yourself. The sensations of safety and warmth in a platonic embrace, savoring the feeling of warm water rushing over your skin in the shower, reveling in the silver glow of a moonlit night are all experiences we might have access to in our day-to-day lives that are potentially bursting with sensuality. Bringing a quality of awareness, attunement, and even allowing for the possibility of awe in each moment can transform our life from rote and ordinary, to a playground of the erotic if we allow for the erotic to mean all experience that have the power to bring us deep sensations of pleasure through the body. These experiences of sensuality are available to us in nearly every moment, whether or not we have a partner, and even if we have experienced trauma that makes explicitly sexual connection difficult.

I have observed in my work with hundreds of clients that developing a healing relationship to our sexual selves is far bigger than just learning to enjoy sexual contact or limit out-of-control sexual behaviors. It is about learning to bring our sexual energy, our very life force, into a balanced relationship with the rest of our being, a task that includes ethics, embodiment, and the elimination of shame.

Supporting psychedelic pleasure is a complicated endeavor. Thanks to the trove of mass media articles redeeming the notion of psychedelic healing, people are coming to view psychedelics more favorably. But while psychedelics have gained respectability for their therapeutic utility, their potential to enhance pleasure remains largely unexplored. How and why did we come to see psychedelics as dangerous disruptors of social order and agents of insanity in the first place? The War on Drugs sought to sear a dividing line into the country between "respectable" citizens and drug users. But the conspiracy against drugs also had a secret agenda, and that agenda had to do with sex.

THE WAR ON DRUGS HAS ALWAYS BEEN A WAR ON PLEASURE

"Public enemy number one . . ."[19] with these words, Richard Milhous Nixon marked the beginning of the United States' formal assault not only on illicit drugs, but the people who use them. The phrase "public enemy number one" referred to the scourge of drug abuse supposedly tearing the fabric of the nation apart in the early 1970s, a problem the War on Drugs supposedly sought to rectify. In reality however, the taxpayer-funded War on Drugs resulted in disaster, including the cruel persecution of Black and Brown people and communities, the dismantling of organized political resistance to state violence, and mass incarceration. Much has been written about the political and racist motives behind the War on Drugs, but what goes largely unmentioned is that throughout the 19th and 20th centuries, the United States' policies on drugs were also an attack on *pleasure*. And by pleasure, I am referring not only to the pleasurable effects afforded by the substances themselves, but also things like the fear of "untamed" sexuality, the so-called sexual "moral corruption" of white women (usually by men of color), and the loosening of sexual mores and traditional gender roles.

Understanding this history is important to the thesis of this book, because if one of the obscured reasons psychedelics, and in fact all drugs, are illegal (or gated by the medical establishment) is indicative of an institutional desire to suppress pleasure and sexual autonomy, then the War on Drugs is also a War on Pleasure. The link between the War on Drugs and fear of pleasure is best illustrated in the orchestrated state suppression of the hippie anti-war "Free Love" movement. The Free Love movement, heavily associated with the use of cannabis and LSD, challenged traditional social structures and gender expectations, and promoted the idea of love as an antidote to imperialist violence. But a look further back into history gives us a glimpse into an even more insidious story, the story about how the fear of sex and pleasure fueled United States drug policy.

Prior to the start of the formal War on Drugs in the 1970s, laws had already been enacted to prohibit various substances feared to draw users into moral decay or sexual abandon. But this is nothing new. Mind-altering substances have always inspired fear and fascination. And wherever colonization and religious extremism took hold, you could bet entheogens in particular would face a swift condemnation. Throughout Mesoamerica during the 16th and 17th centuries, sacred texts were burned that contain information on visionary rituals that were then lost to the world.[20] Throughout the New World, cults that used psilocybin mushrooms or mescaline-containing cacti were stamped out, their members facing persecution by Christian colonizers. By 1720 the use of peyote was banned by Spanish oppressors in Mesoamerica.[21]

While the central reason that the Catholic Church sought to ban the use of visionary plants and fungi was primarily about spiritual control, namely ensconcing the institution of the church as the only conduit to a divine experience of God, the historical record implies that the Aztecs, at least, may have been using sacred mushrooms for other pleasures. A main source of information about psilocybin mushroom use in the New World springs from the Aztec culture who referred to the mushroom with the juicy moniker "teonanacatl," the flesh of the gods. In Andy Letcher's exceptionally well-researched and entertaining book, *Shroom: A Cultural History of the Magic Mushroom*, he describes an account by the friar Diego Durán based on an Indigenous source that details the distribution of psychoactive mushrooms at the coronation of an Aztec king in 1481 causing users to "rejoice and grow merry and become somewhat tipsy." Letcher speaks of the "evident delight with which Aztecs took mushrooms to accentuate the pleasure of dancing" as thoroughly modern.[22]

Subsequent centuries of repression of the use of sacred plants in the New World sought to end spiritual practices linked to their consumption. But at least one source suggests that these plants and fungi may have been used for other purposes too, including fun. Since the historical record has largely been destroyed as mentioned above, it's impossible to know if pleasure was a reason ancient cultures might have used these medicines. Since the pursuit of pleasure seems to be a universal human experience, it's hard to imagine that pleasure did not play *some* role in the use of sacred plants and fungi in many cultures, even if it was a happy byproduct of practices centered on healing, spiritual development, or community ritual.

In the United States today, we are still living with the legacy of the modern history of persecution in which the repression of sexuality and pleasure are latent motivations for enacting drug prohibitions. In my opinion, what united arguments against drugs in the United States from the 1870s onwards was the widespread fear that drug use would cause sexual promiscuity, incite sexual violence, and (perhaps most terrifyingly) cause white women to mix with Men of Color who would then lure them into sexual relations. I believe these persecutions had one aim, to curb sexual contact and by extension, pleasure.

This theme can be traced throughout the history of the attitudes and policies surrounding a variety of substances, ranging from the psychedelic to the anesthetic. The first anti-narcotics ordinance in the United States for example, was passed in 1875 targeting opium dens, venues in which people actively sought to experience the pleasure that an opium high induces. Notably, this ordinance against opium not only served as legal basis to justify unrestricted raids and searches of premises owned by the Chinese, but also sought to curb another sources of pleasure: sexual relationships between Chinese men and white women associated with opium dens.[23]* Ironically, by the late 1800s, sixty

---

*The formidable Dr. Carl Hart makes brief mention of these social dynamics in his deeply personal exploration of the racist history of the drug war in *Drug Use for Grown Ups: Chasing Liberty in the Land of Fear.*[24]

percent of opium addicts were not those lured into dens, but instead women prescribed opium by their doctors to treat "female troubles" such as menstrual cramps, uterine issues, and nervous conditions.[25]

The case of the Native American use of peyote represents a parallel, yet unique, attempt at prohibition. Americans of European descent occupy the unceded land of Indigenous Americans. Unlike the Chinese, Native Americans could not be sent "home," so spiritual control (repressing of their right to access their sacred medicines) was used a means not only to force them to assimilate, but to prevent their supposed influence on promoting the "unbridled sexuality" it produced in young girls. In his book *The Peyote Effect, From the Inquisition to the War on Drugs*, Alexander Dawson describes moral panic that ensued as a result of the belief that "secret agents," spreading peyote across western reservations, would undermine the "protection of Indians and their development into the citizenship of the country." Dawson cites testimony given to the United States government that cites "the effect of peyote on morals . . . especially is this true with regard to sexual matters. A number of young girls, some of whom had been attending school, have gone bad under the influence of peyote." Further "scientific" testimony claimed peyote "produced visions that could not be controlled, unbridled sexuality, and an experience that had long lasting effects."[26]

Likewise, the prohibition of cannabis was explicitly linked to fear of sexual relationships between Black and Brown men and white women. Harry Anslinger, the first capo of the Federal Bureau of Narcotics (who also has the distinct honor of being the man who made a career out of personally tormenting singer Billie Holiday) is quoted as saying, "There are 100,000 total marijuana smokers in the U.S. and most are Negros, Hispanics, Filipinos, and entertainers. . . . This marijuana causes white women to seek sexual relationships with Negros, entertainers, and any others."[27] Such historical evidence should give us pause and prompt questions about other motivations for drug prohibition here in the United States. Certainly, there is not one answer to this question, but many. While the massive failure of the War on Drugs has sparked increased interest and support for changing drug policy in the United States, it is equally important to ponder the many covert reasons for drug bans, such as public fear of unbridled sexuality and interracial sexual contact as a means to repress sexuality and pleasure in general.

Certainly, it's impossible to engage in a historical examination of drugs, sex, and pleasure without discussing the social implications of the Summer of Love and the hippie movement. The 1960s represented a time in American culture where young people were pushing back on the sexual, moral, and social norms that had pervaded the post-War years in the United States. The massive consciousness shift of the hippie movement challenged firmly held assumptions about the social roles of women and men, the social order of different races in the United States, and the way people could engage in sexual relationships. In *The Hippies and American Values*, author Timothy Miller references a Time Magazine article from 1967 that outlined the hippie ethos, "Do your own thing, whenever you have to do it, and whenever you want. Drop out. Leave society as you have known it. Leave it utterly. Blow the mind of every straight person you can reach. Turn them on. If not to drugs, then to beauty, love, honesty, fun."[28] This consciousness shift was heavily influenced by two powerful chemicals that came onto the scene during the sixties and changed the world: LSD and the Pill.

The hippies inherited a world from their parent's generation that largely suggested sex should be within marriage (certainly for women), it was your patriotic duty to fight just wars (WWII standing as an example of what may constitute a war worth fighting), and living a life bound by convention and conformity was assumed. The Free Love movement arose as a tidal wave of change. In the midst of all this, the birth control pill was introduced to U.S. markets, giving women far more reproductive control than they had ever had before, and by 1965 twenty-seven percent of American women were on it.[29]

During the Free Love years, you have a rising anti-authoritarian sentiment anchored in opposition to the Vietnam War, mixed with an appetite for sexual freedom. All this happened in a moment when women have exponentially more control over their bodies thanks to the Pill. Radical activist of the era, Peter Coyote, produced a quote that sums up what was perhaps a collective sentiment, "I was interested in two things: overthrowing the government and fucking. They went together seamlessly."[30]

It is against this backdrop that LSD makes its entrance from stage left (stage left being a Sandoz laboratory where the scientist Albert Hoffman accidentally synthesized and ingested a substance in 1943 that would change the world and psychedelic history forever, and send him on the world's first LSD trip). LSD first is considered a powerful tool for therapy to treat alcoholism, depression, and interestingly, to mimic and study psychosis.[31] But the "moral panic" around LSD really doesn't take hold until it begins to creep into the counterculture and act as the trippy rocket fuel for a sexual revolution.

To tell a more robust story about LSD, American culture, and the hippie movement fully would be a book itself (and many good ones have already been written, such as Jay Stevens' *Storming Heaven: LSD and the American Dream* and *Acid Dreams: Complete Social History of LSD, The CIA, The Sixties and Beyond* by Martin Lee and Bruce Shlain). I'll keep my analysis brief and germane to the argument that the War on Drugs was indeed a War on Pleasure, although it is essential to make mention of the fact that by excluding this more fully fleshed out analysis of LSD's influence on American culture, I am also excluding its very dark chapters such as the role LSD played in the brutal murders perpetrated by the Manson Family. Moreover, the 1960s afforded women more sexual autonomy while still falling short of offering them greater political autonomy and financial equality. Problems that "turning on" with LSD clearly didn't solve.

Social scientist Miranda DiPaolo writes, "While the discourse on illegal drugs and marginalization is often focused on cannabis, cocaine, and heroin, I contend that LSD is left out of the conversation too frequently and that it, too, was criminalized in order to target a specific group of people."[32] Who was it intended to target? The hippies. A concerted effort was made in the media to vilify LSD and cast an image of the drug distinct from its use in therapy, but instead its association with a group of long-haired, flower-clad people who wanted to expand their minds and liberate their sexualities from previously constricting social norms. The hippie pleasure revolution was comprised largely of people who detested war and embraced values of equality, peace, and sexual autonomy. While the media-generated rhetoric about the dangers of LSD included scare tactics like such as the untrue assertion that it damaged chromosomes, caused insanity, and uncontrollable impulses,[33] I believe the covert reason that LSD was so heavily stigmatized was because it was the catalyst that shifted minds precisely towards these qualities of non-aggression and sexual autonomy.

Rachel Nuwer's book *I Feel Love: MDMA and The Quest for Connection in Our Fractured World* provides a riveting social history of MDMA which serves as an even more poignant and contemporary example of how the fear of people using a substance for the purpose of pleasure can precipitate a severe governmental response to its use that is not grounded in either science or common sense. Nuwer writes floridly of the salad days of MDMA before it was placed on the U.S. government's restrictive Schedule I, making it both illegal to possess and inhibited access to therapists who had been previously using MDMA primarily as a safe and successful adjunct to couple's therapy. She describes the availability of MDMA-enhanced massage, exclusive nightclubs where MDMA usurped alcohol as the enhancement of choice, and gatherings where human connection ruled.[34]

Nuwer cites Alexander "Sasha" Shulgin's own notes after ingesting MDMA. Nuwer quotes him, "I feel absolutely clean inside, and there is nothing but pure euphoria . . . Everyone must get to experience a profound state like this. I feel totally peaceful. I have lived all my life to get here, and I feel I have come home. I am complete."[35] Shulgin is considered the modern godfather of many psychedelic substances, having discovered novel compounds he most certainly used personally for pleasurable purposes. For reference, see Shulgin's opus *PIHKAL: A Chemical Love Story* which is peppered with stories of the Shulgin and his wife Ann using phenethylamines such as MDMA, 2C-B, and other novel chemicals for sex, connection, and simply exploring the limits of their own hearts and minds.[36]

Shulgin resynthesized MDMA in his lab from a forgotten chemical shelved by Merck in 1912 (a story I will expand upon in chapter six) and reintroduced this substance, considered by many to be the undisputed apex of psychedelic pleasures, to the world. During the 1970s and early

'80s, MDMA enjoyed wide use both in therapy, and in nightlife and personal explorations by users explicitly for the purpose of pleasure. But as MDMA's reputation for pleasure grew, so too did the government's determination to restrict it.

Up until this point, it seems inevitable that MDMA, once an unscheduled substance that permeated both social life and therapy just below the surface, would be cracked down upon once it began to proliferate as a drug of sensual joys. What makes MDMA's story so devastating, and so eye-opening, is exactly how that crackdown happened. Fueled by Reagan-induced drug hysteria, the case of MDMA was brought before a DEA judge tasked with reviewing the evidence on the substance and determining its fate. The DEA judge determined that MDMA indeed had documented therapeutic benefits and low potential for abuse. He recommended MDMA be placed on the less-restrictive Schedule III which would have enshrined its place for medical accessibility. And then, in what is perhaps the most lucid example illustrating how the War on Drugs was less about health and safety than it was a War on Pleasure, the DEA took this determination and said, "You know what? Nah. Therapeutic benefits? Don't care. If people are using it to have fun, it must be banned." And banned it was. It was MDMA's fate to land on Schedule I, the most restrictive category suggesting there was no accepted medical use and a high potential for abuse.[37] Many people knew better.

It is beyond the scope of this book to tell the full and fascinating social history of any of these substances. But it is incumbent upon us to question the narratives we receive about substances, sex, and pleasure, and exactly why these substances have been so vilified in the first place. It is worth noting in summary that the War on Drugs is, and historically has been, largely aimed at narcotics, not psychedelics. And likewise, the people who have suffered most because of the War on Drugs have not been psychedelic users, but instead Black and Brown people and other marginalized communities unfairly targeted and arrested for the use of other substances even though these populations use drugs at about the same rate that white Americans do.[38] Perhaps it's time to use the momentum that psychedelics have gained in terms of mainstream acceptance and leverage that toward a more just drug policy regarding *all* substances that would benefit the people most unjustly harmed.

THE LONG ROAD HOME TO YOURSELF
My Personal Journey of Healing Trauma

It was my own healing journey from sexual and relational abuse in childhood and sexual assault as an adult, as well as my professional therapeutic work with survivors of sexual and relational violence, that inspired me to write this book. For me, it is not theoretical, it's personal. With all this discussion of pleasure, it must be noted up front that when severe sexual or relational violence has occurred, we cannot just wish it away, ignore it, and move on to pleasure. We must take the time to process and accept what has happened to us and grieve what we've lost, or in some cases, never had. I wish that simply taking a psychedelic medicine would catapult us to a state of blissful and complete healing, but it doesn't work that way. The terrible things that have happened to us must be felt, witnessed, and grieved. Community and safe relationships are often not enough to do the job. We might need therapy or other forms of healing with a skilled professional who has the capacity to witness our pain and apply clinical techniques to help our body move through it. There is no ecstasy without first feeling the grief. But in my practice as a psychotherapist, I began to question the medical assumption that healing is the mere remission of symptoms of trauma, anxiety, or depression. True healing is, in fact, so much deeper than that. Healing is coming to a place where we are connected to ourselves, other people, to hope, to accountability, to our bodies, and to the Earth; to a life worth living. Psychedelics can be wildly helpful tools for enabling such connection and thus supporting our ability to heal from acute trauma. We know this from the proliferation of research into their therapeutic potential. But the wider view for which I'm arguing does not stop there. It includes the creation of psychedelic community ritual, sensuality, sexual liberation, and joy, all of which are accessible to us when we are willing to feel and confront the traumas in our past.

I gravitated to the professional practice of psychotherapy and the specific populations with whom I work not only to help others but to find healing myself, to make myself an experiment in healing and benefit others simultaneously. Like many survivors, I sought out traditional psychotherapy as a first step in my own healing process. I had a few very lovely therapists, trained predominantly in psychodynamic approaches to treatment; in other words, therapy that centers on talking and making meaning or garnering insights about your past. While their attunement, caring presence, and being able to tell my story to a compassionate witness was helpful, I recognized that there had to be more. I craved a deeper healing, a more experiential way of processing feeling, which is how I found my way to somatic psychotherapy and psychedelics. As my own healing path unfolded utilizing psychedelic medicines in ceremonial contexts, I began to develop techniques to support trauma survivors going through the process of healing their hearts and bodies.

I became fascinated with the emerging field of psychedelic integration psychotherapy, a type of therapy that helps clients prepare for and make both meaning and use of what they experienced during their psychedelic journeys. I wanted to develop techniques specifically to work with survivors of relational and sexual violations. These were the early days when there were not a multitude of programs and educational resources on psychedelic integration for therapists. Instead, therapists doing integration therapy were evolving our work based on peer-led best practices and personal experience. Typical approaches to psychedelic integration I was encountering in the field generally consisted of just talking to the person about what they had experienced and helping them to find ways of applying the lessons of their psychedelic experiences to their life. Surely, it *is* helpful to have a knowledgeable and non-pathologizing therapist who can help you understand and make meaning of what can be fantastical, scary, or indescribably beautiful experiences. But if talk therapy hadn't helped me heal trauma without psychedelics, why would it be the only appropriate support for psychedelic work?

I started to develop my own techniques by analyzing what helped *me* deal with intrusive memories of abuse. What helped me to stay embodied when I was activated or dysregulated? What helped me to remember and sustain the gains I felt in the days immediately following a plant medicine ceremony? Most of all, what kept me soft and kind to myself and others during this healing process? I came to understand that psychotherapy was a phase of healing, but that healing could continue and expand to community, relationships, and the deepest expressions of joy. My vision for psychedelic healing does not seek to diminish what professional psychotherapy offers. The clear boundaries and techniques to help the body process and release emotion can be a vital first step in the healing process. But medical contexts can also keep survivors in cycles of dependency and reenactment, especially when the treatment they are receiving is primarily focused on the trauma itself. I've worked with many psychotherapy clients over the years who have essentially become professional patients seeing therapist after therapist, often reenacting the trauma of not being helped, understood, or saved from childhood abuse. These clients languish in therapy because they have been *insufficiently supported in imagining who they might be without their traumas*. I don't believe this pattern is a conscious choice not to heal on the part of the client. But more that it is their hurt and scared inner child who, even in being not helped adequately or misunderstood by their therapists, has found the only context in which anyone ever *tried* to help them. Their inner child parts aren't going to give that up! So they continue until the therapist and client are finally deadlocked, stagnant, and the client feels abandoned and disappointed, causing further trauma.

The belief that trauma heals only in the clinical realm has kept many clients tethered to unsatisfying experiences with therapy and therapists they eventually come to view as withholding, inadequate, or ill-equipped to provide the reparenting or robust, reparative relationship for which the client is looking. While psychedelics can be helpful in creating a context in which terrible memories of trauma can be reexperienced and reprocessed, they can also put a survivor into a direct state of bliss, sensuality, and good feeling. Harnessing positive feelings is the antithesis of how many therapists approach work with trauma survivors. Psychedelic experience can be a superhighway to feeling good. And feeling good heals. After all, as trauma expert Janina Fisher explains, "(we) must address the *effects* of the traumatic past. Being able to tolerate remembering a horrific experience is not as important a goal as feeling safe right here, right now."[39] When we can feel safe, we can open up to the beauty of our relationships and the beauty of our world.

One common feature of psychedelic experiences, with virtually all psychedelic medicines, is that in circumstances where our body is indeed as safe as it can be (meaning we are with people attuned to our needs and boundaries whether as guides or companions, the substance we are using is known to be safe from adulterants and administered at the correct dose, and we are in an environment that is a safe container to hold us) the psychedelic experience itself can induce feelings of not only pleasure but also of feeling a secure sense of inner peace and safety from the inside out, which can provide stark relief from a traumatized nervous system hyper-attuned to the threat of harm. In my work with psychedelic integration clients who are also trauma survivors, I have seen firsthand that this synthesis of feeling good and feeling safe can be extremely healing.

No one should have to heal alone, and indeed, loving secure connections with others are essential for healing. While therapists can be crucially helpful in providing relational safety, tools for processing trauma, and a container for insight to take hold, the deepest expressions of trauma healing actually occur when you are living your life fully. Therapy can be a powerful venue for healing. But so can a forest, or an art studio, or a winding highway before you on a road trip. I also hope you'll consider that healing may be an act that unfolds over a lifetime, and that while trauma may be part of your story, it is never your whole story. You are more than what happened to you that you couldn't control. The moment you feel your bare feet on the earth and the sun on your face is a radical act of healing. Exploring the sheer pleasure of the warm water of your shower can be a revolution. Exploring the sensuality of movement in a human body can be an epiphany.

Childhood sexual abuse, rape, incest, and other forms of power-driven, relational violence are easily identified by most as sources of sexual trauma. But to fully understand the nature of trauma, we must broaden our conceptualization of trauma so that it actually encompasses many more of us. Not to pathologize a large part of the population. Just the opposite. Expanding our understanding of sexual violence and its aftermath allows us to understand that the negative experiences that impact our sexual self-perception occur on a spectrum from family, social, and religious shame, and poor sex education, to more overt forms of sexual violence. Growing up in a culture steeped in the sexual shame that springs from the influence of Christianity in shaping cultural attitudes toward sex, experiencing the unwholesome reality of the sexualization of children and objectification of women, unhealthy gender socialization that deprives men of a range of feeling is also sexual violence. Societal forces—for example fatphobia, in which people are shamed for their body type, or sexual harassment, in which (usually) women are preyed upon sexually for example—harm our sexual selves. Virtually none of us grow up with positive mirroring and holistic support around our sexualities because it simply does not exist broadly in our culture. So I'm a trauma survivor, yes. But I ask you to consider, might you be one as well? Did you grow up learning your body was a sacred vessel for exploration and pleasure? Did you experience shaming and judgment for the way you wanted to express your gender, your sexual curiosity, or feel the pressure of compulsory femininity or masculinity? Perhaps this is the first moment of realization that sexual violence, meaning any act that harms one's sexuality, has touched your life as well.

THE GIFT OF PERSPECTIVE

In March of 2023 I had one of the most profound experiences of my life, seeing my grandmother, the archetype of kindness and safety in my life, through her death process. I thought seeing her breathe her last breath would be devastating, and it was. But it was also ecstatic. Seeing this woman of such strong spiritual conviction leave her body while holding her hand filled me with a palpable certainty that there is something beyond our existence in our body, but also that joy and connection were paramount to a good life. In the days following her transition out of her body, consensus reality morphed in mystical ways. I could feel her presence. I would ponder a question and hear her speaking to me. Western psychology might call this bereavement-induced psychosis. But I understood this to be a genuine spiritual experience many people before me had experienced. Was her spirit really speaking to me? (If so, she seemed to be doing just fine.) But when we contemplate psychedelic realities, what does *real* mean? I had a deep spiritual connection with my grandmother, I had internalized her so deeply, that of course she was talking to me. Was it "her" as in some transcendent self speaking from beyond this world? Perhaps. Or was it a manifestation of my own mind's connection to her? Does it matter? I don't think it really does, because it was the connection to her I needed to feel to see me through my acute grief.

About three months before she died, she handed me a giant stack of pictures from my childhood. This stack contained several surprises. First, that the childhood I had spent hours of psychotherapy obsessing over, combing through the worst moments, also contained great happiness. My brain, in its attempt to organize my experience and optimize me for survival as an adult, had prioritized the suffering. But there I was as a child, seemingly having lots of fun! That was part of my story too. Not just the abuse I experienced. The other surprise was that mixed into these hundreds of photos was a picture that must have ended up in the wrong pile. I peered at an image of an infant in an incubator on the first day of life. "That isn't me, I don't think," I puzzled. It was a picture of one of the people who caused me the worst torment and violation during my childhood on the day of their birth. There they were. A helpless baby in a crib totally new to the world before any pain had been caused. At one time, this person who had hurt me so badly was just a baby. A baby wanting love and connection and security. What a gift that was. May I be so lucky that for the rest of my life I can aspire to remember that everyone who has caused me harm was once just a baby in a crib crying out for love. That was my grandmother's last gift to me. The gift of perspective.

CONNECTING WITH THE PLEASURE OF THE PRESENT MOMENT

Sacred Valley, Peru

My partner and I had already been traveling through mountains and ancient cities for days when we arrived in a small town in the Andes. The town is flanked by Inka ruins and antique waterways, its streets a narrow labyrinth of giant stone blocks hoisted into place without anything to hold them but the sheer mathematical perfection of their construction. The town itself was dusty and brown, but the winding streets were filled with the color of gorgeous woven fabrics, the rainbow skirts of the women, and the pinks, yellows, and reds of the ponchos and hats on the men. The sky, a cloudless radiant blue. My partner and I had an appointment to meet with a medicine person recommended by a friend. Not a retreat center, not a person who can be found through an internet search. We were told what street to find and to walk as far as possible toward the mountain. There, we could find him in a small shack surrounded by towering cacti. *He's also on WhatsApp if you get lost*, we were told. You know, ancient, but also modern.

When we arrived, we were greeted by a smiling man with an ageless countenance, long black braided hair, and gleaming teeth. He explained in a patchwork of English and Spanish that he worked with the healing medicine *huachuma* and that if we wanted he would hold a ceremony for us in the mountains and how much it would cost. We were told not to eat any more food until then and to meet him again at seven the following morning. From there we would hike up into the mountains and drink the medicine. "Huachuma medicine . . . beautiful," he said, grinning and nodding reassuringly. We went on our own way to a bustling marketplace to find fruit and other things to bring with us the following morning, including toilet paper. (When I asked about bathroom facilities the answer was simple: *mountain*.) What drew me to this remote town in Peru was not a conscious intention to heal the sexual and relational trauma I had carried for so many years. At that point, I believed I had already done the heavy lifting in healing my trauma in the many plant medicine ceremonies I had done with skilled facilitators with medicines like psilocybin mushrooms, ayahuasca, and even other experiences with huachuma prior to finding myself in the Andes.

During these earlier medicine ceremonies, I had experienced night after night of witnessing and reliving some of the worst moments, and feelings, of my life. Sometimes in these ceremonies the reexperiencing of trauma was accompanied by my adult self entering the picture and protecting my child self, protection I was not afforded as a child when I most needed it. Sometimes these ceremonies would connect me to the perspective necessary to re-narrate the story that had existed within me for so long about my trauma. And yet at other times I would have somatic reactions so massive they appeared to be grand mal seizures allowing my body to release energy and fear that had been trapped within it for decades. These experiences with sacred plants brought me back to life. Made me human. Reconnected me with the parts of myself I most wanted to forget or ignore. The tender parts, the vulnerable parts. These medicines had already shown me that it was safe to feel things besides just anger. I was able to feel a connection to the child part of me that had been banished so far into the background of my existence. This child was a danger and an inconvenience. Moreover, this inner child would, at times, take over my life and relationships, and I despised this child for their needs. Their need for safety made me, the adult, vulnerable, and I hated them for it.

Prior to these intense experiences with plant medicine, nothing had made any significant difference in my life in terms of trauma healing. Not professional success, not positive relationships, not therapy or intensive meditation retreats. Not even time. That's not to say that those things didn't help. I believe they kept me afloat. They maintained me. But I always felt something dramatic was missing. When something in your life is fundamentally missing, or perhaps never there, that state becomes your normal. Many trauma survivors don't even know what their personality is without their trauma. What was missing from my life was a capacity for joy, to be present, *to feel good*. To most people I probably seemed to function quite well, but the measures I had to take to keep the intrusive memories of trauma at bay, to soothe my terror of abandonment, to quell the nightmares that plagued me most nights, to contain an internal world that operated in extremes swinging wildly between over-functioning and quietly falling apart. Because most of the people in my life praised me for being high-achieving academically and artistically, and I did a decent job at masking my dysregulation, the effect was that of being a ghost. A half-person. A being with a smiling face but a broken heart. It's been my experience that when you offer most people the opportunity to engage with your smile but not your brokenness, they take you up on it.

The very last time I participated in an ayahuasca ceremony, which up to that point had been profoundly helpful in my healing, the medicine spirit spoke to me and gave this direction: "Go receive teachings from San Pedro. I have nothing else for you at this time." San Pedro. The medicine known as the guide for healing the heart. And so it was that I found myself in the high Andes, with the vague notion that there must be something left for me to heal and San Pedro would be the spirit guide to help. But I had no idea of what was missing or what I was in for, of how deep healing could actually go. I had no idea what it even meant to be fully alive in a human body. But I was about to learn.

Huachuma medicine, otherwise known by the Spanish colonial name San Pedro, contains the active ingredient mescaline, a chemical cousin to the phenethylamine MDMA, and is an ancestral medicine of the Q'ero people of the high Andes Mountains, the direct descendants of the Inka. It is also used in different ways ritually in Ecuador and Bolivia. The transition from the Quechua name *huachuma* to San Pedro came when Christian colonization and oppression forced the ecstatic practices with the cactus to adapt. Huachuma's name was now Christianized and its ritual use conducted in secret.[40] Under Spanish colonization, its new code name became San Pedro because it's none other than Saint Peter who holds the keys to heaven. It proliferates on the mountainsides and valleys of scorched grass. Its straight columnar body can grow over fifteen feet tall. These, I was told, are the really old "wise" cacti, and during rare times it can blossom a white flower crown, the Grandfather King of the mountains. Huachuma has been largely overlooked in clinical psychedelic research (probably because the "trip" is twelve to fifteen hours, a sensual monster who really lives up to the phrase "all night long") and he is often overshadowed in popularity here in the West by his more famous plant spirit cousin, peyote.

Grandfather Huachuma is also believed to be one of the oldest psychedelic substances to be consumed ritually with archeological evidence pointing back to at least 1200 BCE at the ceremonial site at Chavín de Huantar where a great stone figure called the Lanzón sits at the center of a dark underground maze.[41]* At the Chavín temple, it was believed that ceremonial participants drank huachuma and wandered through the tunnels in blackness illuminated by the hallucinations induced by the cactus making a neon psychedelic filigree around them until they came upon the Lanzón sculpture, part human, part jaguar with a head wrapped in serpents. He holds a giant, phallic cactus pointing to heaven, with rolling eyes, and a grimace.

My journey to meet Grandfather Huachuma that day was very different from the ancient devotees at Chavin, but I would now be touched by the thread of ritual that ran through all the generations who came together with this medicine in nature for healing. It was early morning and the mountain sun hadn't yet reached its maximum intensity. The air was thin and cold as we ascended the side of the mountain to an Inka ruin site. I felt the full capacity of my thigh muscles and lungs as we pressed forward at high elevation to the top of the mountain, a great beast of stone jutting toward heaven, speckled with crumbling ancient fortress walls. Our peak was encircled by higher mountains capped with snow and lower ones textured with green trees and black rock.

Our guide burned Palo Santo, a sacred wood that gives off a sweet smoke, fanning it around the outstretched arms of my partner and I to clear us of unnecessary energies and attract good spirits. He offered us the medicine. It was a large glass of bright green liquid the consistency of snot with an electric, bitter taste. I decided quickly and intuitively I liked the vibe our guide projected. He hung back, playing his flute or drum. I felt attended to without being encroached upon. He had the

---

*To give some historical context, one of the world's oldest religious scriptures, the *Rig-Veda* of the Hindu faith, which has its own controversial history in psychedelia, was composed around the same time.

air of being devoted and humble, trusting the relationship between the medicine and the pilgrim. Over the preceding years I had met many, many medicine facilitators, usually white people serving ancestral medicines from outside of their culture, that relished giving long introductory talks, doing "healings" on people, *and if you were really lucky*, "channeling" what they thought was wrong with you and what you should do about it (according to them, of course). Here on the mountain there was no speaking, only gentle drum beats carried through the wind like a prayer. It was quiet enough to let the medicine speak for himself.

The thing about huachuma is he demands patience. It can take hours to feel an effect from the medicine. He gently rises in your system, first emerging as waves of warm energy coursing through your body. These waves then begin to manifest as undulating rainbow colors outlining the things in your environment. If one aspires to experience very large doses of this medicine, the body takes on a quality of being both alive and pulsing with vibrance, but also heavy. Mythical animals or spirits might show themselves. But, in my experience, you never fully lose your sense of time and place as you can with other psychedelic medicines, you are opened up to seeing other layers of reality in this world, the energy emitted from each living thing. With San Pedro, it becomes abundantly clear that all things are living.

The other thing I've found to be true of Grandfather Huachuma is that he talks to you directly, telling you exactly what you need to know. No interpreting mysterious symbols or trying to discern opaque messages from creatures lurking in inner space, just clear guidance. On this day huachuma told me many things, among them: "You need to leave New York City. If you stay there you will get sick and there will be nothing I can do to protect you." That was August of 2019, before any of us knew the plague of COVID that was yet to come in 2020. Thankfully, I listened and was privileged enough to be able to relocate to the rural farmhouse where I now live.

So, there I was on the side of a mountain with only my partner, our guide, and a large roaming group of alpacas grazing and spitting languidly. The surface of the mountain facing us zipped with color and the outlines of warriors charged across the surface. I wondered if these images were inherent to the land itself and had been revealed by that mountain to many generations of people who sat there before me. My body coursed through with energy matched by the vibrancy of the world around me, each blade of grass, each surface of stone possessed by spirit, animated, alive. I glanced over to see my partner staring out at the same mountain with a satisfied look and shaking their arms now and again releasing the psychedelic shivers. Were these spirit warriors just mine or did they also see them? I later learned they just felt really happy, no spirit warriors. I had no idea how long we'd been there or how long it had been since we'd spoken. My mind was somehow incapable of being anywhere but right on that mountain. I wasn't really thinking about anything. I was just existing in peace. And that was something momentous.

If you are a seasoned reader of psychedelic books, or have had any number of your own psychedelic experiences, my story so far might seem fairly bland. "Person sitting on a mountain in peace," doesn't exactly read as the most riveting of trip stories. But the many experiences of huachuma medicine I've experienced over several trips to Peru all echoed a similar experience of this specific day.* Because on this day, there was no trauma, there was no pain. There were no intrusive thoughts, rushes of anger, or impulse to flee. And most of all, my body belonged to me. For hours, I sat on that mountain doing little besides *feeling good in my human body*. This amazing body that had carried me through life and protected me from some of the most extreme harm.

"This is my human body that belongs to me and *it feels so good*!"

"*Right?*" Grandfather Huachuma said back to me, as if he had known all along. It was better than feeling good. It was a profound state of peace and bliss. Deeper than anything I had ever experienced.

It was from these experiences that I learned the lesson that forms the premise of this book as well as my life; trauma can heal not only through the direct confrontation, reexperiencing and reprocessing of traumatic memories, or by exposing oneself to triggering stimuli until

---

*I've described several of these experiences in different publications and public talks.

your nervous system finally relents as is common of certain contemporary trauma therapies, but can also be healed by offering ourselves safety, embodiment, pleasure, and joy. Perhaps had I not had these earlier experiences in ceremony with ayahuasca and other healing plants, this glorious opening to embodiment would not have been possible. I had no idea before now that the deepest healing would not come through therapy (psychedelic or otherwise), effort, desensitization, or hard emotional work. It would come from the play of shadows and light on a mountain side. It would come watching the figure eights of soaring birds. It would come through the simple and radical act of feeling good right now, in this very moment, an act of sensual rebellion.

Yes, psychedelics are substances that can shift perspective, perception, and somatic experience. But the concept of "psychedelic" is much bigger than that. Like my story of witnessing my grandmother's transition from her body, "psychedelic" can also mean allowing both the big and little moments in life to move you, to transform you. Waking up to the power in nature and the power in human relationships is psychedelic. Orgasm can definitely be psychedelic. Love, an altered state, can be psychedelic. Trauma blocks our capacity to be in the here and now. To open up to the pleasure of this present moment. As Frank Anderson puts it in his wonderful book, *Transcending Trauma: Healing Complex PTSD with Internal Family Systems Therapy*, "I believe in a fundamental and universal truth: Trauma blocks love and connection, and healing our wounds provides access to the love and goodness that is inherent in us all."[42] Psychedelic indeed.

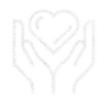

2
Psychedelic Sexuality
Turn On, Tune In, and Connect

Give to me sweet sacred bliss
Your mouth was made to suck my kiss
　　　　"Suck My Kiss" by Red Hot Chili Peppers

WHAT DOES IT MEAN TO CULTIVATE an authentic, honest, and erotically healthy relationship to our sexuality? How could it be that an aspect of self that is so fundamental to our personhood could simultaneously cause so much inner conflict and be the locus of confusion for so many people? Sexuality is an omnipresent cultural phenomenon, and yet we are constantly being implicitly and explicitly told the "right" way to be sexual, how sexual we are allowed to be, and swiftly punished when we step over that line. Developing a healthy erotic identity in early life is a nearly impossible task in a culture steeped in things like religious shame, the commodification and commercialization of sexuality (which tells us what kinds of bodies are acceptable to love, and instructs us in the acceptable manner of *how* to be sexual), and avoidable suffering and confusion resulting from the absence of meaningful sex education and positive sexual mirroring for children.

One social response to this predicament can be found in the movement toward "sex positivity"—in and of itself a wonderful concept—that champions sexual autonomy, pleasure, and erotic self-acceptance.

However, even the "enlightened" politics of sex positivity can lead to harm when these principles are used to promote yet another standard that speaks to the "right" way to be sexual. The expansive values of sex positivity, an exponentially better approach than what the vast majority of us have inherited, can be co-opted in a way that is devoid of ethics, emotionality, decenters meaningful attachment, and fails to include a genuine appraisal of the risks and rewards of opening oneself up to the deepest way we can share our body and spirit with another person. In the midst of all this, what approach might we develop to sex and sexuality that actually serves our growth and wholeness?

This chapter will endeavor to explore the ways psychedelic experiences can impact and mold our sexual self-perception and relationship to others, describe the interplay between psychedelics and our erotic consciousness, as well as formulate a psychedelic philosophy of sexuality shaped by the values of personal and cognitive liberty, sexual ethics, and erotic love I refer to as Psychedelic Sexuality. The perspectives offered in this chapter are drawn from over a decade of therapeutic psychedelic integration work and psychedelic-assisted therapy sessions with clients looking to develop a more holistic and healthy relationship to their sexualities, as well as my own journey of healing after sexual trauma. However, this chapter is also intended to provide a gentle counterpoint to the current psychedelic discourse on sexuality which seems to exist in a curious dichotomy between New Age visions of cosmic orgasms and modern tantra, or radical sex positivity that abandons the sacred as an aspect of our erotic identities by situating sexual relationships solely in the realm of the political to the exclusion of other facets of eroticism.

My vision of Psychedelic Sexuality includes:

- Celebrating sexuality and pleasure as a birthright; all human beings have an inherent right to pleasure, to a positive relationship with their own sexuality, and to exploring sexual difference.
- Acceptance and respect for all bodies and challenging internal and external expressions of racism, ageism, ableism, and fatphobia.

- Acceptance of our own sexual identity and the sexual identities of others.
- Acceptance of our own gender fluidity and gender diversity in others.
- Including spirituality or a quality of sacredness in our sexual self-perception, connections, and expression, whatever that means for the individual.

Psychedelic Sexuality is both a conceptual framework that describes the mindset of acceptance, curiosity, dignity, and respect for the sexuality of ourselves and others, but it can also describe the features of the psychedelic experience that might support the cultivation of these qualities in our lives. I believe psychedelic experiences, when grounded in an intention for personal erotic growth and sexual acceptance, have tremendous potential to heal our relationship to our sexuality. The specific ways psychedelics might support us in making a shift toward erotic heath is backed up by the existing clinical literature on personality change. These changes include:

- Increased openness, cognitive flexibility, and decreased neuroticism about our sexuality and the sexuality of others.
- Increased empathy and interpersonal connection in relationships.
- Increased mindfulness and presence with pleasure.
- Connecting a quality of sacredness to our sexuality.

PSYCHEDELICS, SEXUALITY, AND PERSONALITY CHANGE

Abundant clinical research suggests that psychedelic medicines show tremendous promise for treating trauma, anxiety, and depression that can disrupt sexual connection and impact sexual functioning. But, here I will focus on several unique outcomes of the psychedelic experience with the potential to transform our sexual selves: the impact of psychedelics on personality that may lead to enhanced erotic health, sexual creativity, and increased capacity to be present with pleasure. In fact, it is precisely the power psychedelics hold to affect personality change that has led them to be regarded with fear by those who view increased tolerance and decreased hunger for dominance as a threat to society. In a recent research paper, José Carlos Bouso aptly points out that it was Timothy Leary's now famous cri de coeur, "Turn on, tune in, drop out" that spoke directly to shifts in personality occasioned by psychedelics that he believed could, on a whole, change society by changing psychedelic users from the inside out.[1] This obviously instilled great fear in those committed to a status quo of capitalism, war, and social control. When I imagine a new vision for Psychedelic Sexuality and sexual ethics, I might amend Leary's dramatic declamation to something like, "Turn on, tune in, and *connect*." In fact, contemporary research into psychedelics supports several observable and consistent shifts in personality that encourage deep connection, and support the development of sexual ethics including increased empathy, openness, post-traumatic growth, and mindfulness that can help us do just that.

One of the most enduring findings related to psychedelics and personality change centers on the personality trait of Openness (one of the so-called "Big Five" personality domains including Conscientiousness, Extraversion, Agreeableness, and Neuroticism). In 2011, a landmark study led by Dr. Katherine MacLean showed that a single "experimentally manipulatable discrete event," namely a high-dose psilocybin experience, paired with preparation and integration in a clinical setting, could shift personality traits normally considered fixed in adulthood. Openness refers to increased tolerance for others' values and views, sensitivity, imagination, and fantasy. The researchers found that when the study participants had a "full mystical experience" while on psilocybin, characterized by feelings of ineffability, transcending time and space, and interconnection between all things, the increase in openness was both greater and endured a year after the experience for those who had mystical experiences than for those who had not.[2]

How does an increase in openness benefit sexuality? Many clients arrive at my practice with very rigid stories about themselves and their sexuality marked by intolerance for their own body and its functioning, a denial of their own desires, and narrow ways they want to experience and control intimacy with others that form as the result of both socialization and trauma. An increase in the domain of openness potentially creates a space to dismantle the stories around our own inadequacy, soften our judgments around the types of erotic play and connection we want, and most importantly open up the capacity for fantasy. The ability to engage in erotic fantasy has two benefits. First, we might begin to break apart the script we've long relied on about the sexual person we are supposed to be, and deepen our relationship to erotic curiosity. Fantasy also allows us, without shame or judgment, to revel in (and reveal) our desires, needs, and erotic wishes.

When we can arrive at a place where our true sexual desires are acknowledged, understood, and accepted by us, we are on a path to greater erotic health. I have witnessed firsthand in my clinical practice, the harm to our psyche that results from disavowing our erotic desires. We may have erotic fantasies we seek to disown because they are viewed as socially inappropriate according to our upbringing or community, or perhaps we simply don't know how to present these fantasies to partners without risking shame or rejection. Cultivating openness allows us to work skillfully with our own erotic shadows, and embrace our own sexual desires. When we can truly accept what is within us, it becomes far easier to find the courage to share our sexual interests with a partner. Failing to master this developmental challenge can lead to severe inner fragmentation that can manifest as compulsive or harmful sexual pursuits, or even highly judgmental attitudes about the sexuality of others.

Increasing openness is not only about enhancing tolerance for our own erotic identity, but it potentially also supports the development of a clear set of sexual ethics that are distinct from the ones with which we were raised that can be practiced in relationships. For example, we might have been raised to believe sex should only be in the context of marriage, but might evolve toward a mature sexual ethic such as only engaging in sexual relationships with full consent and respect rather than in a particular relationship structure. We might also consider acting with empathy, respecting the sexual boundaries of others, and being affirming of sexual practices and interests that are different from our own as sexual ethics. As sex therapist Jack Morin put it in his classic text, *The Erotic Mind: Unlocking the Sources of Sexual Passion and Fulfillment,* "the erotically-healthy person develops a clear set of ethical values that possess intrinsic personal meaning and applies them in the sexual arena." Morin goes on to discuss the concept of *right sexual conduct*. He describes a nearly universal predicament that we can be "dismayed to discover . . . that our early moral training was so fundamentally anti-erotic that it's of limited use to you now." He further points out that the authoritarian and repressive moral guidelines handed to us by dominant religions or cultural norms that emphasize sexual control and repression generally have quite the opposite effect. As he puts it, "prohibitions have a way of increasing one's fascination with the very acts they seek to suppress."[3]

If we cannot rely on our previous moral conditioning to shape our adult sexual ethics, then we are required to step into a deeper level of inquiry about our sexual behaviors that must include sustainable, heart-centered, and emotionally healthy sexual practices that are consistent with our personal sexual ethics and boundaries developed through introspection. The critical ingredient to embracing more sophisticated sexual ethics is an open mind and the capacity to ask hard questions of ourselves. But our sexual lives do not exist in clear-cut reality where there are always easy rules to follow (remember, it's the rules that got us into this mess in the first place). Sexual relationships exist in a shifting landscape of emotions, desires, and previous sexual imprinting. It is for this reason that there is another trait known to be bolstered by psychedelic experience which must exist at the very core of our ethical stance and sexual decision making: empathy.

Literature reviews point to numerous studies of classic psychedelics like psilocybin and LSD, both in and outside clinical settings, that suggest users experienced increased emotional empathy which strengthened pro-social behaviors and relationships.[4] Another study exploring the ritualized use of ayahuasca found that openness and extraversion may increase, while neuroticism may decrease in participants polled after ceremonially facilitated ayahuasca retreats.[5] One particularly touching study observed that for long-term survivors of HIV, some with extreme histories of childhood abuse and stigma, when given group therapy and an individual psilocybin session, experienced psilocybin as a "catalyst for reconstructing their identities from rigidly centered on their past traumas to more flexible and growth-oriented life narratives."[6] So, if psychedelic experience has the potential to leave us more empathic, less neurotic, more open and flexible, how might we apply this in a meaningful way to our erotic identities?

Healthy eroticism must have at its foundation the quality of empathy for both yourself and for your partners, and curiosity about how our past trauma and socialization have given us inadequate tools to navigate our sexuality. So many clients who have come to my practice over the years struggle with their sexual relationships because they cannot square how to get what they want from their partner (for example more or less sex, kink, or sexual variety) with genuine empathy and understanding of their partner's needs, desires, and boundaries. Psychedelic experiences can help us not only tap into a quality of universal love, but at their best, also put us in touch with genuine tenderness for others. Because our sexual relationships are so often the ones in which our drive to get our specific needs met carries the highest emotional stakes, they are also often the same ones in which it is the hardest to experience genuine empathy.

Embracing empathy for our partner means that we have to take on the work of healing our youngest and most vulnerable parts *of ourselves* that crave approval, stimulation, unconditional attention and care, instead of enacting these needs in the sexual arena at the expense of the safety, autotomy, and connection in our relationship. Foundational to the concept of Psychedelic Sexuality is the idea that pleasure is a birthright. But with any right comes responsibility. It is my belief that psychedelic experience offers a potential for growth so that we might undertake the responsibility for our own healing to make us erotically available partners who are also capable of knowing and stating our own boundaries, while simultaneously honoring the sexual uniqueness, needs, and limitations of others. And to do so with kindness.

Mindfulness, according to Jon Kabat-Zinn, one of the leading voices to have popularized the practice in Western culture, is "awareness that arises through paying attention, in the present moment, non-judgmentally."[7] The practice of mindfulness has its roots in Buddhist and Hindu spirituality, but has been secularized (for better and worse) into modalities such as Kabat-Zinn's Mindfulness-Based Stress Reduction, which have found their place in the canon of empirically based psychotherapeutic techniques used for anxiety, depression, trauma, and pain management. The thinking behind mindfulness is that attunement to the present moment cultivates qualities helpful to reducing negative affect and ruminative thoughts. One of the standard measures utilized in research on mindfulness, the Five Facet Mindfulness Questionnaire, outlines *Observation* (being able to watch our inner and outer experience), *Description* (how we perceive and label experiences), *Aware Actions* (our attention to the present moment), *Nonjudgmental Inner Experience*, and *Non-reactivity* as the different facets of perception that can be cultivated through mindfulness practice.[8]

Mindfulness is also fundamental to the practice of sex therapy. Perhaps the most famous sexological duo of all time, Masters and Johnson, pioneered a form of therapy called Sensate Focus that helps people struggling with sexual issues to tune into the sensations in their body, and work with thoughts as they emerge during sensual stimulation, fundamentally, a mindfulness practice. While engaging in a series of progressive touch-based exercises, the process aims at "managing or eliminating performance expectations for any specific emotion, whether it be pleasure, relaxation, or arousal."[9] As it turns out, our inability to be present with pleasure is not only a pervasive sexual experience, but impacts desire, sexual response, the ability to orgasm, and sexual self-esteem.

In her phenomenal book, *Better Sex through Mindfulness, How Women Can Cultivate Desire*, Dr. Lori Brotto situates women's sexual issues in the context of a stressed-out world obsessed with multitasking, when in fact, the opposite is needed for robust and fulfilling sexual response. She writes, "Brain-imaging studies show that distraction and inattention impair our ability to attend to sexual cues. Even in a highly sexually arousing situation, our brains may not be able to pay attention to sexual triggers that are necessary to elicit sexual response.... It's as if the body is in the present, but the mind is elsewhere—lost in thoughts, memories, or plans."[10] Who can't relate to this? On one hand, we may be consumed with the mundane, allowing our to-do list to take over the bedroom. But this lack of mindfulness can also show up when we are fixated on our body's appearance during sex, or monitoring our own sexual responses. For trauma survivors, this experience can come in the form of flashbacks that drive a wedge between the safe connection of the present moment and the horrors of the past.*

A recent meta-analysis of thirteen studies on psychedelics and mindfulness found that "the ingestion of psychedelics is associated with an increase of mindfulness specifically relating to the domains of acceptance, which encompasses non-judgement of inner experience and non-reactivity." In fact, this systematic review looked at studies relating to substances as varied as psilocybin, 5-MeO-DMT, and ayahuasca in clinical, naturalistic,† and ceremonial settings and found clinically significant increases in mindfulness existed across the board after psychedelic ingestion. They further stated that certain studies suggest that gains in qualities such as awareness and non-judgmental inner experience tended to persist when measured days, weeks, and even months after taking a psychedelic.[11]

There are an abundance of ways that increased mindfulness brought about by psychedelics might enhance sexual experience. The ability to be present with pleasure, to stay connected to the body, to relax the parts of us that monitor sexual experiences for the "right" response are all potential outcomes that bolster the quality of sexual interaction through mindfulness. Heightened mindfulness also offers the possibility that sex can become less about achieving a certain end goal, and instead help us to be fully absorbed, alive with the sensations in your body in the present. Mindfulness additionally fosters a quality of present-moment awareness that can support us in avoiding sexual

---

*Sexual trauma and psychedelics is a topic so big it will be the chief focus of the next chapter.
†"Naturalistic" refers to a non-clinical setting, in which the researcher records the behavior of subjects in real world settings.

experiences that are unwanted, too intense, or even triggering as we become not only more aware of, but also present with our own needs, boundaries, and limits as the experience unfolds.

A recent research study presented another striking finding about sex and pleasure: people are simply having less of it. The study examined sexual frequency of nearly ten thousand subjects between 2000 and 2018 and found that for nearly all demographics and relationship statuses, people were doing it less. While these numbers alone don't say much, it was the discussion of possible reasons for these shifts in behavior that struck me. The authors hypothesize that it is not pornography or longer working hours that accounted for the downward trends in sexual connection, but more likely that increased stress, depression, and anxiety could play the biggest role. Additionally, the authors speculate that the ubiquity of smartphones and the decline of real-world skills in human connection may contribute to the erosion of sexual relationships.[12] As it turns out, the unrelenting stress of our modern world has put us out of touch with the very thing that can give us increased well-being, energy, and connection: a sex life worth wanting.

It is also worth noting that research on sexuality often focuses on one metric, frequency. In other words, "How much sex are you having?" The question that is often lost is "How do you feel about the sex you are having?" Clients have often come to my practice with the goal of increasing sexual frequency, when they don't even enjoy the sex that's currently available to them. Why would you want more of something that you feel as though you have to endure, rather than savoring? The first time I saw iconic sex researcher and therapist Peggy Kleinplatz teach I was struck by her obvious, but revolutionary conceptualization around this issue. To paraphrase, *if you want people to want sex, you have to have sex that's worth wanting.* Cultivating sex that's worth wanting means we need to know what it is we want, be willing to ask for it, and to approach sexual connection with an attitude of exploration and joy, all skills I believe are supported by the shifts in personality occasioned by psychedelics.

Psychedelic Sexuality is not about having to dismantle our limits to become a more sexual person, nor is it about aspiring to a model of so-called sexual freedom that meets some outside standard of the right way to be sexual. In fact, becoming your best sexual self might mean making time for genuine connection in your life, *especially* with yourself. For many of the female clients with whom I've worked, the ultimate expression of sexual freedom is not being more outwardly sexual or erotically game, it's saying no to sex they don't want. Psychedelic sexual ethics means honoring the sexual person you are, including the aspects of ourselves that reside in places of shame. However, Psychedelic Sexuality might also mean stretching out of the comfort of other activities—video games, television, social media, and even pornography—and finding the self-energy to show up in our relationships and in the world. For so many of us, it's easier to embrace leisure than it is to embrace real pleasure, because real pleasure demands (and requires) our genuine presence. The call of a psychedelic sex life means stretching past the places we hide and dare to feel deeply. Whether that deeper expression of our genuine self is a strong "No" or a "Hell yes," we are called to be our most authentic selves if we want real enduring satisfaction.

THE DEVIL YOU KNOW
The Case of Ben

Ben came to me seeking help integrating an experience on psilocybin mushrooms that he told me "stirred up a lot of disturbing stuff about me I don't know what to do with." Ben had been curious about having a psychedelic experience, so he did what any curious seeker might do: he got some mushrooms and he tried them. He set up his home in a way he thought would be inviting, made a music playlist, and took his mushrooms. A lot of them. The whole bag in fact. He described a kaleidoscopic experience that included visions of him having sex with demons, witnessing sexual acts with children that disgusted him, and seeing himself as a devil enacting coercive contact with others. He was terrified that all of this lived inside him and that actually, somehow, he was a sexual deviant, only held in check by a thread.

When we dug into Ben's sexual history, it was sadly not unique. He was one of many gay men who had fled bullying and rejection in his community in the Midwest and was embraced in the gay scene in New York

City, where he was viewed as desirable and wanted. So wanted in fact that he was overwhelmed by sexual partners constantly being on offer while he struggled to find a boyfriend with whom he could make an emotional connection. Ben had years of therapy and felt he put his internalized homophobia to bed, so to speak. But he also remembered the reaction of his religious relatives who all of a sudden wouldn't let him be unsupervised around his younger cousins after he came out. That still hurt.

Ben felt caught between the world from which he came that rejected him, but also felt uncomfortable in the New York gay scene, which felt to him superficial and at times compulsive and dark. When we started to unpack his psychedelic experience, Ben was able to get in touch with a part of him that *did* fear a gay devil was alive in him and that his religious relatives were right, he was a demon in hiding. But he also feared becoming a sexual (party) monster that could do things to others without remorse. Through our integration work, Ben was able to resolve his fear that he was an unsafe person, and instead grieve as he put it "that he went out of the frying pan and into the fire." He left behind a world that hated him for his sexuality and fell into a world that expected him to be unrelentingly sexual. He was so hurt and disappointed that the gay world he was able to access did not feel safe or healthy.

A few months later Ben checked in again for more integration after another self-guided psychedelic experience on a lower dose of mushrooms where he was able to process his feelings of hurt and extreme grief through to completion. He excitedly shared that he was starting to date someone who felt genuinely interested in him. And he saw himself as someone worthy of someone's interest, loveable. At the conclusion of our integration work, Ben shared that ultimately, psychedelics led him to deeper self-acceptance that meant rejecting both the religious shame that had been put on him as well as the unrealistic sexual expectations he encountered in New York. He found both his yes, and his no.

SEX ON PSYCHEDELICS?

I'm going to come right out of the gate with the one question that inevitably comes up at every panel, each public talk, and in private conversations when I share with friends or colleagues about the topic of my work, yet enjoys a near total absence in clinical research: What's the deal with sex while *on* psychedelics? Is it a good idea? Should I do it? Is that what you help people do? It seems that most experienced psychonauts have strong opinions about their favorite medicines to combine with sexual experiences, and are keen to know what I think about it. In fact, people love to share their psychedelic sexual experiences when given the opportunity. For some, psychedelics can enhance the depth, sensation, and mystical quality of a sexual experience in ways that are transcendent. But remember, sex itself, when approached mindfully and awake, can be an altered state, a medicine. Being fully present, embodied, and alive in a consensual sexual experience is just about as psychedelic as it gets whether or not a substance is involved. The combination of sex and psychedelics can potentially lead to deeper connection, shared mystical experience, and expanded pleasure, but there are some very important considerations and harm reduction measures that need to be implemented first.

I'd like to share a perspective on sex and psychedelics that comes from my own experience of healing sexual trauma. The process of healing from sexual trauma for me happened in stages, the first of which is common for many trauma survivors. I sought out high stimulation relationships, situations, and misused substances, especially alcohol, for two purposes: to feel something, and simultaneously avoid feelings and sensations I did not want to feel. This is in fact a healing stage. At the time, it was my way of surviving when I would have otherwise been numb, depressed, or alternately totally overwhelmed with unwanted thoughts or sensations stemming from earlier trauma. I was often dissociated during sexual experiences. Yet, I yearned for connection and love that I pursued through relationships. But when sex actually happened, I was often offline entirely, unable to really feel pleasure in my body, and became rapidly bored with sexual partners. When I began the process of healing my trauma during ceremonial psychedelic experiences, I first had to confront the terrible things that had happened, and truly process them. I had to feel all the big feelings of rage, sadness, and grief. But then, these experiences began to shift toward pleasure, joy, and connection with myself and the Earth. I was healing something in myself lost during my childhood: the capacity to play, feel free, and be embodied. It wasn't explicitly sexual, but it was incredibly sensual.

When I met my partner, the person to whom I'm now married, I really wanted to be able to experience pleasure with them. From my individual healing work, my body was ready to trust my own judgment about my wants, needs, and partner choice. Trauma was no longer a beast I had to either avoid or suppress. I knew my partner was attuned, caring, and loved me deeply. Rather than wanting to include psychedelics with sex, I instead found that what I really wanted was to bring my psychedelic sexual healing to our intimacy without the use of substances. I wanted to feel what transcendent, mindfully focused, connected sexual experiences really were with someone to whom I felt a safe attachment. The addition of substances to sexual experiences was a way I had previously escaped from feelings I wanted to avoid, to experience increased sexual energy, override my body telling me "no," and to promote an inner narrative that I was a sexually sophisticated and adventurous person. What I really always wanted was to feel alive, safe, and loved. My psychedelic healing led me to a place where I no longer needed substances to enhance, avoid, override, or feel. I could be present with pleasure right then and there in every moment. I could fall in love with my own body, my own pleasure. *Love became the medicine.*

I believe this is an important perspective when the prevailing depiction of psychedelic sex is sex on psychedelics. In fact, sex on psychedelics can be overwhelming or unpredictable for some rather than pleasurable. For me, trauma healing with plant medicines helped to restore pleasure, healthy eroticism, and sensuality to my life. It was a gift I had inside of me all the time. Sober sex, which I had never before been able to tolerate, became the deepest psychedelic experience I could imagine. No substance needed. This story illustrates that for some people combining psychedelics and sex is a powerful healer. But for me, it was the healing I attained through psychedelics that allowed me to become an erotically healthy person.

That said, people have been getting high and having sex just about forever. For people who engage in the practice of using psychedelics to enhance their sexual connection with a partner, new dimensions of eroticism, connection, and sexual mysticism can open up. If using a psychedelic substance during sex is something you are interested in exploring, I encourage you to first consider your motivations. Would adding such a substance to this experience genuinely add a dimension to it that would be relationship or satisfaction-enhancing? If this sex involves a partner, are they a safe person who can respect your boundaries and voice their own? Do you have experience with the substance you'd like to explore during sex so that you can generally know what to expect in terms of the effects, duration, physical sensations, and other somatic aspects? What do you expect will be enhanced by adding an entheogenic dimension to this experience? If you are interested in exploring sex on psychedelics, the following topics are ones to consider to reduce relational harm and optimize pleasure.

Know Your Substance, Know Your Dose

Knowing your substance means you have had experience using the substance in a non-sexual context, you are familiar with its effects, and that to the best of your ability that substance has been tested for harmful adulterants. If I could express one sentiment about psychedelics and sex in a giant blazing neon sign to make you pay attention to it:

> More substance does not necessarily make a better experience.

I really do get the allure of blowing your mind out on psychedelics and having really cosmic sex. But honestly, starting with very low doses of medicines that allow you to stay anchored in the present, aware of what's happening to your body, and attuned to physical limitations (including possible physical injury) is vitally important. No one wants a sex injury when they're high. Remember, mindful sex energy itself is medicine, and should be thought of the same way you might think of combining any two psychedelics; you want a thorough understanding of the way each medicine feels before you bring them out to play together.

Psychedelics and Consent

A fundamental ethic that forms the foundation of Psychedelic Sexuality is enthusiastic, ongoing consent. But navigating consent while actively on any substance is challenging if not impossible. Although recent robust media coverage of campus sexual assault mostly involves the use of alcohol, the developing national conversation about altered states and the nature of consent apply just as much to the use of psychedelics. One psychedelic golden rule you should observe is to negotiate sexual consent in a sober state and continue to respect and abide by those boundaries for the duration of time you are feeling the effect of a medicine. Often, with a foundation of trust firmly in place, consent can be navigated in an ongoing way during a sober sexual experience, but this is not one of those times. If you agreed to certain boundaries before ingesting a medicine, those are the boundaries you keep for that experience. You can always have another experience, or do that totally adventurous thing when sober. In fact, if your perception of your sexual boundaries change during a psychedelic experience, it can be helpful to note that so you can later try to understand more about the feelings that led you to consider more open boundaries.

Respecting your sober sexual boundaries prevents sexual harm or regret for yourself, and potentially, sexual harm to others. It's helpful to understand there is an inner negotiation between what you may want and what feels true to you in a psychedelic state versus a sober state. Certain psychedelic substances, particularly entactogens such as MDMA, can open up new windows of relational possibility, softening defenses, and promoting more flexible thinking about what might be possible in a relationship. It is generally believed that increased connection and empathy engendered by entactogens and many entheogens paves the way for better communication and relationship negotiation. But not always. In some unique integration cases, I've worked with clients who have agreed to changes in relationship structures (say, from monogamy to non-monogamy) only to later feel that MDMA had played a role in the decision they made in the moment that later had to be re-negotiated in a sober state, creating painful feelings of betrayal. I've also worked with individuals who engaged (or more precisely acquiesced) to unwanted sexual behaviors because their increased state of empathy made them not want to reject the pursuer.* In these complex situations, it may not be the case that one party is deliberately seeking to violate consent, or manipulate the psychedelic experience to achieve a certain end, but genuine consent is impacted by psychedelic-induced feelings of empathy and closeness leading to sex that would perhaps not otherwise would have been wanted.

One teaching from my Buddhist training I've found particularly useful when navigating this relational space is that compassion must be mediated by wisdom. Feelings of compassion and openness must be tempered with a more sophisticated analysis of what is actually skillful in a particular relationship or situation: the application of wisdom. For example, one partner may feel like they are being open, accepting, and generous to agree to sexual experiences or shifts in relationship boundaries while in a psychedelic-influenced state. But if these agreements or changes are not built on a sustainable foundation that includes informed, sober consent, the time and space to work with the parts of us that fear change, and the ability to reconsider all of the factors involved in a decision about our sexuality or relationships, the chances of an emotional backlash are high. An old psychedelic rule of thumb is to not make any life-changing decisions within two weeks of a big medicine experience. I would take it further. Psychedelic experiences can transform us by giving us the direct experience of the softening of our inner defenses which can be a great thing for in-depth healing and change facilitated by an integration process. But safely integrating psychedelics into a sexual relationship also means paying attention to how and why these inner defenses have developed and how they protect us. Overriding our defenses and boundaries might seem perfectly right while on psychedelics, but can create massive emotional blowback later.

Your Body Will Keep the Score

It is helpful to know that your body may not function as it normally would during sexual experiences. If you have equipment that normally

---

*This is actually one of the most common reasons heterosexual women report they have sex they do not want: to spare the feelings and ego of their male partners.

gets erect, that just may not happen. Likewise, orgasm can be delayed or impossible. This is especially common with MDMA, one of the love drugs par excellence. (Notice I said *love* drug, not sex drug.) It is helpful to understand this and plan an experience more around sensual pleasure, connection, and stimulation, than centered on the achievement of resolution in the form of genital arousal leading to orgasm. Remember, it's about the ride, not the destination.

Even more importantly, while psychedelics can help heal sexual trauma, they can also cause sexual trauma memories to emerge unexpectedly, which may present both psychologically (memories of abuse) and somatically (activated body states relating to past abuse). It is essential to know that while psychedelics can bring us into the present moment of pleasure, unprocessed trauma can rear its head during a psychedelic experience. Having an emotional first aid plan for yourself, including talking with your partner about how they can support you should difficult feelings or memories emerge, is highly recommended for everyone, but particularly people who are aware of their sexual trauma history. Which makes my next point so important . . .

Partner Choice: Or, Please Don't Go Home with the First Cute Burner You See

I hate to break the news to you, but psychedelics do not make you a good person. If you are someone interested in using psychedelics to look at yourself in hard ways and *become* a *better* person, entheogens hold tremendous promise to support your journey. But psychedelics themselves do not make you more evolved, more spiritual, or more ethical. In fact, in some sad cases they seem to very much make certain people more narcissistic. The topic of people who perpetrate sexual harm will be discussed in great depth later in this book. There are people out there who try to introduce psychedelics on dates to encourage sexual experience that would not normally happen, that use their access to psychedelics or psychedelic spaces to impress people, or even pressure partners to take psychedelics to override consent. I strongly advise that if you want to experience the fullness of what sex and psychedelics have to offer, do it with a trusted partner with whom you already have a working sexual relationship, or develop a working sexual relationship with a partner interested in exploring this with you before you do so.

PSYCHEDELICS AND QUEER IDENTITIES

To be queer is to inhabit a space between, to be liminal. It is a state of existence between worlds, seen and unseen. Throughout history, to be queer is to inhabit the role of the outlaw. Queerness is intrinsically sacred as we are special beings imbued with the power of shapeshifting. To understand the relationship between queerness and psychedelics, we can examine queerness as a concept related to a philosophy of psychedelics, and also explore how queer people uniquely use and benefit from psychedelics. Queer people carry aspects of self that remain hidden and secret for fear of rejection, bullying, and shame. But these aspects of self may metabolize into a great source of power. To be queer means that we carry pain. But it is that very same pain that can deepen our relationship to Spirit and uplift us. Queerness is a liberatory state. Psychedelics are vehicles for transportation to other realities, a space between worlds, and also tools to bring us back to ourselves. Their use often must exist in shadows or in secrecy. Despite the explosion of mainstream acceptance, the psychedelic user focused on freeing their own mind or relating to pleasure remains in the fringe. Psychedelic experience defies our attempts to pin it down or explain it in words. Psychedelics are allies in expansion and connection. When queer people and psychedelics meet, magic is made.

It is first helpful to define "queerness," which is no easy task. The LGBTQIA+ community is comprised of a large, diverse group of individuals, and there is no single consensus within this community on what the term "queer" means. What follows is my working definition of queerness based on my lived and professional experience as a queer person and queer therapist, the reflections of my colleagues who are scholars studying psychedelics and queerness, and personal relationships with progressive queer activists.

While "queer" is a label that often overlaps with LGBTQIA+ (lesbian, gay, bisexual, transgender, queer/questioning, intersex, and asexual) identities, they are actually not the same thing. Many gay or lesbian people do not consider themselves queer, and there are many queer people who hold identities not specifically represented in the LGBTQIA+ acronym. A person who identifies as queer might do so on the basis of the relationships they engage in, say a person who dates people of all genders. A queer person might identify as queer on the basis of their gender identity or gender expression; perhaps it differs from their gender at birth or they have no gender at all. Queerness can be about relationship structures as well. A person might consider themself queer because they do not conform to the expectations of heteromonogamy in how they share intimacy.

In recent years, the term queer has expanded even more and can mean not only people who are outside of the sexual margins, but outside of society's acceptable margins generally, including neurodiversity (the emerging theoretical framework of "neuroqueering" seeks to understand the matrix of neurodiversity, sexuality, and gender) or even spiritual practices such as witchcraft. (Witches are now pretty queer too, if they choose to don the title.) Although this is a very liberal use of the term "queer," which most often (but not always) points to people who are marginalized on the basis of sexuality or gender identity or expression.

But the one common thread that unites all of these disparate groups of people has little to do with sexuality, gender, or the many "othered" identities. Queerness is the synthesis of an identity marker that society traditionally rejects as different or aberrant, often gender or sexuality, a willingness to embrace that difference, and a political stance that is dedicated to the liberation of all oppressed people everywhere regardless of their identities. Queerness is *not apolitical*. So my personal working definition of queerness, consistent with progressive activism, is that it is a self-applied label (if one chooses to label themselves at all) that relates to identities that society considers outside of mainstream acceptability, engages position in the world to stand for the liberation, acceptance, and empowerment of all oppressed people, and, most importantly, being queer is something queer people celebrate about themselves. Queer psychedelic writer Bett Williams, author of the phenomenal book *The Wild Kindness: A Psilocybin Odyssey* put it best when she said, "Queer is a realm of being that is personal, political, spiritual even, and like psychedelics, the form it takes is dependent on cultural context. Queer has always been whatever we decide it is."[13]

I sat down with psychotherapist, author, and queer community activist Justin Natoli, JD, LMFT to dive deeper into the unique relationship between queer people and psychedelics. Justin and I first met at the Psychedelic Science conference in 2023, and it was as if the heavens opened and a being of radiance, intelligence, and spiritual depth (not to mention a tremendous sense of style) appeared. Justin is one of the leading voices developing a queer perspective on psychedelic healing through his clinical work, public speaking, and writing. Justin added some further texture to my definition of queer. "Queerness is absolutely political because whatever gets labeled queer tells us more about the society doing the labeling than the people who carry the queer label. Queerness is broader than just gender and sexual orientation. Queerness might mean all the parts of ourselves that don't fit neatly into the boxes and categories that society considers normal. But the whole concept of normal is an illusion because there's no one way a human is supposed to be. We're supposed to be different. Some people's differences just happen to be labeled as queer based on whatever *status quo* that society is trying to preserve."

How can psychedelics be of benefit to queer people and communities? Even queer people in relatively safe and affirming environments can carry internalized homo and transphobia, can moderate aspects of their presentation and affectation to fit into or achieve safety in straight work or social environments. They may be vague about their relationships, subject to harassment (including physical violence), and are often in the position of having to downplay aspects of self to make others comfortable. Ask anyone who has repeatedly had to tolerate being called the wrong name or referred to by the wrong pronoun and make a gentle correction with a smile on their face. Or worse, keep quiet entirely. Psychedelic experience can not only help heal the pain and trauma queer people carry, but bring them to deeper levels of self-acceptance, release shame, and allow them to live fully empowered lives.

Justin elaborated further, "Queer people are taught that our body's natural aliveness is a problem, so we create a filter where our body has a desire, our body has a way it wants to express itself in the world, and instead of just allowing that energy to flow freely, there's now a filter that says, 'Hey, let's wait a second. What are the consequences of this? Is this safe to do?' This puts shackles around us, around our ability to really explore and express who we are. It creates shackles of fear, shackles of shame, that prevent us from accessing our authentic self and personality. One of the things that psychedelics do so well is open our heart and remove that filter of shame and fear to explore within ourselves. We can really get to know the unique beings we are. Society pathologizes the most beautiful aspects of our uniqueness because they don't fit into the boxes of what it considers normal."

To say that there is a checkered relationship between the medical system, the very place we seem determined to situate psychedelic healing, and queer people would be putting it mildly. While psychedelics themselves might be liberatory tools, they have the potential to cause great harm in the hands of researchers, therapists, and doctors in service to a medical system that at best dehumanizes people, and at worst has abused and discriminated against queer people. If you think that statement seems extreme, a 2020 survey conducted by the LGBTQ Research and Communications Project found fifty percent of transgender people, and sixty-eight percent of transgender People of Color, had been denied medical care, abused, or mistreated by their health care providers.[14] A recent study showed that LGBTQ adults were exponentially more likely to have negative experiences with health care resulting in worsening health than their straight counterparts, and that they were less likely to receive health care altogether to avoid discrimination.[15]

This information is an important backdrop to consider whether psychedelic healing will feel safe and accessible to queer people when situated within the current health care system. Historically, there is a hidden legacy of harm perpetrated against queer people by psychedelic scientists and clinicians that must be illuminated and considered to understand the foundation upon which current psychedelic research is built. Alex Belser and Ava Keating explain, "The history of psychedelic clinical research is rife with 'conversion therapy,' a practice intended to heterosexualize and otherwise conform queer people into hegemonic sexuality and gender norms through the combined application of psychedelics and homophobic propaganda." They continue, "Conversion therapy is most adequately described as a form of clinical abuse; it instills shame and self-rejection."[16] In fact, some of the most beloved luminaries of the early psychedelic movement were involved in the practice of psychedelic conversion therapy, including Stanislov Grof who believed homosexuality was a "neurotic behavior" that was the result of birth trauma.[17] This occurred in the same cultural moment when Timothy Leary's claimed that LSD was a "specific cure for homosexuality."[18]

The history of psychedelic conversion therapy must be situated in its historical context. It is important to note here that homosexuality was once considered a disease to be treated, codified in the first Diagnostic and Statistical Manual (DSM-I) in 1952, where it remained until its removal in 1973. Back then, homosexuality fell under the umbrella of "sexual deviation" alongside pedophilia and sexual sadism including rape, assault, and mutilation.[19] In a particularly cruel twist, when the diagnosis of homosexuality was removed from the DSM, it was replaced by disorders related to being *distressed* by being a homosexual.

Some of the applications of psychedelic conversion therapy historically are coercive and shocking. One particularly heartbreaking story is described by author Zoë Dubus in the book *Queering Psychedelics, From Oppression to Liberation in Psychedelic Medicine*. Dubus details the use of high dose psychedelics as a form of "shock treatment," to "cure" two young boys of homosexuality in a French hospital in the 1960s. They were given astronomically high doses of up to 1,200 mg of mescaline and 800 micrograms of LSD after these youth, fifteen and eighteen years old, were criminally convicted of "indecent acts" in court.[20] But other stories of psychedelic conversion therapy are harder to reconcile. Rather than treatments inflicted on minor children without consent, adults distressed by their identities would seek this treatment voluntarily at places like the Hollywood Hospital.[21] This raises difficult ethical questions about self-determination in treatment. If a patient avails themself for psychedelic conversion therapy, is it ethical?

Before I address the question of ethics, let me address the question of efficacy. A recent position statement by thirty-seven scholars asserts that (non-psychedelic) conversion therapy is "ineffective and likely to cause individuals severe physical and mental pain" and lacks medical validity.[22] Andrea Ens notes that in historical cases of psychedelic conversion therapy it is "impossible to make definitive statements on treatment outcomes . . . based on the limited primary sources available." However, she goes on to describe at least one case of voluntary psychedelic conversion therapy at the Hollywood Hospital in the 1960s that seemingly ended in a successful treatment, namely, a homosexual man ended treatment, found a girlfriend, and was living happily. A year later the same man was receiving non-psychedelic conversion therapy treatment at another facility, struggling and living a socially isolated life.[23] We know conversion therapy does not work. One cannot change their sexual or gender identity with psychedelics or through any other means. (Although anecdotally, I have worked with dozens of clients who came to greater *acceptance* of their sexuality and gender identity through psychedelic use.)

As to the question of whether psychedelic conversion therapy is ethical, if voluntary, I will share this. While, to my knowledge, the harmful practice of psychedelic conversion therapy is no longer administered or promoted by Western practitioners within the medical model, underground practitioners (meaning people serving psychedelic medicines extra-legally) still do receive requests for this treatment. I spoke off the record to an underground practitioner with over twenty years of experience who shared in a personal conversation that he has received requests from gay men from fundamentalist religious backgrounds for psychedelic work aimed at orienting them to heterosexuality. The practitioner, of course, declined the requests suggesting that, in his view, a client's right to self-determination does not trump his commitment to do no harm. To me this seems obvious.

While we can offer some grace to historical figures who practiced psychedelic conversion therapy given that it was codified as a disease at the time, we cannot erase the legacy of harm done. Today, people struggling with their sexuality due to a lack of social support, religious conditioning, or discrimination may still believe that psychedelics can change their sexuality because of the powerful knowledge that psychedelics can and do shift major personality traits as outlined earlier in this chapter. But is the answer to this problem honoring a client's wishes for conversion therapy or offering them sexuality and gender-affirming care, support, and perhaps even treatment?

While Western psychedelic practitioners from within the medical model may not be using overt conversion therapy today, that does not mean that there are not still questions as to whether Western medicalized psychedelic care is safe for queer people. It is also essential to acknowledge the erasure of queer people from psychedelic research and name the ways psychedelic research has traditionally excluded the queer experience. Research studies often do not even ask questions that would help differentiate responses to psychedelics in queer people, and have failed to recruit queer research participants, so we really don't know if there are indeed differences that can be illuminated through study. Assuming that queer people want or will benefit from therapy offered by straight and cisgender therapists is a huge misstep, and there is a lack of qualified queer professionals in Western psychedelic research.[24] Moreover, Western psychedelic research has often relied on a "gender dyad" of therapists in study settings, meaning a male and female therapist duo. Queer scholars have pointed out that this "promotes retrograde conceptualizations of masculinity and femininity . . . and privileges cisgender therapists and disenfranchises trans, non-binary, and gender non-conforming from the psychedelic clinic room."[25] As it turns out, the Western psychedelic world continues to have a lot of work to do to create safe, affirming care for queer people.

This book is laced through with examples of how psychedelics can help us tell new stories about ourselves, dismantle rigid inner narratives, and connect with pleasure. What queer people really need are the spaces in which to come together for healing and connection. In an essay for the book *Queering Psychedelics*, mentioned above, I describe a vision for queer psychedelic healing.[26] This vision includes:

- Spaces for healing that are held by communities rather than presided over by figures of authority

- Accepting the psychedelic experience as it is, whether or not it leads to decreases in depression, anxiety, or increases in functioning
- Including play, artistic expression, communal music-making, and storytelling in the psychedelic experience itself
- Allowing for the free expression of gender presentation and embrace of shape-shifting identities
- Creating new ritual forms relevant for this moment in history that support healing for all people
- Celebrating erotic energy as intrinsically valuable to our identities and life force

During the process of writing this book, I've spoken to many psychedelic therapists, researchers, underground guides, and activists. When I bring up community models of healing as the possible ideal, especially for people with marginalized identities, people are interested, but are quick to point out the potential obstacles. In my conversation with Justin Natoli, a different perspective on the potential of community-oriented psychedelic spaces for queer people emerged.

> Psychedelic research scientists say that the mystical experience is the conduit of healing in psychedelic-assisted therapy. That's half true. I think the other half of the healing is through the community. This is especially important because of the wounds of shame, of being in the closet. Many of us carry the trauma of believing our own unique essence is a problem rather than a gift. The antidote to this shame is interconnection. It is realizing that just by being our essential selves, we have something valuable to contribute to the tribe. This can't happen in the way that psychedelic-assisted therapy is currently being studied and practiced, where there are one or two therapists and an individual client. Nothing can really replace the ceremony of people who gather together to share these experiences. It's these community psychedelic experiences that are the most powerful. It's the way that they've been managed indigenously for thousands of years, and it's really the way that queer people are going to get the

most healing out of psychedelic work, because it is this community aspect that provides such an essential element of the healing.

Perhaps, if we truly wanted to make meaningful reparations for the harm caused to queer people by the early psychedelic medical establishment, we could put the power to create and hold community spaces for our own healing into our hands without legal risk or medical obstacles.

Psychedelic experiences have the power to speak directly to our hearts and help us not only to *think* new things about ourselves, but to *feel* new things about ourselves. Healing and wholeness is about accepting and embracing all that we are. Like the concept of "queer," the notion of "psychedelic" is also about being in the space between. The psychedelic experience is of this world, but it is also of something much greater. It is generated from within you, but is undoubtedly also something expansive and sacred that is beyond ourselves. Thus, the psychedelic experience is a queer experience by its very nature. Bett Williams put it best in her pithy comment, "Psychedelics are queer, just saying!"[27] In queer psychedelic community, we can call back the parts of ourselves that have been disowned, shamed, or hidden, and embrace these aspects of ourselves in love. The early attempts at psychedelic conversion therapy, of course, failed. You cannot change someone's sexuality or gender identity, nor are they disorders to treat. Psychedelics do not heal things that are not in need of healing. They can, however, help us connect to and accept our personal uniqueness.

PSYCHEDELICS AND POLYAMORY

When we envision the cultural associations linked to psychedelics during the 20th century, perhaps one of the most common tropes is "Free Love." Since the psychedelic cultural renaissance of the 1960s, these medicines have been both venerated and reviled for their presumed power to dismantle the socially imposed standards for romantic relationships, namely, a heteronormative, dominator-submissive relationship between one man and one woman only, and open the possibility for relationships that are more egalitarian, sexually experimental, and free. But this movement also left a vacuum in its wake. If there wasn't a specific path to follow, meaning monogamous marriage and children, what did we have?

One relationship orientation which has gained visibility and legitimacy in Western culture since the 1990s is polyamory or conscious non-monogamy (CNM)/ethical non-monogamy (ENM). The word polyamory is derived from the rhetorical mishmash of Greek *poly* meaning "many" and the Latin *amor* meaning "love." It refers to "having multiple loving, often committed, relationships at the same time by mutual agreement, with honesty and clarity,"[28] and although CNM/ENM are terms that are often used synonymously but can also refer to multiple relationships of varying levels of commitment, both models nonetheless strive for transparency and seek to involve the informed consent of all people involved. These "open" relationship structures can be hierarchical with one relationship receiving priority, or more equanimous without any relationship being prioritized over another, sometimes referred to as relationship anarchy.

Over the past decade or so, popular articles and panels have tackled the question, can psychedelics make you polyamorous? This question rests on the assumptions that psychedelics engender feelings of expanded love, potentially reduce feelings of jealousy and increase interpersonal security, and generally liberalize people's belief systems. But I venture to think perhaps when it comes to psychedelics and polyamory, these articles and panels are asking the wrong question entirely. Instead of wondering whether psychedelics can *make you* polyamorous, what if instead we were to explore whether psychedelics could support the tools needed for being in multiple relationships with devotion, security, love, and ethical care?

The success of any healthy sexual relationship depends upon things like clear agreements, boundaries, and transparency. However, because non-monogamy involves multiple people, in order to ensure the true consent—by all partners involved—to how sex and the relationship will be handled, a commitment to such practices is critical. For people in a polyamorous relationship, such agreements often center on how much time is spent with other partners, how those relationships are codified, and sexual boundaries related to both health precautions and emotional needs.

In my many years of working with clients who are either opening their relationships, or are seeking support in maintaining open relationships, the act of establishing relationship agreements and boundaries is usually the least of it. Here is where I think the current discourse on psychedelics and polyamory often misses the boat. There has to be more to the story than just being able to communicate clearly and manage feelings of possessiveness and jealousy when they arise. The much deeper and more complex terrain is how you manage your own emotions and relationships when you are in love with two (or more) people. How do you stay grounded when the intense sexual desire of a new relationship could easily consume the presence you might bring to more established, securely attached (and usually less activating) relationships? How do you confront every part of yourself that whispers comparisons about lovers in your ear, and actively honor the individuality of each person you love? And most importantly, how do you cultivate the emotional maturity and wisdom to be thinking, at all times, about what is actually best for all of the people involved in this relationship, not just you.

This chapter previously described how psychedelics can engender qualities of openness and empathy that are certainly supports to the conscious and ethical practice of polyamory. But successful poly relationships are not only about being open, flexible, and kind (although it certainly helps). Solid, passionate, and sustainable multiple relationships also rely on perspective, spiritual maturity, and the cultivation of secure attachment. Attachment theory has certainly become a buzz word that has found its way into the popular psychological consciousness. My clients mention it constantly when trying to understand and describe their own behaviors in relationships. Simply put, classically, attachment theory posits that the quality (and more granularly, the *nature*) of an infant's connection to their caregivers in early life molds their capacity to form secure attachments as adults. More contemporary thinking on the matter suggests that our adult experiences also heavily influence how we make and maintain emotional connections.[29] Certainly, my anecdotal experience of speaking with many sex and relationship therapists suggests that many still hold the view that polyamory is an expression of pathology that grows from an avoidant attachment style (meaning, people who avoid or even fear deep intimacy in romantic relationships) and amounts to diversifying sexual partners to avoid being truly close and connected to any single one, whipping oneself into a constant state of avoidant stimulation without any deep substance. I disagree. In fact, research has shown that people who practice polyamory are more likely to be securely attached (where deep intimacy and connection comes easily) or anxiously attached (where an individual might crave affirmation of intimacy and safety).[30]

And now the juice . . . psychedelics are often thought of as connection-enhancing. Ask any couple you know doing MDMA together this weekend and you'll quickly get an assessment of the perceived attachment benefits. But classic psychedelics like psilocybin have also been shown to increase feelings of connectedness not just to specific people, but on a larger scale, to the world itself. A recent study found that anxiously attached people, when given psilocybin and psychotherapy in a group context, experienced reductions in attachment anxiety. Most fascinating, anxiously attached people were more likely to have a full mystical experience that includes sensations and perception of being connected to something greater than oneself, perhaps due to being hardwired to crave feelings of attachment. Higher attachment avoidance was a predictor of a more challenging psychedelic experience. The researchers conclude that psilocybin may actually help people alleviate feelings of attachment insecurity for months after ingestion, opening up new avenues for adult healing, and to becoming a secure attacher.[31]

How does this relate to the practice of polyamory? Poly relationships—like monogamous ones—are fundamentally successful or not based on our capacity to be rooted in our own sexual ethics, mature in our approach to love, and securely attached to our partners. Secure attachment allows for breathing room, both in a relationship and in our own mind. It allows people the space to be themselves and not to have to meet every one of our needs perfectly, because when we are securely attached, we fundamentally feel able to attend to our own emotional needs while valuing support and connection from partners. Secure attachment is of particular importance when it comes to polyamory, because it allows us to feel stable and empowered when we are in varying degrees of romantic love and sexual passion with different people at different times. All of this to say, whether or not psychedelics can help support a polyamorous relationship depends on how you look at it. You certainly don't need psychedelics to create an interest in having sex with more than one person. People have done a fine job of that themselves given that infidelity continues to be a central reason people end relationships. Perhaps there's a better way? Perhaps the better way is doing the work to be grounded in our own erotic morals, able to attach securely in our connections to others, and to cultivate compassion and clear communication with our partner. Then, if you touch someone who is not your partner and they spark joy . . . well, I think that puts you in a pretty good position to decide what you might do next.

The shadow side of psychedelics and polyamory occurs when psychedelic use is presented as justification that one partner is more evolved, and that the partner reticent about having an open relationship is simply too rigid, too fearful, or insecure. "If only they could see that all love is abundant in the universe, they would just be ok with me fucking this person from Tinder!" Unfortunately, that's a therapy session I've sat through one too many times. Fear and insecurity are completely understandable responses when someone is asking for a sudden, drastic reframing of your relationship structure. What good is it to connect to expanded feelings of universal love and abundance if you don't have compassion for the person with whom you're already having a relationship?

Much like psychedelics themselves, polyamory can be a gateway to progressive ways to love, to parent, to share resources, and to connect. It can be practiced with the utmost ethics and care. However, it can also be a label that is used to justify not only harm in relationships, but held over reluctant partners as evidence that they are not spiritually or emotionally mature enough to be ok with what's happening, as opposed to acknowledging that they have real concerns about the impact non-monogamy might have on their relationship. I want to be abundantly clear, whether it's polyamory, ethical non-monogamy or monogamy, it's not about the relationship structure. It's about consent. Does this relationship truly work for everyone involved? Can everyone involved collaborate on a workable situation where perhaps stretching your emotional comfort zone is necessary, but it can be done with discussion and empathy?

Another concept gaining traction is that of radical monogamy. As a person who has been deeply involved in poly relationships and communities my whole adult life, I found this concept to be a breath of fresh air. The vast majority of us grow up with the idea that monogamy is the only legitimate relationship style. Many of us are even raised with pervasive examples that show us possessiveness and jealousy are signs of deep love. Other relationship styles such as polyamory and conscious non-monogamy serve as legitimate alternatives to monogamy. But can monogamy be practiced in a different way? Journalist Nick Levine asks the question in this way, "Can monogamy be a choice you arrive at—after considering your own agency and options—rather than a blind expectation?"[32] I would say yes. A truly "psychedelic" approach to relationship structures is not that they have to look a certain way, but that the form of relationship you are choosing is supportive of your own spiritual growth, personal values and ethics, and respectful of the needs of others. It is not about how it appears outwardly, it's about whether genuine love and respect exist at the core. That's the best of what psychedelics (and relationships) can offer us.

PSYCHEDELICS, BDSM, AND OVERCOMING SEXUAL TRAUMA
Transgression to Transformation

Sociologist Corie Hammers asks the question, "What does it mean to repeat—to repeat in order to move through?" Hammers' work explores the dynamics in queer BDSM communities in the United States, specifically trauma survivors who engage in reenactments of trauma during BDSM play.* In her essay, "Reworking Trauma Through BDSM," she

---

*Albeit, this is not the reason all, or even most, kinky people engage in the practice of BDSM. The primary reason people engage in BDSM is pleasure.

elaborates on S/M's "suffering pleasures," and "the generative, productive affects/effects borne from these reenactments." Hammers goes on to outline that these kink scenes are not repetitions, but rather *reenactments* that embrace the role of consent and performance to rework trauma. She argues that sadomasochistic reenactments of trauma contribute to a sense of control and power over trauma, and that this redoing "corporeally and psychically reworks the traumatized body as it reassembles trauma's negative affects."[33]

BDSM (bondage/domination, dominance/submission, sadism/masochism) is the label given to the practice of consensual, relational, intentional act of exploring power over, power given, and intense stimulation for sensual pleasure. It also plays a role in the healing of certain sexual trauma survivors who engage in reenactments of trauma in order for the body to process through experiences of actual violence, orchestrating scenes in consensual ways with trusted partners. As Hammers notes in her essay, the key missing piece in many psychotherapeutic approaches to healing trauma is the body.[34]

I believe there are many underexplored correlates between BDSM and ceremonial psychedelic experiences. Psychedelic experiences in ceremonial settings almost always include a facilitator who holds the responsibility for creating a safe container for orchestrated, consensual surrender. There are often elements of performance: specific clothing, music, accouterments and tools, and ritual. But most importantly, there is submission. One cannot have a full psychedelic experience without the willingness to surrender to the medicine and trust the facilitator to make sure the body remains safe. Once consent is given, once the medicine enters your body, you can do nothing but go through. Resistance will not serve. The experience cannot be stopped. It must be endured (and perhaps also enjoyed).

BDSM shares many of these same elements. Specific clothing is worn that heightens the performative aspects of the interaction between dominant and submissive (or the "top" and "bottom"), and, in a healthy BDSM session, informed consent always precedes the commencement of any BDSM "scene." The transformative nature of the experience occurs in the interplay of the sensitivity, attunement, and responsibility of the dominant who is entrusted with finding exactly the right balance between stimulation and safety, and the willingness to give over power and surrender to sensation on the part of the submissive. When conducted in a deliberate and consensual way, these scenes of fantasy stimulation, humiliation, or role-play facilitate transformation through transgression of roles, norms, and personal histories. Healthy BDSM must also always include a discussion of risk, harm management, and boundaries. It must also include aftercare and integration of the experience. All crucial elements that parallel psychedelic ceremony.

Because BDSM and psychedelics are both taboo topics in our culture, and because psychedelics are undergoing a shiny, new image resuscitation washed clean of the redolence of the Free Love era, bringing the two together may be seen as controversial to some. But both are acts that can be deeply sacred and offer the opportunity to move the body through trauma, not from an intellectualized perspective, but through the experience of direct feeling and affective release, provided the intention brought to the experience is growth. Both can offer participants the experience of initiation, of offering up physical comfort and power for higher purpose, and the opportunity to attain higher consciousness.

Both BDSM and certain psychedelic experiences can be understood through the lens of "suffering pleasures." When we consider both, the experiences themselves might be intense to the breaking point. But it is in the surrender, the going through, the release, that pleasure later takes hold, or, arises simultaneous to the suffering.* Many who engage in these acts of intentional overwhelm do so because they create a space within where trauma was once rooted, and in that space, room to feel. These experiences ask of us, where exactly is the line between suffering and pleasure? What does it mean after control was taken from us, to volunteer one's autonomy to another person or to a non-human sentience in service to healing? Dominant narratives about psychedelic healing and sexual healing would have us believe that conventional Western medicine, which is rife with power structures and power-over

---

*I have spent many nights violently puking into a bucket while also seeing the most incredibly beautiful visions imaginable during ayahuasca ceremonies.

relationships that are most often never discussed, is safer somehow than what can transpire in the context of ceremony and ritual. But it is often in these theaters of transgression, ones in which people have the most power over the container, that they access the means in which to fully heal.

However, it must also be acknowledged that many, if not all of our relational and social problems have at their core, both the human impulse to play with power and/or the desire to have power over others, depending on the context. When not practiced with love, respect, and an intention to use sensation and intensity as a transformational tool, BDSM is simply another form of violence with a high aesthetic. When people are drawn to facilitate psychedelic experiences for others, that is, to hold the power of the medicine without the pure intention to be in service to healing, playing with medicine is just another way of asserting dominance. The most important thing is a genuine appraisal of our intentions. Both BDSM and psychedelics—as parallel practices—offer the opportunity for growth, change, and deep healing through transformational experience. But only if love is at the foundation.

PSYCHEDELICS, SEX, AND SPIRITUALITY

The deepest expression of Psychedelic Sexuality is finding our path back to spirituality, whatever it means for you, and integrating the sacred into our erotic identity. For many of us, the harm done by oppressive religions, devoid of a connection to the Earth and obsessed with distancing us from a direct relationship with the divine, hell bent on framing our life-force—our very erotic vitality—as something to be repressed and controlled, has done so much harm that the space between sexuality and spirituality can seem insurmountable. But even for the most agnostic, sexual climax often is accompanied by the ecstatic invocation, "Oh god, oh god, yes, yes, oh god." This is the god at whose altar I gladly worship. A god of connection, a god of love, a god of pleasure and holy bodies whose name we rapturously call at the height of abandon. Can psychedelic experiences help us find our way home to this god?

Sex therapist Gina Ogden was a pioneer of bringing together the erotic and the spiritual in her work. She writes, "Spirituality means a sense of direct, personal connection with the Divine (however one defines Divine). . . . in terms of sexuality, the spiritual involves an intimate connection with one's self, one's partner, and/or a power that is beyond one's self."[35] It also means dismantling ideas of what is sacred and what is profane. A quick Google Images search for "sex and spirituality" yields pictures of people gazing into each other's eyes, engaging in modern tantric practices. Fine. That is a perfectly wonderful expression of sexuality and spirituality for some people. But sacred sexuality can also be the high ritual of leather communities, the bending of gender norms and sexual roles, and most fundamentally, the simple practice of being fully present and connected with someone you love, giving and receiving pleasure. These are all holy acts if the intention is there for them to be sacred.

Why is there such a tremendous gap between our sexuality and spiritual lives? One foundational reason is the trauma sustained by many from the oppressive teachings and social control inflicted by organized religions. The teachings of most Western religions promote a vicious paradox; to be good means first to be heterosexual, second to adhere to traditional gender norms, and third to withhold and repress our erotic energy and maintain "purity." Then, we are meant to find a relationship sanctioned by said religion and blossom into a person who is sexually knowledgeable, eager, available, and most importantly *generative*. What once must be withheld, now must be given freely; withholding sex means we are not living up to the contract of our relationship, even if it means having sex we don't want. I've worked with many individuals and couples from religious backgrounds who arrive to therapy in middle age after marrying young, without any sex education or sexual experience, often fundamentally loving each other, but without knowing themselves as sexual people and resenting what they feel they've missed. In my practice, they often ask the question "Should we be non-monogamous?" They believe non-monogamy might be a way of having ethical sexual variety or saving a flagging relationship, which it seldom does. But the problem is rarely about monogamy or non-monogamy. It is actually about grieving the lost opportunity to develop in a sex positive environment, the opportunity to learn what feels good to you sexually, or even how to practice consent in a relationship.

It is not possible to overstate the emotional damage that this type of socialization inflicts upon people. Very often, healthy individuation in this context forces one to make an almost impossible choice: Do I honor myself? Or do I stay connected to my family and community? And sometimes, an even more painful one: Do I stay in my marriage? I have a career's worth of experience working with struggling LGBTQIA+ people for example, who—due to the oppressively religious environment of their upbringing—had to go as far away from their home of origin as possible in an effort to simply be themselves. But this is not just an issue that impacts sexual minorities. Purity culture, a term that refers to standards within certain religious sects that require sexual abstinence before marriage, deprives *everyone* involved of the right to pleasure and sexual autonomy. In order for people who were raised in sexually repressive environments such as these, to begin healing this trauma, we first must approach our own narratives about sexuality and spirituality with curiosity, so that we may begin the process of understanding how religious and societal conditioning around sexuality and spirituality may have impacted us.

The next great disservice I believe some organized religions do to our sexuality is by promoting the view that God, Higher Power (or Wider Power, as I like to say), Universal Consciousness—whatever language works for you—is not accessible to us directly. A hallmark of organized spiritual belief systems is that the priest, guru, or pastor, nearly always male, sits in a place of authority between us, and as such, acts as a third-party intercessor sitting between ourselves and our direct personal experience of the divine.* When we are repeatedly taught that religion consists of rules to be followed or that damnation is undoubtedly our fate, and that our only means of speaking to our Wider Power

---

*One great example of this—mentioned elsewhere in the book—is Spanish colonizers who (rightly) viewed Indigenous use of mushrooms as a "mortal threat to the authority of the church" because it afforded users direct access to the divine, bypassing the middleman (the priest) competely.[36]

is through an intercessor, we are denied the opportunity to cultivate a direct connection to the divine. This is a deep wound, a hole that a personal relationship to spirit is just waiting to fill.

Likewise, it feels important to acknowledge that many Western spiritual seekers interested in consciousness and ritual gravitate to Buddhism or other Eastern esoteric traditions. I was one of those people. I began practicing Buddhist meditation in my early 20s, far before I ever had a serious interest in psychedelics. I will forever be grateful for the training in mindfulness and compassion that I learned in the context of Buddhist sanghas. This fundamental training gave me a working relationship to my own mind that has continued to serve me well as a therapist, a seeker, and a human being. But it can be extremely hard to separate what is acceptable in the context of a religious practice originating outside own culture from practices that are indeed abusive. I learned, to my incredible heartbreak, that sexual abuse can be pawned off as "enlightened spiritual practice" by unscrupulous religious leaders in any religion.

Over the past number of years, allegations of sexual abuse, coercion, and financial exploitation rocked the Buddhist world. Teachers—more than teachers, *gurus*—in a variety of different Buddhist schools used their power to manipulate and abuse young students into sexual relationships of vastly unequal power under the guise of spiritual practice. I coped with years of rage at this betrayal. I stood by with astonishment watching people I once respected defending the actions of teachers who used their position of power to rape their disciples. I somehow expected that people training their minds and following the ethics of Buddhist dharma teachings would be more outraged when they learned about these abuses. But the spell of influence wielded by a "guru" has the power to exert a rigid hold on the parts of us that crave a parental or god-like figure. It can feel incomprehensible that spiritual wisdom can co-arise with abuse. And yet, we've seen just that happen in nearly all religions, as well as in psychedelic and other consciousness communities.

It was a very long time before I was able to pluck the gems of dharma I learned in my training—and they are indeed stainless gems—and separate them from a modern Western Buddhist culture, which is, in my opinion, just as washed in toxic and harmful behaviors as the religions I had rejected for those very same reasons. And to learn the hard lesson that perhaps we are living in a cultural moment in which we are called to a difficult task, which is to stand in our own power rather than handing it over to institutional structures and/or individual figures of authority. It could well be that we are entering an era in which more and more people are forging profound relationships to personal spirituality rooted in respect for the Earth, sexual autonomy, human rights, and love, while the counter-power of religious supremacy continues to be used to justify violence and oppression. I don't think it's a coincidence that psychedelic consciousness, the normalizing of the use of entheogens for serious spiritual work, as well as community-based psychedelic practices are emerging as helpers and guides in our collective healing process toward a new spirituality.

How exactly do psychedelics help us to develop a personal connection to the divine? Psychedelics have reliably been shown, particularly at high doses ingested within the context of intentional ceremonial or therapeutic settings, to occasion mystical states of consciousness and the directly felt presence of divine love, interconnection to all beings, and deep spiritual truths. I believe that through the practice of psychedelic integration work, we can use these experiences to cultivate a link between our sexuality and spirituality, leading to profound healing. Research also shows that psychedelics impact our spiritual belief systems in ways that promote positive changes in functioning and mood. A recent study surveyed 866 respondents engaging in psychedelic use in a ceremonial context to measure shifts in metaphysical beliefs. The researchers found significant shifts away from a materialistic worldview. In fact, it was more common than not for so-called "hard-materialists" to become more accepting of spiritual perspectives. Moreover, these shifting beliefs were correlated with positive mental health changes and improvements in well-being.[37] A thread that runs through much of the emerging psychedelic science is that in both controlled and naturalistic settings, people who have "full" mystical experiences, including a sense of being outside of time, a sense that all is one, feeling that you experienced something profound and holy, and (my favorite) *oceanic boundlessness*, enjoy lasting shifts out of depression, cancer-related anxiety,[38] as well as discontinuation of tobacco use and other substance use.[39] The list goes on.

However, psychedelic science has consistently tried to toe a difficult line maintaining scientific standards while acknowledging the mystical as a crucial part of the psychedelic experience. Mysticism is a topic once relegated to the dusty annals of humanities departments. Not a topic for serious science. And yet, the concept of the "mystical experience" is peppered through nearly every emerging study on psychedelics and mental health. While I want my clients to experience reductions in depression and anxiety, or to find the inner strength to shift away from harmful substance-using behaviors, what happens when we take our relationship to the divine and put it in service of measurable results? In my view, the psychedelic experience and its powerful capacity to connect us to the divine is a birthright, whether or not one continues to experience depression or smoke cigarettes. There are powerful reasons to cultivate a relationship to spirit even if it doesn't constitute a clinical success story.

I believe entheogenic experiences that include a feeling of connection to spirit, interconnection of all beings, the self as divine, and psychedelic love can help us to develop a relationship between spirituality and eroticism, and guide us in cultivating a quality of sacredness in our sexuality and sexual relationships. Based on my clinical work with both sexual trauma survivors and people looking to heal inner religious conflicts related to sex and relationships, several key themes have emerged:

- Psychedelics can engender a sense of the body as sacred and promote a connection to the divine.
- Psychedelics can help people reconnect to the spiritual aspects of their sexual identities free from religious shame.
- The act of taking a psychedelic medicine is introducing a non-human sentience into your body which is a deep act of union and intimacy.

Common thoughts that plague many of us (especially survivors of sexual trauma) are negative self-referencing beliefs about our lovability, worth, and goodness, are often internalized in the form of "I'm dirty," "No one will want me," "I'm broken." These internalized beliefs not only shape our inner worlds, but also impact our personal relationships. Psychedelic medicines can help us cultivate a direct relationship with the sacredness of an already-perfect self.

Sacred plant medicines such as ayahuasca, psilocybin mushrooms, and huachuma all are thought to have plant spirits. In other words, a personality or an essence that is sentient and can come to our aid in the context of ceremonial ingestion to support our healing. It is common to hear practitioners refer to "Mother Ayahuasca," "Grandfather San Pedro" (or Father P, as my dear friend and I call him) or "los niños" referring to the spirit of the mushroom. This can also be true to the personal experience of people who relate to the "spirit" of MDMA or ketamine. This animist view of psychedelics can be harnessed for the transformation of internalized destructive beliefs about our sexuality. Plant medicine practitioners often report the "felt sense" of a divine presence in ceremony. Experiencing divinity through the self, or inseparable from the self, presents a direct challenge to the perception of the self as deficient or broken.[40] This certainly comports with Gina Ogden's notion of "an intimate connection" with "a power that is beyond one's self."[41] The journeyer may come into direct relationship with a sense of divinity, receive information about their healing path, and most importantly, feel the loving presence of a plant spirit conspiring to help them heal. My psychedelic integration clients have described this quality as feeling as if they are not alone with their trauma for the first time, or experiencing a loving presence within that acts as a guide to their inner work. Feeling a loving divine presence within you is incompatible with beliefs that one is dirty or unloveable. Likewise, these directly felt experiences of the divine have the power to reconnect us back to a sense of childlike wonder and facilitate a relationship to the sacred that can be supported and nurtured in our lives into individual spiritual practice.

Here's where things get really exciting. If sacred plants have distinct, sentient spirits often attributed unique characteristics who are conscripted to guide us in our healing, what does it mean to take that into your body? The act of taking a sacred medicine means not only to take the divine within you, but to allow a non-human sentience to enter you in a union unlike anything one can experience with another human. This medicine enters your mouth and rides in waves through your body. It affects your thoughts, your vision, your self-perception. It speaks to you. It anchors you in your heart and mind. It walks with you through dark memories and flows through you in ecstasy. What in heaven and earth could be more sensual than that?

By bringing together psychedelics, spirituality, and sensuality, we are called to see "entheogens," a term that refers to sacred plant medicines and literally means "to take the divine within," as part of a new mystical practice where nature is our church and ecstasy is our prayer.

In fact, this may have been the case all along. I will mention two examples of highly disputed, yet very interesting theories, both of which notably seem to support not only a more unified concept of psychedelics, spirituality, and sensuality, but also illustrate how organized religion can seek to exert control by denying the individual right to spiritual autonomy, installing itself instead as authoritarian intercessor between seeker and source. Author and classical scholar Brian C. Muraresku argues that psychedelics played an important role in early Christian sacraments. Muraresku points to "compelling evidence for the ritual use of psychedelics in antiquity" including at the Temple of Eleusis in Greece, dedicated to Demeter and Persephone, which was a spiritual center of the ancient world. Notably, the secrets of the rituals practiced there were guarded not by men, but by women. He argues that the ancient sacramental drink *kykeon*, derived from a fungus known as ergot (from which LSD was also synthesized), had psychedelic properties that induced mystical visionary experiences.[42] Muraresku argues that these practices trickled into early Christianity during a time when the practice was outlawed and had a more gnostic bent. What could have inspired the early adherents of Christianity to risk death for their beliefs? Muraresku, who calls his work "the pagan continuity hypothesis with a psychedelic twist,"[43] also argues that the act of receiving the Christian Eucharist—a ritual in which believers ingest bread and wine that has been transfigured into the body and blood of Christ by a priest—may have had its origins in these early rituals, implying that

that the Christian Eucharist itself may be of psychedelic origin.[44] It just might have been a psychedelic Eucharist ritual that actually let these followers of Jesus experience divine love in a big way.

Author Mike Crowley makes parallel arguments in his book *Secret Drugs of Buddhism: Psychedelic Sacraments and the Origins of the Vajrayana*. After painstakingly examining sources such as art, texts, and archeological evidence, Crowley claims that the Hindu god Shiva, described as having a blue throat and one leg, is "simply put . . . an apotheosis of a blue-staining (i.e., psilocybin-rich) psychedelic mushroom." He later argues that the Vajrayana rituals practiced by Buddhists in the tantric arm of the religion were also secretly psychedelic rituals. He describes how Chogyam Trungpa Rinpoche, one of the first Vajrayana Buddhist teachers to make an impression in the United States and Europe during the 1970s, stated that when he began to teach the Buddhist dharma and tantric practices to Western students there is one element he would omit. Crowley speculates that this omission was the *psychedelic* tantric practices thought to be dangerous in the hands of Western students (who were, at that time, mostly hippies.) But the sacramental substance *amrita* of Buddhist practice, was, in fact, psychedelic.[45]

In a moment when Western tourists are stampeding to South America for a chance to experience psychedelic healing rituals originating from cultures that are not their own, is it not a time when we can reflect on what it might mean to forge a personal, mystical, earth-based, and more holistic relationship to sacred psychedelic sexual healing? I argue that the sacredness of psychedelics is derived only in part by the medicine itself. It also comes from the sacredness of the container we create around their use and the sacredness of our connection to others. I invite you to imagine what it might mean for you to marry this quality of sacredness to not only our respective sexualities, but to our relationships. After all, sex and spirituality meet in the beautiful space where we choose to honor the holiness of ourselves and our partners. Might we invite ceremony, ritual, and divinity into our sex life? I believe we can, and it does not require anything but allowing for the unfolding of the sacredness that already resides within us.

THE POWER OF PSYCHEDELIC LOVE

How do we form and nurture a psychedelic sex life? For me, it has very much to do with perhaps the hardest word to define, the easiest to misunderstand, and yet one that acts as a non-negotiable foundation for conscious sexual relationships: love. Western culture, steeped in notions of romantic love, often linked to ownership and jealousy, as well as the withholding and offering of sex as an expression of love, as opposed to say, a means through which to signal our love for another, we've lost the real meaning and power of erotic love. If the erotic is understood to be a life force within us rather than simply a sexual or libidinal drive, then to *make love* is to share our very essence with another person, generating erotic power together. Whether we want to share that essence joyfully with many people, or direct it intensely at very few, when sex is undertaken with love, it is not only impossible to dishonor our own body, it is unthinkable to use it to harm someone else.

One of the most powerful feelings linked to every psychedelic medicine when taken in nearly any context with conscious intention, awareness, and preparation, is love. The call of a psychedelic sex life is to ask ourselves: is what I'm about to do in service to my growth, honoring the body and spirit of my partner as well as my own in alignment with my sexual ethics, and an expression of love? I believe through personal experience, and in bearing witness to the vastly diverse sexual experiences of my clients, that this love can be within marriage or committed partnerships, in casual sexual interactions undertaken with joy and consent, in the dark corners of kink clubs, or in the embrace between sex workers and their clients. If we dispose of the notions of romantic love most of us were raised with and instead ask ourselves, "Can I fall in love with this person in this moment, and interact with their body with dignity and respect?," we are on the right path. To answer this question authentically, we must be willing to take an honest inventory of our own sexual healing and be honest with ourselves about whether our sexual desires are in service to our growth, or to limiting feelings of heartbreak, poor self-esteem, power-seeking behavior, compulsive behavior, or avoiding sensations related to trauma. This takes a tremendous amount of self-awareness and spiritual maturity, which is why sexual relationships are often the site of so much harm.

Psychedelic Sexuality invites us to nurture our own sexual uniqueness, to honor the sexuality of others, and to act in service to love at all times. It's a very tall order, but one I believe is possible when we use these medicines to support our own healing, and restore ourselves to a relationship with our sexual vitality that is healthy and grounded in ethics. Pleasure can heal us. Pleasure can be the path to a joyful relationship with our spirituality, sexuality, and self. The question is, are we ready to receive a love that big?

3
SEXUAL HEALING

A Psychedelic Approach to Understanding Sexual Violence and Sexual Dysfunction

Is it possible to experience pleasure when you can't even experience yourself?

AMITA SWADHIN, FROM *PLEASURE ACTIVISM*

IF WE ENDEAVOR TO EXPLORE how psychedelics can guide us to a life of meaning, joy, and increased pleasure, it's essential to examine what prevents us from accessing those things in the first place. One very important reason why we struggle to find enduring sexual pleasure and sexual self-esteem resides in a misunderstood topic: the impact of sexual violence. In this chapter, I will explore the repercussions of harmful acts, both dramatic and subtle, that shape the basis for our sexual response, our sexual self-perception, and inform the narratives we have about ourselves and our relationships in order to discern what role psychedelics might play in healing these burdens. But to really understand sexual violence and its aftermath, the trauma held in the body long after, we must form an expanded definition of these terms that serves a more nuanced understanding.

I believe that relieving us of the definition that many hold—even therapists—that sexual violence must be an overwhelming, violent event like a rape, or secretive, chronic violation like childhood sexual abuse actually liberates us to move away from having to fit trauma and sexual violence into the framework of pathology and instead look at the real impact of life events, both interpersonal and systemic, that prevent us from accessing pleasure, self-esteem, and embodiment in our lives. Through this lens, we can define sexual violence as any act that harms a person's sexuality or sense of sexual self. Trauma is the lasting impact of those events.

> Trauma is any experience that overwhelms our capacity to cope or disturbs our sense of safety in our bodies, in relationships, or the world in an enduring way. Trauma disrupts a steady sense of self, connection to the earth, and to community. Trauma impairs our ability to be present with pleasure which is our birthright.

Sexual violence exists on a spectrum, as does sexual trauma. Being shamed for the number of partners you've had—whether by a friend, pastor, doctor, or even your partner, for example—is a form of sexual violence, but an assault such as a rape where the body is physically violated and a survivor may even fear for their life, is a far more severe form of sexual violence. They are both sexual violence, but they are not the same. The level of healing necessary is not the same either. Understandably, the traumatic impact of these two examples represents the spectrum on which trauma is held in the body. A person who experienced sexual shaming may hold destructive sexual narratives, poor self-esteem, or other characterological traits that prevent them from having access to pleasure and a healthy relationship to their sexuality. A survivor of repeated childhood sexual abuse, on the other hand, may experience severe symptoms such as hypervigilance, dissociation (being "not there," detached from the present moment), somatic symptoms (pain during sex, headaches, or panic attacks), or have intrusive memories of abuse. In other words, the events of the past can cause severe inner fragmentation of the psyche and disrupt a survivor's life holistically. Serious trauma occurs when the nervous system simply cannot metabolize the events of the past, so at times they are experienced as happening right here and now.

PSYCHEDELICS AND HEALING SEXUAL TRAUMAS

I will not undertake to explore the neurobiology of the traumatized brain, or the neurobiological shifts occasioned by psychedelics in the treatment of PTSD. Instead I will address this topic from a psychospiritual perspective centered on sexual autonomy, human rights, personal and clinical insights, the dismantling of systems of oppression, and pleasure activism. Multiple research studies with diverse psychedelic medicines including MDMA, ketamine, psilocybin, and ayahuasca have explored how psychedelic-assisted therapy can ameliorate PTSD-related symptoms such as depression and anxiety in clinical and research settings. The emergence of psychedelic-assisted therapy treatments comes at a moment where we are experiencing epidemic levels of sexual, political, and systemic violence. The standard non-psychedelic treatments for PTSD such as SSRIs (which dull all emotions, not just those related to trauma) and Cognitive Behavioral Therapy or prolonged exposure therapy (in which a traumatized person must endure trauma-related stimuli until they are "desensitized" from a fear response) are lacking. In fact, forty to sixty percent of people undergoing these treatments don't respond adequately.[1] I would venture to say there are many reasons for this, not the least of which is the inhumanity of exposing and re-exposing a traumatized person to a terrible memory. These therapies can be like psychic surgery with no anesthesia. It's no wonder that they are often not well-tolerated.*

Psychedelic-assisted trauma treatments, by contrast, work because the medicine can help extinguish fear and arousal related to trauma,

---

*I have personally found that somatically oriented therapies such as Somatic Experiencing, EMDR, sensorimotor psychotherapy, and Internal Family Systems (IFS) present more compassionate, effective, and tolerable alternatives.

increase feelings of trust in the therapist or guide, or by affecting memory reconsolidation (allowing new thoughts, feelings, and stories about trauma to be felt and integrated). MDMA, a substance commonly used in the treatment of trauma, is helpful in reducing fear of anxiety-provoking memories and may increase the capacity for trust and attachment while increasing emotional empathy. Ketamine, a dissociative anesthetic that targets the glutamate system in the brain (as opposed to the serotonin system impacted by both SSRIs and most psychedelics), is now commonly used as an alternative to SSRIs for the treatment of depression due to its capacity to enhance neuroplasticity and its unique impact on the brain. This increased neuroplasticity, a term referring to how neurons can be provoked to form new connections which in turn shifts how thoughts are organized (something I will explore in more depth later), along with the inner emotional and mystical experience ketamine offers, can also be optimized in the context of trauma therapy to encourage the formation of new ways of looking at the self and induce experiences of euphoria or feelings of spiritual connection. In my ketamine-assisted psychotherapy practice, I have seen incredible results for trauma survivors simply because the medicine takes their fear response "off line" long enough for us to actually work on the trauma, and later for new information about the self to be integrated in a deep way. The classic psychedelics, such as psilocybin mushrooms and LSD, have been shown to promote emotional empathy, divergent thinking, mindfulness, and acceptance while also creating neuropsychological shifts toward decreased depression and anxiety.[2]

Clearly, evidence supports that psychedelic medicines are broadly effective tools to treat depression and post-traumatic symptoms. But how may psychedelics help heal the trauma-based inhibitions of erotic aliveness? I discussed this question with Dr. Jeffrey Guss who has been a personal mentor and is a friend of mine. Dr. Guss is deeply intelligent, funny, self-reflective, and if I may say so, the owner of the best funky shirt collection in all of psychedelia. Jeff is, simply put, a psychedelic OG. He is a psychiatrist, psychoanalyst, and psychedelic teacher and trainer for a new generation of therapists working with these medicines after being involved in many years of groundbreaking research on psychedelics for cancer-related anxiety and other indications, as well as working to bring the worlds of psychoanalysis and psychedelic therapy together.

Dr. Guss offered this:

There are two main narratives in this, and both integrate the neuroscience of psychedelic action with psychoanalytically described mechanisms of that action. First, psychedelics alter the activity of the Predictive Processing functions of the brain. As a way of understanding consciousness, Predictive Processing describes that we are always predicting what will happen to us, and must do this to not have to figure out our existence anew at every moment. We watch to see how correct we are by paying attention to information coming in from each moment, and seeing how well new information matches what we predict. A little surprise—a tiny bit of novelty or a wrong prediction—keeps life interesting. Too much novelty makes life feel overwhelming, and not enough surprise makes us feel bored. But importantly, we don't perceive the information of 'now' impartially. We come into each moment with our 'priors,' experiences of what we expect the world to be, and who we are in it. In psychoanalytic language, this would be called transference; how prior experience shapes what we expect to happen, and more deeply, what we pay attention to, what we ignore, what we cannot perceive, and what we cannot stop thinking about.

Another neuroscience construct with utility for understanding psychedelics and sexuality is the Default Mode Network (DMN). The DMN is a connected assembly of brain locations that function to maintain a coherent, recognizable narrative "self" as its primary product. When you are thinking about yourself, and telling yourself a story about yourself, who you are, what your past means about the present and the future, the DMN is active. The DMN is intimately linked to language and is in a mutually reciprocal and creative relationship with what are called defense mechanisms. For a trauma survivor, this activity can be marked by some severe psychological problems including dissociation (not being aware of present-day information, affective dysregulation), or overarching defenses (seeing others as unsafe, threatening, unreliable, malevolent, absent, or abusive.) These defenses are useful in preventing any further abuse from anyone. This guarding against more damage has a great cost: it screens out the possibility that some people could be safe, boundaried, reliable, and even a source of comfort, welcome excitement, connection, and sensual pleasure. The DMN may be very effective at establishing an entire realm of life as inherently dangerous. It can declare that erotic arousal, of any sort, is linked to danger, victimization, disgust, fear, and aversion.

But how exactly does a reduction in Default Mode Network and Predictive Processing priors open a special healing opportunity for trauma survivors? He continued:

Psychedelic consciousness is marked by reduction in the generation of these predictive "priors." During psychedelic experiences the activity of the DMN is softened and at higher degrees of psychedelic effect, rendered silent. Language signifiers are lessened, affective and somatic information becomes foregrounded. Thus, there is less prediction of what will happen, more openness to surprise, and a sense of the present as interesting and safe. Thus the world can be seen with more openness and possibly more trust, and less dissociation and self-protection. This action opens up the possibility of recovering lost erotic aliveness, and/or allowing for the possibility of a new experience, especially if the psychedelic journey is undertaken with a particularly safe guide, or an attuned erotic partner. In this way, new internal working models for relating to emotional and sexual intimacy can be experienced, and then learned. Far from talking about traumatic events using language and memory like much conventional psychotherapy does, psychedelic experiences offer an almost magical transportation to a playground of experimentation. You can try things out, enjoy the edges of pleasure that threaten a feeling of loss of control as mostly safe, intense in a good way, and most of all, offering an experience of healthy aliveness with just a touch of risk in place of dissociative or avoidant deadness.

What can we draw from this information upon reflection? Psychedelic experiences have multiple vectors of action that offer potential for erotic healing and post-traumatic sexual and relational growth. This growth is not only marked by changes in brain function, but—when carefully managed by a trusted companion or guide—can be witnessed in the relational aspects of the psychedelic experience itself. And lastly, the time following the experience allows for present-moment awareness, empathy, curiosity, intense erotic arousal, and self-discovery.

Using psychedelics in the treatment of sexual trauma must be understood as a multi-phased approach. It is dangerous to assume that a person with severe sexual trauma, such as being sexually abused by a parent, can simply attend an ayahuasca ceremony, "embrace joy," and somehow roll back years of emotional harm in the nervous system. Some survivors of severe trauma require professional help, whether that help be through conventional or psychedelic-assisted psychotherapy. Feelings of pleasure cannot substitute the hard work of experiencing, feeling, processing, and accepting terrible things that have happened to us. Relying on the help of a therapist trained to be present in these moments of excruciating feeling and grief can be necessary.

However, when it comes to the issue of trauma, most forms of trauma-focused psychotherapy, both psychedelic and non-psychedelic, stop and are declared successful when certain quantitative benchmarks of symptom reduction are met, such as the reduction of depression, anxiety, or dissociation. But healing, *real healing*, encompasses more than not having flashbacks or a cessation of depressive symptoms. It must also focus on fostering a life worth living, one that includes joy, embodiment, and connection to our creativity and vital sexual life-force. This is where psychedelics shine. A new, expanded model for a psychedelic, pleasure-inclusive approach to healing trauma is possible which makes access to these medicines crucial, even when a survivor might no longer meet the criteria for a mental illness like PTSD.

If sexual harm is healed in stages, what are those stages and how can psychedelics support us during each step of our healing? Psychedelics are uniquely useful, and experienced differently during each phase of healing sexual trauma. It is also important to understand that "psychedelic" is an umbrella term that encompasses radically different medicines, different types of settings, and therefore different paths to healing. They are not all the same, and each is not equally useful for different survivors. People distrustful of the medical system are unlikely to heal within it. Likewise, people fearful of the unmonitored nature of sacred plant medicine ceremonies, or put off by ritual, might thrive in a clinical context. But I do believe there is a common trajectory for healing sexual trauma that threads through the psychedelic experience whether it be in a therapist's office, a research study, or sacred medicine ceremony undertaken either as part of a community or alone.

PSYCHEDELIC STAGES OF SEXUAL TRAUMA HEALING

What follows are a description of healing stages survivors might experience when addressing sexual trauma through psychedelic work. The emotional and somatic processes outlined in these stages often occur during a psychedelic experience. These stages can also be a guide for integration work after a psychedelic experience.

Stage 1: Feeling

Feeling, for the sexual trauma survivor, is complex. Survivors can experience feeling too much, not feeling enough, feeling at the wrong time, or having the "wrong" feeling about a perfectly safe person or situation. When sexual trauma survivors come to traditional forms of therapy, they can often fear that they will not be able to access the emotion needed to process trauma due to dissociation or numbness, or they are afraid they will be consumed entirely by the enormity of their feelings, and may therefore avoid "losing control."

Psychedelics can help sexual trauma survivors through intense feeling states in two distinct ways. Psychedelics in the phenylamine branch of the pharmacopeia, specifically MDMA, can often induce pleasurable sensations in the body, downregulate parts of the brain such as the amygdala that signal danger, encourage feelings of trust, and support a survivor by increasing their ability to tolerate memories, sensations, and triggers related to trauma. These medicines act as a psychological "warm blanket" to make the intolerable tolerable. However, if we switch gears to the tryptamine branch of the psychedelic family, medicines like psilocybin mushrooms or ayahuasca can have a very, very different effect. These medicines often amplify the experience and sensations of trauma. Simultaneously they have the power to induce a feeling of connection to a benevolent force outside of ourselves protecting our emotional work. And then again, sometimes not. That may sound scary, and it certainly can be, but these medicines can guide us through the full expression of very intense emotions, the reliving of horrible traumas, or the re-narration of a story of trauma, all for the purpose of extracting and reprocessing what has long been stuck in the nervous system. A survivor may feel excruciating feelings all the way through to completion, or be able to enter the world of the past to protect their child or younger adult self from horrible wrongs, or even intervene psychically in a previous act of violence. Whether the medicine a survivor chooses to work with amplifies or ameliorates traumatic sensations or feelings, each can be a vital support in the processing of intense feelings through to completion so they are no longer trapped in the nervous system, lingering artifacts of the past. The above generally must be experienced first in the healing process. It is worth mentioning that in these early stages of healing trauma there might be little pleasure to be found. Since the main thesis of this book is that pleasure heals us, it's helpful to state clearly upfront that there are times when we first need to walk through the fire of our pain and discomfort to have later access to the deep healing pleasure provides.

Stage 2: Witnessing
When sexual violence occurs, it is by nature relational. The relationship may be between a survivor and someone who assaulted them, or a survivor and a whole family or community that harmed them. The cruel paradox of sexual violence is that despite this, the act of harm is something we experience very, very much alone. And it often begets further loneliness as survivors can struggle to form and maintain trusting rela-

tionships. In the process of psychedelic healing, witnessing has multiple meanings. It can mean that the survivor goes through a process of being witnessed by a therapist or facilitator during a psychedelic experience as they feel through the intense feelings and grief related to trauma (which is why it is essential to have a guide or therapist equipped emotionally to do that job), or they might be witnessed by a healing community if the work occurs in the context of a group. But unique to entheogens, the survivor using psychedelics to heal might feel the medicine itself/himself/herself is a witness to their process. This is especially true for medicines such as ayahuasca, where people engaging her for healing reliably report the presence of a forceful spirit. Now, it's above my pay grade to frame this presence of spirit as a psychological convention, primed by the way participants are prepared for ceremonial psychedelic work.* But it is most certainly my personal belief that these spirits are very much real. The act of being witnessed, and indeed of the survivor witnessing their own feelings, creates connection where there was none before. When these experiences are held by an "other" in ways that are ethical and safe, they can also provide a blueprint for trust in others, and challenge the inner narrative many survivors carry of being alone, unloved, and unlovable for their feelings.

Stage 3: Accepting

My colleague, trauma therapist Laura Mae Northrup, who you'll hear from in more depth later in this chapter, commented to me that she has some concerns about the concept of the "corrective emotional experience" that is often described as a healing factor in psychedelic-assisted therapy. This concept of the corrective emotional experience rests on the premise that if you didn't have a loving caregiver, the therapist can provide the experience of being loved and cared for, thus "correcting" any deficits one may have experienced in early life. Laura states that, "while it can be powerful to have an experience that one has profoundly

---

*Participants may have been "primed" by the pervasive use of terminology such as "Grandmother Ayahuasca," or hearing the reports of other participants, which may color their interpretations.

needed, and that can offer significant repair, healing from trauma is also learning how to suffer and grieve what did not happen. If you didn't have a mother, part of healing is feeling that loss and accepting it. . . . leaning too heavily on the corrective emotional experience the therapist runs the risk of depriving their client of that necessary grief and promising a role that they will not consistently fill."

Acceptance, in psychedelic trauma healing, is the process of grieving what you did not have and coming to a place of acceptance, which in turn, frees us to be present in the life that is possible now. Certainly, traditional psychotherapy has the same objective for the healing of trauma; while the intense and accelerated emotional process of psychedelic healing can, for some, make this process more intense, it can also be faster. Psychedelics not only expedite emotional processing, but also tend to imbue perspective. This perspective can help sexual trauma survivors to see, feel, and tolerate how things were for them in the past, in order for them to move into the present moment. As I shall discuss more in depth later, I believe that acceptance is also tied to making meaning. When we accept a terrible thing that has occurred in our lives, we are also willing to see it as a chapter that connects to the wider view of who we are. We might not like what happened to us, but psychedelic experience might help us to consider whether our experience of trauma could make us more compassionate, wise, or to be of service to the world or ourselves in some way. The process of accepting our past trauma is about reorienting ourselves to our own narratives. We can never undo the past, but by accepting what has happened we can potentially start to view it as a transformative event that, while remaining terrible, unjust, or exploitative, can also be an affirmation of our own strength, resilience, and grace. In other words, a tremendous source of personal power.

Stage 4: Releasing

The process of releasing sexual trauma can be emotional, symbolic, or somatic. It's often all of these. I would venture to say that all psychedelic medicines I've helped clients integrate, from MDMA to psilocybin mushrooms to LSD, have the potential to create an inner experience of symbolic release. This may be a literal vision during the psychedelic experience of releasing the traumatic event. It may be a symbolic act such as releasing a stone into a stream or burning a letter to an abuser that can be part of the integration process and undertaken in a meaningful ceremonial way. But release can also be a pure somatic process such as shaking, vomiting, crying, screaming, often with no conscious memory or connection to the trauma itself. Psychedelic experiences can help the body take the lead. The conscious mind can be out of the way enough that other, often profound ways of expressing all suddenly become available. A survivor who has held decades of pent-up rage might shake and vocalize, suddenly able to let the body do what it has been afraid to do in ordinary consciousness with tremendous healing impact.

Stage 5: Embodiment

Embodiment can occur at any stage of healing trauma, but it is often most accessible to us after the intense processes described above have taken place. Embodiment means first being able to notice the body. Sexual trauma survivors are often so disconnected from their body they struggle to feel anything at all. Some may be overwhelmed by feelings and sensations. Embodiment is the process of coming back to inhabiting a human body. Psychedelics (and again, here I'm speaking generally as I believe all psychedelic experiences can encourage qualities of embodiment) can not only help us connect with the body without the sensations of trauma, but can help us to connect the state of being in a body, period. Interestingly, certain psychedelics such as higher dose ketamine or 5-MeO-DMT to name a few, can temporarily make us lose connection with our bodies. However, when the medicine subsides and survivors reenter their bodies, it can be in a new way. Using the breath, sensing the body in space, whether against the furniture a survivor may be situated on or simply feeling connected to the earth, are all ways of anchoring back in the body.

Stage 6: Restoration of Pleasure

Coming home to pleasure is the most overlooked stage in the psychedelic healing of sexual trauma. When emotions have been felt, when negative stories about the self are challenged, when real acceptance has occurred, it's tempting to believe that healing is done. But the loss (or transformation of) trauma symptoms can be experienced as lost aspects of identity, leaving some survivors to feel a black hole inside. What goes in the place of these symptoms and ways of being when they are suddenly gone? Pleasure. Connection. Joy. Being present in sex and in our bodies. So, how can psychedelics help us to achieve this kind of outcome? First the psychedelic experience itself, despite my prior description of being paraded through scenes of previous trauma or vomiting out long-held emotions, can actually be quite pleasurable! All of these harrowing things can happen, but they often give way to relief, good feeling, an afterglow, and an increased sense of connection. We go *through* in order to transform. By transforming our relationship to trauma, we also transform our suffering into pleasure, our isolation into connection, and even our depression into satisfaction. Opening the path to pleasure is the deepest level of healing, one that goes far beyond managing memories and symptoms. It is the way we cultivate a life worth living.

PSYCHEDELIC INTEGRATION STRATEGIES FOR SEXUAL TRAUMA SURVIVORS

The following chapter in this book will explore the process of psychedelic preparation and integration through the lens of sexuality in detail, but first I will touch on some specific integration topics and techniques for sexual trauma survivors. Pleasure itself is the very foundation of my integration practice with sexual trauma survivors. What does it mean to have pleasure as a foundation? It might mean that we view the hard and often excruciating work of healing in service to a very big payoff: the restoration of a connection with our bodies, with our sexuality, and to the joy of being an empowered person in our relationships and life. All psychedelic integration work for sexual trauma survivors should include support in crafting a vision of who that survivor might like to be, as a person no longer encumbered by trauma. Psychedelics can often encourage connection with qualities of wonder, awe, embodiment, and joy. Walking these qualities into our lives—choosing joy—is a culmination of the healing process. Here are some specific approaches to integration that can be helpful in using psychedelics to facilitate healing from sexual violence so that we can access true pleasure.

Making Sense of Traumatic Memories

In my experience, if a trauma survivor forms an intention to work with past sexual trauma during a psychedelic experience, it is very likely that trauma will emerge within the context of the work. With more "lucid" medicines like MDMA, this can often happen at the will of the journeyer or with the prompting of a therapist or guide. With many of the classic psychedelics like LSD, psilocybin, and ayahuasca, the material can emerge in complex symbols, fragments of memory, and even confusing pseudo-memories (memories that are conflations of conscious memories with the additional of fantastical or inaccurate details). In the case of medicines like 5-MeO-DMT, often described as lacking a symbolic narrative, instead linked to expanded affective states, journeyers can either experience intense reliving of trauma sensations, full somatic releases in the form of shaking or vocalizing, or full ecstatic states. It is not usually the question as to *if* trauma material will arise, but *how* it arises that should be the focus of the integration process.

A useful integration practice for survivors is journaling or verbally recalling as much as possible to help consolidate the experience after a psychedelic journey. Details in psychedelic experience can be extremely dreamlike. What seems like you can never forget can fade quickly in the following days. In the context of psychotherapy, having a session the day immediately following the journey is helpful, but it can also be helpful to write everything down, audio record it, or speak it aloud to a trusted person who consents to hearing about the trauma if the integration process is more self-directed. Look for emerging themes, and make careful note of any images, feelings, or narratives that were helpful, confusing, or incited curiosity. It is particularly important during this preliminary phase to notice details such as whether the trauma was reexperienced directly, whether it was observed from outside (and if so whether from a safe distance or within the experience itself), and if any other figures real or imagined were players in your inner cast. As mentioned previously, it is common, particularly with sacred plant medicines, for a survivor to experience the spirit of the medicine presenting as a protective force or ally. You may also have support from ancestors, guides, or resource figures from your life. This will be particularly useful in the subsequent meaning-making phase of integration and should be noted.

This recalling can help garner insights simply because we are translating a psychedelic experience that is felt directly and usually experienced through symbols into words. Even the process of verbalizing, much like sharing a dream, can in and of itself make themes and features stand out that were not immediately clear. For survivors who are not inclined to write, I have assigned them to make a pictogram or illustrations of their experience. Drawing significant symbols or scenes, a storyboard, or other visual representation is equally helpful to recalling and consolidating psychedelic experience.

Somatic Work

Another facet of psychedelic trauma healing is the release of trauma directly from the body or the experience of otherwise overwhelming emotions all the way to completion. These emotions can be rage, disgust, fear, to name a few. When sexual trauma occurs, especially in childhood, the body can enter a protective dissociated state.* Psychedelics can make sensations associated with trauma come flooding back in full force. However, this does not have to be a terrifying or fully overwhelming experience; when witnessed by the session guide, shaman, group of participants, or even the inner world of ancestors or plant spirits providing a safe space for the emotion to be fully felt, the survivor can revisit state in a more tolerable manner. It can also be the case that no clear emotion is arising. The survivor may instead experience seizure-like shaking, purging (vomiting, retching, spitting), or engage in loud

---

*A "dissociated state" is when one becomes disconnected from their thoughts, memories, and bodily sensations. While dissociation is a protective mechanism (the brain's way of protecting someone during a traumatic event), it can persist long after the trauma, recurring to again protect a survivor during moments of stress or overwhelm, making it difficult for the survivor to be fully present and alive in the current moment.

vocalization. These may not be linked to any specific memory, but may instead be the body ridding itself of sensation long stuck in an unprocessed state.

What do we do with these big emotions and feelings in the integration phase? First, we can make an inner inquiry as to whether we feel that whatever this sensation or emotion was has indeed been fully released. It's helpful to note that when in a safe place and with the psychedelic medicine acting as a support to your process, I believe the body knows and has always known exactly how to clear what it doesn't need from your inner system. Survivors can also try what I call "controlled releases" after a psychedelic experience. For example, if the survivor experienced the body shaking out trauma during a psychedelic journey, this same action of "shaking out" can be turned into a tool for healing in their everyday life. For example, when the survivor notices difficult feelings arising or feels triggered, they can shake it out, vocalize it out, or otherwise move it out of the body. In this manner, the survivor gives the body resources to help it return to equilibrium. In the context of psychotherapy, when distress arises in a session, physical movement can be used as a technique to return someone into their window of tolerance. If the somatic sensation linked to trauma was felt to completion during the psychedelic experience, it is possible it will have to be felt to completion in the presence of a compassionate witness again, often taking place in a therapist or other somatic practitioner's office in a sober state. It is common that after profound trauma, especially that occurred in early life, somatic release during a psychedelic experience can be genuinely healing, but the body may need to repeat that process of release many times. This does not require undergoing more and more psychedelic experiences. Survivors can use the somatic "blueprint" of the physical release they experienced during a psychedelic experience as a model for how the body can release the sensations related to trauma more holistically in their ordinary state of consciousness. This kind of physical resourcing can also be used to help survivors gain a window of tolerance by assisting the body to know that it can feel, and it can release.

Another aspect of the integration process that can be helpful for coming back to the body is sequencing the sensory experiences of the psychedelic journey. Tracking each sense memory (what was seen, heard, felt, and/or smelled), can be a link back to peaceful, insightful, or exuberant states. If recorded music was used during a psychedelic experience, listening to it again while tracking the sensory experiences of the journey can be useful. It can also work the other way. After a particularly challenging ayahuasca experience, a client entered my office and experienced near total panic after smelling an incense scent that reminded them of the ceremony space. Sexual trauma often entails a slew of sensations, smells, or visual images that so overpower the nervous system, the survivor can become disconnected from their senses to block out stimuli that can re-trigger traumatic memory. Mapping the full sensory experience after psychedelic work can be a starting point to supporting survivors in letting the world come alive for them once more.

Meaning-Making, Reprocessing Trauma, and Deconstructing Harmful Narratives

Whether you are a survivor trying to understand how your trauma fits into the bigger picture of your life, or are a therapist supporting clients in making meaning of their experiences, relating meaning to trauma is a complex process. In my clinical work I've observed that psychedelic healing can offer accelerated access to perspective, resilience, and curiosity that encourages meaning making and positive self-image in the aftermath of sexual trauma. I have also witnessed psychedelic facilitators, neo-shamanic contexts rooted in wellness culture and New Age spirituality, or pseudo-spiritual figures promoting a reframing of trauma that can be destructive to healing. Examples of this include: "You need to be grateful to the person who abused you so you elevate to a higher plane of spiritual consciousness;" "The abuse didn't really occur. All of life is an illusion;" "You stay stuck on this trauma because you see yourself as a victim;" "Karmically, you called the abuse to you for your own evolution." I wish I was making this up. This stuff really gets said.

If a survivor *independently* arrives at any of these narratives, that can be approached with curiosity and careful evaluation as to how it might support their healing. Forgiving a perpetrator or seeing abuse as part of a spiritual unfolding process may be an essential shift in inner narratives toward wholeness. However, when this commentary originates from a facilitator or transpersonally oriented therapist, it is tantamount to gaslighting and can result in re-traumatization of survivors. An act of invalidation, it is every bit as destructive as being told by a parent, "You just have to get over it," or, "Just move on." Survivors may also be encouraged by such misguided practitioners to act as if they are "spiritually evolved" beyond their trauma in order to stay connected to a community, to a particular facilitator, or be praised by their peers.

This phenomenon is linked to a concept often discussed in tandem with integration practice called spiritual bypassing. Spiritual bypassing is when spiritual practice or beliefs are co-opted to avoid dealing with inner pain, past trauma, or even systemic injustice. In his book on the topic, Robert Augutus Masters characterizes spiritual bypassing as "avoidance in holy drag."[3] People engaging in spiritual bypassing will often use the persona of a spiritually evolved person to distance themself from their own trauma and need for healing work, and often have a lot of unsolicited advice about the healing of others. For example, a need to feel rage after trauma may be shamed as not being "high vibration," or that the act of attempting to navigate messy human emotions is indicative of an "attachment to ego." It is essential to normalize that the feeling of messy emotions is essential to the work of healing. Anger, fear, and grief, far from being "lower" emotions, are every bit as functional and spiritual a part of our process as forgiveness and transcendence.

One study about the influence of childhood sexual abuse on the perception of self by adult survivors identified themes that can be helpful to understanding the meaning-making process in psychedelic integration. The authors of the study note that the healing of sexual trauma involves "integration and reinterpreting past experiences in ways that give meaning to the past while at the same time realizing it is possible to alter the present," and identify different facets of self-perception common in the aftermath of trauma: the worthless self, the self as unknown, and the potential developing self.[4] Many survivors who seek therapy, mutual support, or psychedelic work live with perceptions of worthlessness or responsibility for their trauma. In my clinical experience, the psychedelic healing process often leads to what these researchers call the "self as unknown" (meaning, self-enquiry of who the survivor might have been if they had not experienced abuse or assault, including wondering what type of personality they might have had), and the potential developing self (who might a survivor be as the process of healing unfolds). Psychedelic integration work to heal sexual trauma can encourage this process of inquiry. Survivors can sometimes feel traits of personality unencumbered by trauma, or even feel their body free from somatic activation. Integration work can build upon these questions about self, allowing curiosity to fuel their process of self-discovery.

Trauma reprocessing can also occur during and after psychedelic experiences. During the integration phase, a way of determining whether a trauma has been processed to completion during the psychedelic experience or needs further processing during the integration phase is to recall an image that represents the trauma and notice if there are any body sensations related to the trauma that are still active. A technique derived from EMDR therapy, this exercise can be used as a stand-alone method of calibrating the integration process. If the survivor still feels activation in the body, such as the stomach flipping or tingling in the limbs, it is likely that the trauma material has been confronted in some way during the psychedelic experience, but is not yet fully resolved. This is a juncture where pausing and seeking out a skilled somatic psychotherapist can be essential. When I am working with clients in integration psychotherapy who have recalled or witnessed past trauma in a psychedelic state, and still experience a somatic charge coming from the traumatic memory, I generally encourage them to pause on using more substances and use somatic psychotherapy techniques to help the body process the trauma through to completion. However, some survivors may be in very supportive psychedelic environments for healing with trauma-trained guides, in which case subsequent psychedelic experiences with robust integration support between them can also help the client process the trauma through to completion.

The deconstructing of harmful narratives about the self is the link between the therapeutic and the sacred. Self-blame for abuse or negative self-referencing beliefs are always a protective part of us trying to prevent more harm from occurring. The belief that we could have stopped past abuse means we can prevent future abuse. If we are dirty or unloveable, for example, we avoid the risk of further rejection or harm. Psychedelics, at their best, can connect us temporarily, and sometimes permanently, with an inner knowing that we are whole, loveable, and worthy. However, that spark of knowing must be supported in the integration process as those protective parts won't concede their role easily! They have a job to do, and that is preventing disaster. In my therapy practice, I have found the compassionate approach of Internal Family Systems a wonderful way of working with protective parts that hold harmful narratives. Internal Family Systems encourages understanding and gratitude for those inner parts of ourselves that have protected us throughout our lives (even though on the surface they do some really mean things like saying that no one will love us, or prompt behaviors like self-harming). When those parts feel seen and appreciated, survivors find more room to question these harmful narratives and build new ones, and more importantly, make new alliances with their protectors to shift them into more functional ways of supporting the survivor.

Whether or not a survivor relates to this as a spiritual process is up to them. For me, I believe that releasing stories that link us to shame, self-blame, and unworthiness is the process of recognizing the inherent sacredness of self. Moreover, survivors may begin to be curious about the transition between the need to acknowledge and sometimes heavily relate to oneself as a survivor, and integrate the experience of trauma into a more holistic picture of identity that is not wholly defined by trauma. Again, this must be a self-initiated and organic process. Telling a survivor not to be so identified with their trauma is abuse. But when natural curiosity arises, when trauma and its aftermath are no longer running the show in our life, we are arriving at a new, more functional place.

I've worked with some survivors who have had so much trauma-focused therapy and other healing work, that they have developed a whole identity, personal relationships, and sense of personal limitations around their trauma. The trauma serves as a double not only to impede them, but also to protect them from having to engage in a fulfilling career, tolerate the ordinary discomfort that can arise even in non-abusive relationships, and tolerate the boundaries set by important people in their life. A part that stays attached to trauma is also a protective part and needs the same validation and gratitude of any other protector. But those protective parts limit us nonetheless. Creating space in integration work to acknowledge the fear around releasing our trauma-identity and the responsibility that comes with it can be a crucial step in the healing process.

In order to advocate for a pleasure-centered perspective on the psychedelic healing of traumas that impact our sexuality, understanding trauma theory and history—especially as it relates to the larger context we live in, for example the impact of things like systemic injustice, misogyny, and violence—provides a useful foundation as we craft a new vision that diverges from the conventional, medical understanding of trauma. Perhaps it's easier to think about sexual trauma just being the effect of very bad things that might happen to us, rather than acknowledge that the enduring wounds we carry are the result of a sex-negative society, poor sexual mirroring in childhood, religious upbringings, and identity-based traumas—such as discrimination, and mistreatment experienced by marginalized groups and other traditionally oppressed communities, to name a few. Acknowledging that so many of us have been traumatized in our homes, churches, schools, and relationships elicits deep grief. If trauma is all around us, how do we ever escape it? Conversely, if trauma is something that touches virtually all of us, then might it be possible to build collective models for healing and social change in which we are all invested that are rooted in social justice, respect, and pleasure? When we see our healing as tied to the healing of all people, we take a step closer to collective action and reclaiming pleasure as our birthright and the birthright of all.

A BRIEF GENERAL HISTORY OF TRAUMA

Few concepts have been as debated and controversial in modern psychology as trauma and its diagnostic correlates, post-traumatic stress disorder (PTSD) and complex post-traumatic stress disorder (C-PTSD). What exactly constitutes sexual trauma? What events are bad enough to meet the criteria as to be traumatic? How is sexual and relational violence unique in its symptom expression and aftermath? What happens when trauma occurs at the hands of a person otherwise responsible for your care or engaged in a familial, professional, or personal relationship with the survivor? As author Staci Haines puts it, "One thing that is so difficult about childhood sexual abuse and other forms of violence that are intimate is that it confuses the need to survive and the need to be connected and love. Instead of these two foundational functions operating together, they are put at odds through trauma."[5] Sexual traumas are violence enacted against the very being of a person on a physical, psychological, and spiritual level, and so they require healing of the body, mind, and soul.

Let's first explore trauma as a general concept. The idea of trauma as a discreet mental illness itself did not begin to gain scientific definition until the mid-nineteenth century at the dawn of industrialization and the invention of the railway system, where accidents were increasingly common and destabilizing, resulting an increasing sense of vulnerability in the public. As Crocq and Crocq describe, "The Industrial Revolution and the introduction of steam driven machinery were to give rise to the first civilian man-made disasters and cases of PTSD outside of the battlefield."[6] A neurologist, Hermann Oppenheim, offered that the Greek word for "wound" does not only apply to a physical malady but could also apply to a psychological wound that is beyond our capacity to adapt.[7] As soldiers from the First World War returned from battle mentally scarred by the likes of technological warfare never before seen or experienced, the idea of trauma as a condition that affected not only the body but also the mind became recognized and accepted.[8]

Trauma has indeed been heavily associated with veterans, and it was veterans who in 1980, more than a hundred years later, would successfully lobby the American Psychological Association to codify a new diagnosis: post-traumatic stress disorder (PTSD).[9] That trauma is associated with both development of the railway industry and war provides insight into how the social and scientific recognition of trauma is linked to the expansion of capitalism. As we aspire to a pleasure-centered approach to trauma healing, the remedy for the moral and physical injury of violence under the forces fueling unbridled capitalism and imperialism may be found in the earth-based, the collective, and reconnecting with the sacred.

While violent sexual assault has always been understood as an identifiable trauma that can lead to post-traumatic stress disorder, the early theories of Sigmund Freud and Josef Breuer give us historical context for how sexual abuse has been psychologically conceptualized. In her seminal text *Trauma and Recovery*, feminist author and trauma theorist Judith Herman tells us that by the 1890s, Freud and his collaborator Breuer were positing a theory around a condition that was nearly universally applied to emotionally dysregulated women: hysteria. Freud and Breuer theorized that extreme responses to psychological trauma could induce an altered state of consciousness they called "double consciousness," which lead to hysterical symptoms. When Freud began to further develop his early theory by interviewing "hysterical" women, he found histories of abuse, incest, and other sexual traumas, leading him to conclude that it was "one or more occurrences of premature sexual experience" underpinning the diagnosis of hysteria. Herman continues, "Hysteria was so common among women that if his patient's stories were true, and his theories were correct, he would be forced to conclude that what he called 'perverted acts against children' were endemic . . . among respected bourgeoisie families. This idea was simply unacceptable." Freud eventually abandoned his theory, instead attributing these stories of abuse recalled by his patients to fantasy.[10] In my opinion, Freud's decision to abandon his original thesis—lest he risk losing his power and status in "respectable" society—is an excellent example of how prevailing social structures are upheld and reinforced even by "men of science;" Freud chose to privilege his own status and professional ambition over advancing clinical thinking about the diagnosis of hysteria, betraying his patients in the process.

The exact criteria and nature of the PTSD diagnosis has evolved and changed through the various versions of the Diagnostic and Statistical Manual, the clinical bible of psychiatric illnesses, over the years. However, clinicians who treated traumatized individuals, particularly when that trauma was relational or sexual in nature, realized there were experiences that did not neatly fit under the umbrella of PTSD, and in the 1990s, a new concept was introduced: C-PTSD.[11] Complex post-traumatic stress disorder occurs when trauma is recurrent and occurs over a period of time, often in the context of a family or community, such as in the case of many childhood sexual and emotional abuse survivors. These sexual traumas are not single, terrible incidents. They are repeated events that may be subtle or dramatic that impact the survivor's sense of self and result in hallmark traits of emotional dysregulation, dissociation, physical symptoms like headaches or pelvic pain, shifts in self-perception, shifting perceptions of the perpetrator of abuse (the perpetrator might have also been an otherwise-beloved parent or family member), difficulty in relationships, and difficulty making meaning in the survivor's life.[12] As trauma therapist and author Erin Carpenter puts it, "While a survivor of a single trauma event (like a rape as an adult) may feel like she is not herself, the survivor of chronic trauma may lose the sense that she even *has* a self."[13]

If it's true that survivors of trauma can lose touch with their sense of self, what broader implications might that have? The physical, emotional, and relational impact of trauma is fairly widely understood in our culture. But what about our spiritual selves? Our political selves? What can we understand about who the sexual trauma survivor is as a person existing in the world? I discussed this with psychotherapist Laura Mae Northup. Laura is a therapist, who, like me, specializes in working with psychedelics and sexual trauma survivors. She's the author of the book *Radical Healership: How to Build a Values-Driven Healing Practice in a Profit-Driven World,* and has also produced and hosted the podcast *Inside Eyes* where sexual trauma survivors tell their stories of psychedelic healing. She has intense, penetrating eyes, and hair that is often streaked with various rainbow colors. When I talk with Laura, I often look up and realize an hour has passed. She's a force of nature.

"Sexuality is deeply related to power. Having an intact relationship with desire, pleasure, and the sensations of the body helps us be personally empowered, and thus politically empowered. Being traumatized at all, but especially being traumatized in a way that is specifically overpowering to one's will and bodily autonomy, disables and damages that person's embodied sense of power. To be made to feel powerless is to be abused in a way that lessens our collective functioning," Northrup explained. I agree. Reflecting on the history of trauma itself, we cannot separate an act of interpersonal violence from the wider societal contexts in which they occur.

But there is another lens through which to understand the impact of sexual violence: the effect on the spirit. For Laura, spiritual health is inextricably linked to our political autonomy.

> Sexual abuse crushes the spirit. An inability to be present and in one's own humanity is a spiritual problem. The inability to be empowered is a spiritual problem. It's a very spiritually wounded place to be in, to not view yourself as a part of humanity, to not allow yourself the things people deserve. And this is a pervasive belief for many sexual trauma survivors, that they are somehow not a part of humanity. In a lot of ways I view spirituality from a very practical place. It's about the mystery and the magic. It's about wonder and awe, and big questions. But it's also about choice and beliefs, and what's of value to us. How we live our lives is a spiritual question, and in this world that is also a political question. There is a life force or spirit in each of us. When there is trauma and no subsequent healing, our life-force is diminished. When trauma prevents us from living meaningful empowered lives, that is a political *and* spiritual issue.

THE BRILLIANT RESILIENCE OF TRAUMA SURVIVORS

What exactly is the prevalence of sexual trauma as it's conventionally understood, that is, sexual assault, childhood sexual abuse, incest, and other forms of overt sexual violence? The epidemiology of the problem is staggering. Over forty-seven percent of women and twenty-three percent of men reported some form of unwanted sexual contact in their lifetime.[14] The statistics for the LGBTQIA+ community are even worse, with transgender people and bisexual women most at risk. Recent statistics from the National Sexual Violence Resource Center reports that for transgender people, nearly half had experienced sexual violence and for those who have been unhoused, engaged in sex work, are People of Color, or have (or have had) a disability, the number grows even higher.[15] If we expand the frame yet again to include all of those who experienced sexual shaming, conversion therapy, lack of sex education, religious judgment, homophobia and transphobia, and those inappropriately sexualized as children, we are now talking about a very large portion of the population.

One way of understanding the aftermath of sexual trauma is to look at how the mind, body, and spirit adapt to such wounds. The literature on sexual trauma survivors most often points to the problems these individuals experience such as interpersonal issues, sexual dysfunction or out-of-control sexual behaviors, poor self-esteem, shame, and substance use as the *result* of trauma. We look at these outcomes as the problem to fix, instead of regarding these behaviors as strategies employed by an elegant and intelligent inner protective system that will stop at nothing to protect the survivor from overwhelming feelings and sensations. Take substance abuse (since this is a book on healing with substances). One study from a drug and alcohol treatment facility found eighty-one percent of women and sixty-nine percent of men in substance use treatment had histories of relational or sexual abuse.[16] In a society obsessed with individual achievement, and also individual responsibility, we tend to look at a person using substances, whether or not the way they use the substance is harmful to them or their community, and attribute their uses to personal weakness.

But a trauma-informed way to understand this type of substance use behavior is that using substances is one of the most effective ways to block out the feelings, negative self-referencing beliefs, and somatic artifacts of trauma. People do it because it works. Traumatized people might also use substances because it affords them a moment of simply feeling pleasurable relief. If we blame individuals, we are ignoring our own responsibility to create safe and expansive, community-held contexts to honor and hold space for healing relational and sexual trauma, as well as creating accessibility to treatments, such as psychedelic interventions, that work. Perhaps it's because that would require acknowledging that it is the people within our very midst—parents, siblings, neighbors, and teachers—that are most often the ones responsible for creating this suffering. In fact, eighty percent of sexual assaults are perpetrated by someone who knows the victim, and ninety three percent of juveniles who experience sexual abuse knew the perpetrator.[17] Turns out, we are not so far from Freud and Breuer after all.

This shift in perspective gives us an opportunity to look not only at the use of psychedelics, but the use of all drugs as it relates to trauma. Psychedelics, in many cases, actually *amplify* the emotions and sensations associated with sexual trauma. For the psychedelic healing of trauma to be effective, a person has to be prepared to go through that experience of feeling the worst of their emotions, which—although potentially uncomfortable in the short run—can then in turn lead to intense pleasure. Whereas the substances we heavily vilify in our society, such as cocaine and heroin (both of which are acknowledged to have medical utility), are generally the ones that are extremely helpful for doing with the mind exactly what they do in the body—numbing and stopping pain. The resilience of the traumatized person exists in being able to find what works to block out overwhelming feelings for as long as they need to, including dissociation, seeking high sexual stimulation, and workaholism. These strategies, however, eventually leave us sick, isolated, and disenfranchised, rarely leading to *actual* pleasure, if further healing is not available.

Rachel Yahuda conducted a fascinating study on the sexual outcomes of people who experienced nonsexual trauma. Yahuda and her team looked at survivors of combat, being the victim of a crime, or vehicular accidents, and studied the impact of these traumas on their sexuality. She references multiple studies that support a correlation between nonsexual trauma and sexual dysfunction. Yahuda explains that sexual dysfunction occurs after nonsexual traumas because of "an inability to regulate and redirect the physiological arousal needed for healthy sexual function away from hyperarousal and aggression circuits." She furthers that the hormonal and neural circuit activation that would normally support feelings of being sexually aroused are already in overdrive due to the effects of PTSD. Instead of arousal, she found these people experienced fear, anxiety, and even flashbacks during sex. She cites further research that suggests the problem may be relational as people with PTSD tend to experience sexual difficulty with partners, but not during erotic self-stimulation (masturbation). In fact, trauma therapists may not even be asking about the co-occurrence of sexual issues when treating trauma survivors without explicitly sexual trauma.[18]

It's unsurprising that in most conventional medical and therapeutic contexts, in-depth questions about sexual functioning and trauma-informed care are not offered. After all, unless they are pursuing a specialty, medical doctors receive less than twelve hours of education about sexual issues during their training, while psychotherapists receive less than nine.[19] Given what I've observed in the psychotherapy field at large, namely, that sexual trauma means rape or childhood sexual abuse, and sexual dysfunction amounts to sexual anatomy not working right, it's no wonder that even people seeking support may find themselves underserved by providers. This is why adopting a sophisticated perspective of sexual trauma and dysfunction is crucial for healing and wholeness.

A Note on Borderline Personality Disorder

A lack of an anchored sense of self is common for people who have suffered early life sexual and relational traumas. Complex post-traumatic stress disorder resulting from sexual abuse is often linked to a series of personality traits known in the DSM-V as "Cluster B" diagnoses, the most stigmatized of which is borderline personality disorder. Progressive trauma therapists have been moving away from these stigmatizing diagnoses, instead preferring to understand these symptoms as the result of repeated traumas. Understanding that so-called borderline symptoms—including unstable interpersonal relationships, tendencies to self-harm including suicidal impulses, and intensely idealizing and then later devaluing the same person—have their roots in trauma is more reflective of the etiology of the client's suffering, as well as less stigmatizing for the trauma survivor. However, trauma survivors with these characteristics often experience intense difficulty in relationships, including the one they have with their psychotherapist. Individuals with these types of trauma outcomes can have, at first, intense positive projections about the therapist which the therapist cannot possibly live up to, or perhaps very distrustful projections. Even a well-resourced therapist can struggle to navigate such projections effectively. A therapist might feel the client's desperation for connection and help, while also getting drawn into what can be a tumultuous inner world of intense anxious attachment, projections, and subsequent devaluation and threats.

Extraordinary caution needs to be exercised when considering psychedelic treatments for certain people with a C-PTSD diagnosis and what is typically labeled as borderline personality disorder. I believe psychedelics hold tremendous promise for symptoms common to this diagnosis such as ameliorating urges to self-harm and bolstering the ability to see people and experiences in "shades of gray" (as opposed to the rigid thinking that often characterizes someone with this diagnosis), and that perhaps not everything is exactly the way it seems to the survivor. However, clinical monitoring for suicidality and managing intense attachment to and projections about the therapist, called transference, are also real concerns. Because psychedelic experiences can be initially destabilizing and require intense integration to regain equilibrium, clients with very fluid and unstable inner worlds need comprehensive support.

I've seen firsthand in my ketamine-assisted psychotherapy work that even a very skilled psychiatrist conducting a medical intake and a competent therapist engaging in preparation sessions cannot always see these traits at first. Because psychedelic-assisted psychotherapy is often short term, when the treatment ends the client can be left feeling abandoned and rageful, even if the therapist consistently prepared the client for this ending. Additionally, psychedelics can cause rapid shifts in perspective which can be experienced as confusing when the survivor's inner world is already the site of turmoil and confusion. It is worth considering what types of special needs psychedelic practitioners need to adopt to effectively work with these sexual trauma survivors. Certainly, the model utilized in research settings where the therapeutic relationship is severed when the participant's involvement in the study concludes can be harmful for people already struggling with unstable interpersonal relationships and feelings of abandonment.

BEYOND PTSD
Developing an Expanded Definition of Sexual Trauma

This brief overview of trauma as it's been understood in psychological thinking from the mid-nineteenth century to the present, and the diagnoses that have evolved to describe the symptoms of trauma, are important to name and understand so we can embrace a new, holistic definition of sexual trauma that is relevant to this book and to a pleasure-focused philosophy of healing. To review, our definition of sexual and relational trauma centers on the impact of systems, events, or interpersonal experiences that affect our self-perception and deprive us of safety in our body, the world, and in relationships, and impairs our ability to be present with pleasure in an enduring way. By embracing this expanded definition of trauma we can bypass the need for survivors to have to justify what happened to them was "bad enough" to be truly traumatic, and instead focus on how a person's inner system, both their literal nervous system as well as their inner system of protective "parts" of self (to borrow the terminology of Internal Family Systems Therapy), copes with the world around them. This allows for a more sophisticated approach to healing that is not pathologizing and is centered on the inner world of the survivor rather than society's need to codify and quantify traumatic events. In the *Myth of Normal: Trauma, Illness, and Healing in a Toxic Culture*, Gabor Maté writes, "Trauma is an inner injury, a lasting rupture or split within the self due to difficult or hurtful events. . . . Trauma is not what happens *to you*, but what happens *inside* you." He continues, "Trauma pervades our culture, from personal functioning through social relationships, parenting, education, popular culture, economics, and politics. In fact, someone *without* the marks of trauma would be an outlier in our society."[20]

Progressive trauma theorists have in fact commented that the emphasis on events and the individual, rather than on subjective and the collective experiences, is rooted in the broader context of Eurocentrism and colonialism. A more accurate approach to trauma decenters the individual response and instead emphasizes the need for a collective and social responsibility to end the social conditions that promote traumatic experience.[21] First Nations author Renee Linklater describes how the term "trauma" itself, as it has been situated in the Western medical system, should be critiqued. She explains, "Using trauma terminology implies that the individual is responsible for the response, rather than the broader systematic force caused by (the state's) abuse of power."[22] Linklater is speaking directly to the experience of Indigenous people, and by extension People of Color, who are subject to the unique collective and intergenerational traumas of European colonization, oppression, and slavery. But we can also extend this thinking to anyone traumatized by institutional abuse and discrimination in employment, health care, and social institutions, including in psychedelics healing initiatives, medicalized or otherwise.

There is a crucial distinction to be made which might seem paradoxical to my argument about the pervasiveness of trauma in our culture: the distinction between trauma and stress. While on one hand I'm arguing that we are well served to expand the definition of trauma, it is also important to detail that uncomfortable or unpleasant experiences are not necessarily traumatic. Trauma is a concept that I believe to be clinically underutilized as a descriptor to understand our experiences and how they impact embodiment, self-esteem, and self-perception. I simultaneously argue that the word "trauma," in certain contexts, is colloquially overused. Reading a story with upsetting content, or hearing a perspective with which you don't agree is not traumatic. It is more accurate to call it arousing or stressful. Researchers Gal Richter-Levin and Carmen Sandi argue that it is "impossible to define a stress experience using only the parameters of the stressor" and describe the distinction between an *arousing experience*, one that activates a detectable emotional reaction and may affect an immediate behavioral response; a *stressful experience*, an experience that activates a substantial emotional response that is capable of impacting future emotional responses but without shifting a person's ability to adapt to future challenges; and a *traumatic experience* which elicits a robust emotional response and induces lasting alterations that are enduring and compromise a person's ability to be resilient.[23] Age, social location,* and previous trauma history can all impact whether an experience is stored as a trauma in our nervous system or not. In a moment when we are bombarded with social media armchair psychology and Instagram mental health memes, naming that bad things can and do happen but are not always traumatic, feels important. Using our expanded definition of trauma, we might also consider whether an event has shaped our ability to experience safety, pleasure, or embodiment in an enduring way.

THE BIG IMPACT OF EVERYDAY TRAUMAS

Aaliyah was a twenty-two-year-old woman who came to her first session of therapy anxious, struggling to make eye contact, and dressed in clothes that were excessive and heavy for the warm spring weather. She initially contacted me because she was interested in ketamine-assisted psychotherapy for what she described as "lots of problems with sex and relationships." She explained that she struggled to trust men, feared being naked in front of a partner, and felt highly anxious at parties and social events where her friends were having fun meeting people to date. Aaliyah found all this confounding because she could not think of any event in her past that had been explicitly traumatic in her mind. During the first few sessions, we took a detailed history of her sexual development and history. When given the opportunity to share her story, she remembered a moment of coming down the stairs in her home one summer morning around the age

---

*The National Council of Family Relations defines "social location" as "the combination of factors including gender, race, social class, age, ability, religion, sexual orientation, and geographic location. This makes social location particular to each individual; that is, social location is not always exactly the same for any two individuals."[24]

of twelve wearing a bathing suit. Her father looked up from his seat at the kitchen table with disgust in his eyes telling her she was too old to be walking around like that and to cover up. He went back to reading, but to Aaliyah, the look on his face said everything. She was a sexual object when she wasn't even trying to be. Her body was a source of danger, not celebration. She wasn't even safe in her own home. Her father, with whom she had a loving relationship, now saw her as sexual, inappropriate, and scandalous. Aaliyah got the message loud and clear that if a man feels sexual toward you, it is your fault, and this message was reinforced at the teen youth group meetings at her church.

During our ketamine work, Aaliyah mostly had very deep emotional experiences of crying, and feelings of sadness and loss. This eventually gave way to anger. She usually asked me to sit in a certain chair in my office the farthest from her, she was adamant she did not want the option for supportive touch such as holding her hand if requested. Her ketamine experiences didn't have much narrative; she didn't see images or have a "journey," but she did gain access to emotion. After a few sessions of processing these feelings of grief and anger, Aaliyah was ready to go deeper. During a session when the ketamine began to wear off, Aaliyah was open to making contact with her twelve-year-old self. In her inner world she entered the room where her child self was stranded, ashamed and confused. We asked her what that twelve-year-old needed from us? "Really," said Aaliyah, "she just wants to go swimming and be a child." She was free.

In our integration work, we explored all of the assumptions about sex and women Aaliyah had grown up with that she had never considered before. She didn't feel ready to date yet, but she did feel ready to wear the clothes she liked and felt less afraid to be part of the world. She no longer imagined eyes staring at her and judging at all times. For Aaliyah, this was real healing. Her healing required understanding the lasting impact of what happened to her, but also understanding the culture and assumptions of her father. She had to form new narratives about herself, her body, and her right to exist in whatever clothes she wanted to wear. The increased cognitive flexibility and experience of emotional release afforded by our ketamine work got her there.

Unraveling our personal stories is sometimes necessary for understanding how little things that seem non-traumatic can have lifelong impact on our relationships, sexual self-perception, and ability to feel pleasure. Living in a society characterized by extreme individualism creates a stage on which we all have to grapple to form any holistic, healthy sense of sexual self. Any act of pleasure under these circumstances is an act of rebellion. Every moment of celebrating your body exactly as it is is revolutionary. Any time you take to feel good is pushing back upon a system that rewards productivity over pleasure, and accomplishment under capitalistic ambition and greed over human connection. Likewise, engaging with the true courage it takes to look at your story and realize that perhaps the sexual mirroring and messages you received about your sexuality were not ideal after all, while still allowing yourself the perspective and softness to recognize that under this system, these traumas are inevitable because we are collectively traumatized. Individual healing can never be complete without addressing the collective healing necessary to cultivate a sexually affirming society that values pleasure.

BODY BETRAYAL
Exploring Sexual Dysfunction Issues

Painful intercourse, difficulty with sexual response including erectile dysfunction, the inability to orgasm, and low desire are some of the conditions that fall under the clinical umbrella of sexual dysfunction. But crucially, it is not a physical condition alone that constitutes sexual dysfunction. It's our psychological distress response that is most important. According to one study, about twelve percent of women reported distress about their sexual functioning, though forty percent reported sexual issues.[25] Some types of sexual dysfunction have a physical etiology related to illness or injury. Examples include poor circulatory or heart health contributing to erectile issues, or hormonal changes leading to sexual difficulty or vaginal pain. Thus, some dysfunction is best addressed by medical providers who can utilize medication, laser treatment, or other interventions to help with sexual issues. But by far, for the majority of clients with whom I've worked in my therapy practice, sexual dysfunction has much more to do with stress, anxiety, depression, the impact of past trauma and sexual violence, and life in a culture that devalues human connection and mental well-being. While I will not make an argument that psychedelic experiences can reliably be helpful in treating sexual dysfunction for people who actually need medical interventions such as hormone therapy or erectile-enhancing drugs, a sexual lifesaver for many, I do believe that psychedelics can be a support in shifting the inner emotional conditions that give rise to many sexual dysfunctions and help optimize sexual self-acceptance, which are the most important factors in having an erotically satisfying life.

At the time of writing, there is no clinical research that has studied the impact of psychedelics on specific sexual dysfunctions such as pelvic pain or low desire (although I've certainly discussed working on projects like this with different researchers and a few companies, so it is likely on the horizon), but there *is* newly emerging research studying psychedelics and sexual satisfaction mentioned later in chapter six of this book. I believe the much more profound application of psychedelic medicines in treating sexual dysfunction issues is in treating the underlying psychological factors. People experiencing sexual dysfunction can carry not only shame, but extremely inflexible stories about themselves, their relationships, their bodies, and their worth, not to mention profound anxiety about not being able to "perform" sexually in a way that is acceptable to them and their partners. Examining distress and harmful self-referencing beliefs is key to successful treatment of sexual dysfunction. I believe the existing research does support that psychedelics can be instrumental in helping us form new sexual narratives and improve sexual self-esteem.

In my work with clients, I've observed certain core emotional themes related to sexual dysfunction including rigid sexual narratives, poor sexual self-esteem, withdrawal from relationships or resistance to pursuing relationships, anxiety, and difficulty experiencing willingness to explore new forms of pleasure. For these clients, their focus becomes "fixing" their sexual issues rather than imagining all of the other ways pleasure might be accessible to them right now. In her groundbreaking work studying optimal sexual experience, Dr. Peggy Kleinplatz found that for her subjects, being physically able-bodied was not necessary for what she calls "magnificent sex." She notes that for some of her subjects, "sex only became magnificent after previous sexual options became impossible. The experience of disability caused the individual to set aside assumptions and preconceptions about sex, which helped open the door to magnificent sexual experiences."[26] Here, we see that it is actually resourcefulness and willingness to experience sex in a new way that facilitates pleasure.

One scientifically supported fact worth mentioning is the massive pleasure gap between men and women. Numerous studies confirm that heterosexual activities vastly benefit men, with men of all sexual orientations experiencing more reported sexual pleasure than women, with the largest pleasure deficit experienced by heterosexual women. Research suggests women orgasm only sixty-five percent of the time with a male partner. This is not because women inherently have more difficulty with orgasm. In fact, women with female partners had a three times greater likelihood of always having an orgasm than women with male partners. There are complex social, physical, and emotional reasons for this. Socially reinforced ideas that women's sexuality is dangerous, men not focusing on the types of sexual activities that actually give women pleasure, and prevailing attitudes that women's reason for sex is ultimately procreation, and the priority of men's pleasure over women's persist to this day.[27] Wouldn't it be a wonderful thing if the empathy that is engendered by psychedelic experiences could actually promote better sexual connection in couples simply through an increase in caring how your partner feels about the sex you are having?

I'd be remiss if I did not mention a major contributor to sexual dysfunction that *absolutely* relates to the potential for psychedelic healing: the use of SSRI medications. SSRI medication (selective serotonin reuptake inhibitors) are a first-line treatment for many mental health conditions including depression, anxiety, and post-traumatic stress disorder. I'm not against their use. In fact, many of my clients have experienced profound relief from depression and anxiety using SSRIs. However, SSRIs have a more than shaky track record as to their actual efficacy. Not only do some studies show antidepressant medications to only marginally edge out placebo in terms of usefulness,[28] SSRIs are both widely prescribed *and* widely known to extinguish libido and cause issues with orgasm and sexual response in as many as eighty percent of the people who take them.[29] Certainly, it can be profoundly distressing to lose your capacity to be interested in sex and sexual responsivity when trying to treat depression or anxiety.

But even more fascinating, authors Brian Earp and Julian Savulescu describe a startling reality in their book, *Love Drugs: The Chemical Future of Relationships*. The authors posit that successful romantic love between partners must include an enduring investment in the feelings of your paramour. They ask the question, *what if you were to take a drug that directly impacted your ability to care about your partner's well-being?* They muse, "Does such an awful-sounding drug really exist? Yes it does. It's called a selective serotonin reuptake inhibitor." The authors go on to assert that SSRIs may blunt "maladaptive feelings of sadness. . . . but for some patients, the ability to care about other people's feelings seems to be blunted as well."[30] At the risk of sounding like a proverbial broken record, why would we opt for ongoing treatments that sometimes help depression, but often impair sexual quality of life for users, while also potentially decreasing interpersonal connection and empathy, when we can continue to develop psychedelic treatments—potentially effective in little as one dose—that do just the opposite? Psychedelics have been shown not only to be incredibly helpful with ameliorating the symptoms of depression and anxiety, but do so by making us more connected to ourselves, to others and the world, not less so. Researchers are only beginning to understand the vastly powerful impact this will have not only on depression, but on sexual satisfaction and functioning.

BODY BLISS
Psychedelics and the Journey Home to Yourself

A later chapter in this book will explore specific psychedelics and their possible application in healing our sexuality and increasing pleasure. But first, we return to Kleinplatz's research. She names eight major components of optimal sexual experiences. They are:

1. Being completely present in the moment, embodied, focused, absorbed
2. Connection, alignment, being in sync, merger
3. Deep sexual and erotic intimacy
4. Extraordinary communication and deep empathy
5. Being genuine, authentic, transparent
6. Vulnerability and surrender
7. Exploration, interpersonal risk-taking, and fun
8. Transcendence and transformation[31]

Kleinplatz, of course, was not thinking of psychedelics and their potential impact on sexuality when conducting her research. But I could not come up with a list more aligned with the transformative qualities of psychedelics if I tried. Clinical research supports that psychedelics have the power to increase empathy,[32] support greater openness,[33] reduce neuroticism,[34] and increase interpersonal connectedness,[35] all qualities that would support a shift towards greater empathy and self-compassion, reducing anxiety, and increasing cognitive flexibility necessary to deconstruct harmful narratives about the self and imagine new realities where access to pleasure flourishes.

What if the greatest gift that psychedelics might actually be able to offer us in terms of "healing" sexual dysfunction, has nothing to do with changing the physical functioning of the body? What if the real healing was actually about diversifying the ways we embrace erotic pleasure, to cultivating a sense of present moment awareness during erotic experiences, to alleviate the distress associated with changes in sexual functioning through the process of falling in love with our body and our partner's body exactly as it is and exactly how it works in this moment? Perhaps we can even come to see the distress we experience around sexual functioning as just another protective part, a part that wants us to have the "right" body that functions the "right" way. Certainly, if a medical intervention will help you change your sexual functioning in a way that increases pleasure, go for it. Hack your sex life with science, by all means. But psychedelic experience can also shape a deeper layer of emotional and spiritual maturity that tells us pleasure is here for you, right here, right now. In this very body.

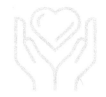

4
Psychedelic Preparation and Integration for Sexual Healing and Expanded Pleasure

Living Ritual

Even a wounded world is feeding us. Even a wounded world holds us, giving us moments of wonder and joy. I choose joy over despair. Not because I have my head in the sand, but because joy is what the earth gives me daily and I must return the gift.

ROBIN WALL KIMMERER, FROM *BRAIDING SWEETGRASS*

THE PROCESS OF PREPARING for a medicine journey, experiencing it, and later processing it to make enduring meaning and change in our life is broadly referred to as psychedelic preparation and integration. This process may be self-guided, it may involve community or a ceremonial facilitator, or it may take place in the context of psychotherapy or coaching relationships giving rise to a wildly expanding clinical focus called psychedelic integration psychotherapy. A team of researchers synthesized themes from thirty psychedelic integration providers and developed a consensus definition of psychedelic integration as "a bridge from the psychedelic experience to everyday life that helps clients make sense of the experience in a personalized way, leading to lasting behavior change and a sense of wholeness or completion."[1] This is a solid foundation for understanding the nature and importance of integration work, but particular issues, considerations, and possibilities come into play when we focus integration on increasing sexual self-esteem, healing from sexual violence, or sexual and relationship satisfaction. This chapter offers a comprehensive approach to psychedelic preparation and integration informed by over a decade of developing tools and techniques for working with sexual trauma survivors, couples seeking enhanced relational quality, and curious seekers working to deepen their sexual self-knowledge and pleasure.

In a fascinating paper on psychedelic preparation and integration, Geoff Bathje, Eric Majeski, and Mesphina Kudowor provide contrast between Western therapeutic approaches to integration that require the identification of specific intentions and utilize formal psychotherapy for support, to Indigenous approaches to psychedelic medicines. They argue that living Indigenous practices which may have thousands of years of history and continue on today, are rooted in community, group, and family; use of spiritual beliefs and traditions; and the use of shamans, with body, mind, and spirit seen as a unified whole. This holistic worldview that strives for balance in the self and with nature, as well as the community settings in which psychedelic use occurs, create a context for the psychedelic experience that shifts the need for codified intentions and integration. Most importantly, they stress that separating psychedelic work into distinct phases, preparation, ingestion, and integration, is likely a product of Western dualistic thinking, rather than an Indigenous perspective that includes community, music, trance practices, and ritual before, during, and after the use of a plant medicine in one unified container.[2]

When we shift our intentions for psychedelic healing from the expectations of the medical model that focuses on symptom reduction, to a holistic model that centers community, family, or relationship cohesion, nature-connectedness, being present with sensations and experiences of pleasure, and centers the value of the experience itself, we are actually creating a new paradigm for psychedelic work distinct from the medical model, and inspired by but different from Indigenous practices. The specific aim of this chapter is to explore how erotic enhancement and increased sexual connection with ourselves and others might be supported after psychedelic ceremonies or even recreational experiences. Some helpful questions you might ask in determining how you'd like to approach psychedelic work for erotic enhancement might be:

- Am I looking to connect more deeply with my partner, or do I really need to connect more deeply with myself?
- Do I want to include erotic stimulation in a psychedelic experience, or is that likely to be overwhelming given what I know about my sexual history?
- Am I having a psychedelic experience with a person or people who are safe, who are committed to honoring my boundaries?
- Can I be committed to not interpreting the experience of another person, and likewise, will my companions refrain from interpreting what they think I need to connect with pleasure?
- Do I have ample access to nature, art materials, nourishing foods like fresh fruits so I can use all of my senses during my journey?

Optimal pleasure-enhancing psychedelic experiences can include opening up to all of the senses.* When we are expanding into greater erotic awareness, it is helpful to remember that psychedelics can facilitate something far, far beyond just sexual stimulation and sensation. The erotic is your life-force, and the way that life-force connects you to the phenomenal world. Think big and think beautiful!

WALKING THE MEDICINE INTO OUR LIVES
Living Ritual

The psychedelic experience is often thought of as a three-phase process beginning with the preparation prior to taking psychedelics, the

---

*I have personally experienced the absolute revelation that a ripe mango can be on medicine.

experience itself, and then the integration phase in which we make meaning, identify themes, and initiate behavioral change. This final phase, integration, is often considered an unfolding process that can continue for years as we let the medicine work in our life over time. In most Western therapeutic models I've encountered, these are treated as three separate phases with distinct practices and aims. While this delineation makes sense, a spiritually-grounded approach to psychedelic work might mean that the "ceremony" starts the moment we make the intention to heal. The container of the psychedelic experience can be each intention, action, and wish including making the decision to pursue psychedelic healing, finding the right context for the work, meeting guides or facilitators, or deciding to self-guide your experience.

Using this framework, once we begin on the path of medicine healing, the ceremony never ends. If we so choose, we enter into a state of *living ritual*. Living ritual means that we keep the medicine work alive by creating a practice where we return to the lessons our psychedelic experience offers us, and continually re-engage with these lessons in our life. Not only for ourselves, but so that the change within us is beneficial to our communities, the Earth, and the next generation of people to come after us. We keep the ritual alive in practice. But, living ritual can also mean that our very life itself takes on a context of sacredness, intention, and purpose that we walk into the world every day. I've often pictured the experience of taking psychedelics like standing in pitch darkness in a room full of treasures and all of a sudden someone strikes a match, allowing you, for a moment, to see the glittering jewels surrounding you. When the acute experience ends, the jewels are not gone. It becomes our work to find the jewels even if they are obscured. To pursue all the glittering possibilities for our life. Living ritual means that we approach each person, each leaf, each sunrise, each sexual experience as sacred in its own way, whatever sacred means to us. We acknowledge the jewels around us. Psychedelic experiences shift perception so the jewels are temporarily on full display. Although these shifts of perception generally end when the medicine wears off, we are called to live the ritual of our existence and the sensuality of the world each day.

If we choose to work with the quality of sacredness in our life, pleasure is the natural outgrowth. I've worked with clients who are deeply committed to social justice or ecological conservation who feel the suffering in the world deeply, emotionally, and constantly. These clients sometimes express worry that allowing pleasure in is betraying their cause, or being out of solidarity with others who are suffering and experiencing injustice. I invite you to consider the efficacy and stamina you might have to take concrete action toward positive change when you can also allow in and are nourished by the beauty around you, feel connected to the magic of other people, and live in gratitude for the gifts we all have in our lives in spite of the suffering around us. By shifting our inner landscape to allow pleasure in, we are engaging in a radical act that in and of itself makes for a better world.

PSYCHEDELIC PREPARATION FOR EROTIC ENHANCEMENT

Finding Your North Star: Crafting Intention for Psychedelic Journeying

One aspect of preparation for working with psychedelics that is nearly ubiquitous in all Western approaches is setting an intention for the experience. Our intention is the North Star for our journey. One image I like to share with clients when supporting them during psychedelic preparation is that the actual medicine journey can be like being in a small boat on a vast ocean. The ocean of experience can be so large and, at times, turbulent, that we can lose sight of where we even are. Your intention is like looking into the night sky and finding the star that can put you back on track. A well-crafted intention is specific enough to help steer your journey, while also being broad enough to allow for surprises, new directions, and revelations. There is an old psychedelic adage, "The medicine doesn't give you what you want, it gives you what you need." So it can be the case that what we are offered is quite different from what we were originally seeking. But having an intention can act as an anchor and mold our experience, and can be a powerful way of distilling our mindset for our journey.

Clarifying our intention for a psychedelic experience can grow from exploring the question, why am I doing this? The reason might simply be to feel good and be connected to your body! Although this reason is certainly not one often touted by the psychedelic medical establishment, in my book (literally and figuratively) it's a good one. If we are called to look more deeply at what drives our motivation to feel good, we might notice a desire for increased sexual satisfaction and well-being, improved relationship with ourselves, increased understanding of our sexuality or gender, and enhanced connection with our partner. Examples of intentions centered on sexuality that are expansive enough to guide us, while broad enough not to stifle us might be:

- I would like to learn how to have a better relationship with my body.
- I'm curious to learn more about my gender and gender identity.
- I would like to explore this sensation I notice when I feel desire.
- I would like to understand the parts of me that are afraid of intimacy.
- I want to explore barriers to pleasure.

Working with the Body: Building Skills for Accessing Pleasure

The somatic and emotional regulation techniques helpful for navigating psychedelic experiences are parallel to ones that help us to have optimal sexual experiences including using breath, tracking of body sensations, mindfulness, and embracing an attitude of curiosity about our experience. The biggest difference between psychedelic work and other non-ordinary states that can arise through the practice of meditation, breathwork, or even during an intense sexual experience is that with these other states of expanded consciousness, if we need to stop we (usually) can! There's little we can do to stop the subjective effect of a psychedelic, but we can learn skills to help us through difficult moments and feelings and to deepen positive ones.

When preparing for a psychedelic experience, particularly if you are aware that unprocessed sexual trauma could arise, there are a number of skills that can be practiced in advance that will support your experience.

- **Breathing**: your breath is your life, it is your foundation. When preparing for a psychedelic experience it is helpful to work with deep breathing techniques in advance that can help resource your nervous system. A helpful exercise is to find a comfortable place to recline like your bed or a comfortable chair. Imagine any tension in your body unwinding. Imagine the furniture holding you can take a little more of your weight. When you feel you have reached the maximum amount of relaxation, try taking ten slow, deep breaths with long exhales. Simple exercises like this remind our body that we know how to come back to a safe, grounded place using our breath.
- **Erotic Unwinding**: another way to train the body to be open, relaxed, and connected to the present moment is through erotic self-touch rituals. Erotic unwinding is a self-pleasure practice that is distinct from masturbation. Create a space for yourself that is safe and comfortable. If it's your bedroom, make it free from clutter. Choose music you like, adjust lighting to be soft. You are then invited to notice what your body might want to do. Perhaps it is gentle movement to the music, perhaps it is lying down. Place your hand on your body where it might feel good, like over your heart or your belly. This exercise does not need to be genitally focused. Notice the quality of contact between your hand and skin. How much pressure feels good? What kinds of touch do you like? Developing this slow and deliberate relationship to your own body builds a connection to our erotic selves. Finding ways to self-touch that feel safe, grounding, and alive can help during intense moments during psychedelic work.
- **Getting to Know Your Erotic Parts**: All of us have parts of ourselves we would rather keep hidden, and also the parts that might be scared, unwilling, or skeptical about a psychedelic experience. If our goal for a psychedelic experience is about sexual healing work or increasing erotic relatedness, we must get to know and

get permission from our erotic parts before taking the medicine. From the perspective inspired by Internal Family Systems, we hold a multiplicity of different parts of ourselves, the most obvious of which are our protective parts. These protectors can be proactive and do things such as cause sexual avoidance. Protectors might be reactive, only coming onto the scene once they perceive a threat. You might see a reactive protective part show up in behaviors like binge eating or heavy drinking. Our protectors will do anything to take a bad feeling away. When we override our protective parts by not telling them what is about to happen, hearing their concerns for us, and getting their permission to take a psychedelic medicine or have a sexual experience, especially with a new partner, things can go wrong leading to difficult experiences.

If we want to work on our sexuality, we can start by asking ourselves when we feel sexuality blocked and how that feeling presents in our body. Maybe we want to experience more desire for example. We can imagine "dropping into" a moment where we have felt particularly blocked or even aversive to sex. Notice where that blocked or avoidant sensation shows up in your body. Imagine then that you can speak directly to this sensation in your body. Notice if in your mind's eye the part has an appearance. We can then ask this part of us why it feels it needs to block our desire. Perhaps it tells us it is afraid we will get out of control and put ourselves in a dangerous situation if we feel desire. Perhaps it believes that desire is bad or dirty. We can fully hear the concerns that this protective part of us holds and acknowledge the ways that part has tried to protect us. We can then tell that part that we are planning to take a medicine that will shift our perceptions to try to access more desire and see if it would be ok to move forward. By conscripting our inner protectors into our healing, we can minimize the possibility that one part of us is very drawn to healing and change, while other parts are rebelling and holding onto old ways of being to keep us safe, making for more inner harmony before taking a psychedelic medicine.

Considerations for Sexual Trauma Survivors

A note for survivors of sexual trauma. All of the above are useful techniques for your psychedelic tool kit, but good preparation work must also prepare you for the unexpected which can mean paradoxical reactions to a medicine. For example, "I took MDMA and all I wanted to do was be alone and inward to myself. My partner was very disappointed," or fragments of somatic trauma memories that may arise such as "I was having sex with my partner and all of a sudden my body started to register something very bad was happening to me even though it wasn't." And very big feelings. Very. Big. Feelings. Whether you are doing medicine work with a guide, therapist, or partner, you both must be prepared to hold space for intense expressions of feelings, and in fact for sexual feelings to arise. You also need to have a plan for taking care of yourself afterward. Imagine believing you can process and express sensations and emotions that may have been bottled up for decades and then go to work the next day? And yet, many people do not have the advantage of being able to take multiple days off from work, have childcare or help at home, or even have a safe place to go. More importantly, we have no model in our society, no community, capable and knowledgeable to care for someone after this type of healing work. Being mentally prepared that a psychedelic experience aimed at healing trauma can be initially destabilizing is a necessary part of preparing the best you can to take care of yourself. Having a therapist, family, and friends who know about your process and are prepared to support you is essential for safe healing.

Sexual trauma survivors may express fear of psychedelics, worrying that they will be flooded with memories and overwhelmed, they will not be able to make the experience stop, or they will be destabilized after the experience. A certain amount of nervousness of the unknown is understandable. But if you are experiencing marked fear, that might be a strong predictor that the psychedelic experience could be difficult or scary. This is a great place to pause and turn to other somatic psychotherapies like EMDR and Internal

Family Systems (IFS), in addition to techniques like Holotropic Breathwork that are more controlled and more easily navigated. You can empower yourself with the knowledge that it is better to go slow and feel adequately prepared for a psychedelic experience than rush into it and risk a destabilizing experience.

PSYCHEDELIC INTEGRATION FOR EROTIC ENHANCEMENT

Making Space for Pleasure

When we consider how psychedelics might increase pleasure and enhance our sexual experience, we must first acknowledge that this in and of itself is a revolutionary act in a culture that is obsessed with productivity. Helpful integration approaches to erotic enhancement and pleasure might first start with identifying the obstacles to pleasure. Common obstacles to the expansion of pleasure are lack of time; roles such as parent, professional, breadwinner, that sap our time to focus on oneself; pressure from partners to offer more sexual availability than we want to give; and the weight of responsibilities we carry. When we look at this list, it feels like the biggest disruptors to being present with pleasure is time and pressure. So the first step we can take in our unfolding integration process is to dedicate yourself to making time and space in your life for pleasure to thrive.

As has been noted, to engage fully with psychedelic healing requires far more time than the acute effects of the medicine last. In some cases, it requires preparation such as a special diet, or psychotherapy work for many days prior to the medicine experience, followed by time to properly integrate. When we are looking to increase erotic pleasure, the key is creating a container in our life for pleasure to flourish. This alone is the best integration advice I have to give. It is helpful to see the acute effects of a psychedelic as just one part, but if you are looking to deepen your relationship to pleasure, it means committing to days, weeks, and months of making pleasure (and perhaps sex) a priority, which means embracing an ongoing commitment to willingness and to creating time for intimacy with yourself or a partner.

Psychedelic experiences are also known to help us reprioritize and look at ourselves in new ways. In our integration process, we might consider what roles we play that distance us from a sense of pleasure and work on creating new relationships to these roles. If we work sixty-hour weeks and don't make time for exercise or to nourish our bodies, we likely won't feel well. A lack of vital energy from overworking or a sedentary lifestyle is like taking our erotic reserves and letting it peter out like air from a balloon. You might ask yourself if significant people, memories, or experiences came up during your psychedelic experience and use these things as guideposts for reprioritizing your life. I've never once worked with an integration client who got the message that the most important thing was to be a regional manager at their job.

If our aim is specifically to enhance erotic pleasure, our body becomes the playground in the integration experience. Creating special space, both metaphorically and literally, to explore sensations, movement, breath, and arousal are wonderful integration tools. If a partner is included in your exploration, slowing down and taking time to really look at each other, to see deeply, to feel touch, connect with warmth are all limitless wells of possibility for erotic exploration. Setting a stage for pleasure might mean having a clean environment and bringing in special things like candles and flowers, or leather and masks. Whichever way you roll!

Questioning Sexual Narratives
This brings us to the next facet of integration for erotic enhancement, which is identifying and dismantling the sexual narratives that prevent us from free sexual expression. Psychedelic healing might lead not only to more self-acceptance, but also to neuroplasticity, a window of time immediately following the psychedelic experience in which the mind enjoys an increased ability to integrate new ideas. Recent research that has rocked the science world has shown that in mice, psychedelics reopened the social reward learning critical period. Critical periods are times when the brain is in an especially susceptible state to new ideas,

concepts, and learning, a period of time often associated with childhood and the acquisition of language, culture, and form the basis for human relationships. First it was documented that MDMA in the context of a controlled clinical environment could reopen these critical periods leading to the rapid ability to reprocess trauma and integrate new ideas.[3] But Gul Dolan's remarkable work showed that *all* psychedelics could do this. The amount of time that the critical learning window was reopened was related to the duration of the subjective effects of the medicine. In other words, short-acting medicines like ketamine, whose effects you might feel for thirty minutes to two hours, opened the critical learning window for forty-eight hours, while longer acting medicines like psilocybin and MDMA with acute effects ranging from three to six hours, opened the reward period for up to two weeks.[4] In my clinical experience, I also believe that very powerful psychedelic experiences that encompass a total loss of self, such as is the case with 5-MeO-DMT, despite its short duration (twenty minutes to one hour) might also offer vast opportunity for sustained change.

How does this apply to integration and pleasure? Well, directly after a psychedelic experience one has the opportunity to literally retrain the brain to be open to and present with pleasure. It is also the moment to take a hard look at the stories you've been carrying around that you are unworthy, your body is flawed, your sexual anatomy isn't right, and tell yourself a new story. When we wake up to the fact that these stories have been self-generated to prevent us from experiencing the pain and rejection of others, and heavily influenced by the social messages we have received about sex and our bodies since childhood, we can see them as exactly what they are. Just stories. Integration can be a time to sit with these stories and be curious with them. Where did they come from? Our parents? A bad sexual experience? From a culture simultaneously obsessed with and shaming of sexuality? I once worked with a client who was told they were not good at oral sex by one partner, so they literally never tried it again with anyone else! This is what I'm talking about.

Naming specific new narratives for yourself about your body, about your relationships, and about your worth can be especially helpful in the immediate aftermath of a psychedelic experience. Likewise, we may carry beliefs about relationships that prevent us from experiencing contentment and intimacy because we both crave *and* fear it in equal measure. When the effect of the medicine wears off, you might aspire to look at your partner with new eyes. A child's eyes. What do you see when you allow resentment and distance to fall away? These moments of looking at someone you love with eyes of compassion, like they are your chosen person, the greatest in the world, is affectionately called by my partner and I "having a love bubble." As an expert in psychedelic integration and consummate professional, I highly recommend having a love bubble as often as you can. It's great.

Body Healing

Developing a friendship with pleasure also means accepting our bodies and using them for our satisfaction. Notice I said *accepting* our body and not *loving* our body. Body images issues are pervasive, particularly among women and people who adhere to feminine gender norms, in my therapy practice. Many arrive with the notion that they must love their body and feel defeated and inadequate when they fail to do so. I believe a more functional approach to our bodies is to *accept* the body we have. This is not to say that people seeking to improve their well-being through gender-affirming interventions to align their appearance with their self-image and gender identity should instead work on acceptance. Not at all. But acceptance might mean that when we have done what we can to tend to our bodies in healthy ways including exercise, feeding our body what it wants to eat, allowing for rest, or for some, gender-affirming interventions, we can focus on all of the sensory joys our body can experience. We can notice the parts of us that fat shame, tell stories about our inadequacy or not enough-ness. It's helpful to remember that those inner voices have been conspiring to keep us in line and make us "good enough" our whole lives, protecting us from shame and rejection.

The act of working with those voices, hearing them, and honoring the ways they have worked to protect us *is love*. If we build upon the definition of love offered by Black feminist author bell hooks in her book *All About Love* echoing the sentiments of M. Scott Peck and Erich Fromm, as "the will to extend one's self for the purpose of nurturing one's own or another's spiritual growth"[5] we can embrace that it is not that we need to love our physical appearance *per se*, or look in the mirror and not perceive anything we wished were different. But the act of working with those parts of ourselves that generate internal criticism, nurturing an alliance with our body, and caring for it, *is* loving it. Engaging in the practice of accepting our bodies *is* the act of loving yourself. Loving yourself is simply embracing willingness to grow. We've already explored the potent role psychedelics might play, mediated by the mystical experience, in helping us to garner the kind of acceptance that can be so helpful in this act of practicing self-love.

Reconnecting with the Divine

Every human being deserves access to a spiritual life. Entheogens have the power to create a direct link between us and a sense of sacredness, higher being, and essential goodness within oneself. The impact of religious trauma and disenfranchisement from organized religions, particularly around the issues of sexuality, relationships, and gender roles, can distance us from a connection to our spirituality. Psychedelic integration work can support us in finding, rediscovering, or reimagining what a spiritual life for us might look like. How we define spirituality is essential. Consistent with our definition drawn from the concept of Psychedelic Sexuality, spirituality is however one chooses to define it and is free from an intercessor that mediates between you and a direct relationship with the divine, making it available to all.

The integration process is an opportunity to rebuild that sense of connection with the sacredness of oneself and the sacredness of the world. However, spirituality must never be used as a means of bypassing difficult emotions that must—and deserve—to be felt and witnessed. Sexual violence often exists in a realm of shame, secrecy, and isolation, while a direct relationship with Spirit connects us to ourselves, the world, and other people. In an effort to keep overwhelming feelings at bay, survivors of early childhood sexual abuse may exist in a state of dissociation and distance even from themselves. When someone is sexually assaulted as an adult, the sense of loss, beholding what human beings are capable of doing to one another, and even a sense of being abandoned by God, ancestors, or protectors might be felt. However, you need not have experienced sexual abuse in childhood, or even identify as having experienced sexual violence, to feel the impact of a culture that disenfranchises our sexuality from spirituality. During integration work, you might ponder what a spiritual connection with oneself and the world might look like, and how you might benefit from reconnecting to these aspects of self.

During psychedelic integration, you might first try to remember aspects of your experience where you felt connected to something beyond yourself. Even journeyers who do not have a "full mystical experience" often sense the presence of ancestors, guides, or plant spirits. For people who are strongly atheistic, or feel comfortable with psychedelic work only because current scientific research promotes psychedelics as a specific treatment for mental health issues, an entry point into the spiritual domain might not be ancestors or plant spirits but instead how they relate to themself, the phenomenal world, or others (therapists, other participants, or guides). The sense of connection to the earth, to yourself, and to others is spiritual. When I'm speaking to a client and they are clearly put off by the concept of spirituality (which does not happen often, but it certainly can), rather than pressing spirituality, I ask about moments of feeling peace, inner wisdom, or connection to nature. Beholding the night sky or a towering mountain is a deeply spiritual experience. Find the language that works either for you, or if you are a practitioner, for your integration clients. There is nothing at odds between a respect for science and a spiritual existence. In fact, the deeper we look into science, the more mystery we find.

When we are looking for a spiritual life not generated from a psychedelic experience but from the psychedelic community, we may encounter some troubling realities. The psychedelic world is infused with people donning the aesthetics of Indigenous cultures, decked out in crystals or yoga gear in an attempt to cultivate the appearance of a "spiritual person." My perspective is that if you are cultivating an appearance that serves to remind you of your connection to a high power or purpose, it's not necessarily a bad thing. But it's also helpful to remember that crystals or a particular style of dress do not make you spiritual. You can be perfectly spiritual in your normal clothes.

As we have seen, psychedelic integration work can be about connecting to a sense of sacredness in the world, in yourself, and cultivating a connection to something bigger than oneself. If a sense of connection or sacredness was experienced during a psychedelic journey, the work is about finding your way back to those feelings after the psychedelic experience is over. That might include practices like altar making, singing, or walking in nature. Much more challenging might be connecting those qualities not only to a general sense of self, but to sexuality. The integration process might use these felt states of connection to the divine, sacredness, and calm to challenge harmful sexual narratives that result from a sex-negative culture such as "My sexuality is dangerous," or "I'm impure." Moreover, integration work can focus on our relationship to our body. If we ourselves are sacred beings, how can our bodies be dirty, gross, or inadequate? Our post-psychedelic experience might be a rich time to question these inner divisions and heal the wedge that shame drives between oneself and the divine.

Returning to Pleasure

We deserve more than just not suffering, we deserve pleasure, embodiment, and connection. The psychedelic integration process can be about coming home to yourself or coming home to feeling good in states of joy, calm, and connection, but even more than that, states of erotic embodiment. One helpful strategy during integration is to map all of the sensations you can remember during your psychedelic experience. Often psychedelic users will have the experience of feeling their whole bodies, sometimes for the first time, without shame. You can explore sensations of tingling or warmth. You might notice how it felt for your whole body to be "online" at the same time.

Another helpful way to create an enduring relationship with pleasure is to notice any inner voices, any "parts," that tell us we are undeserving, that pleasure is not to be trusted, or even that it is dangerous. We can notice these parts that create an obstacle to feeling good in our body and engage in an inner inquiry as to what they fear might happen if we feel pleasure. For many of us, feelings of deep shame that surround our sexual feelings and erotic pleasure originate from childhood. Certainly this is the case for childhood sexual abuse survivors who may have experienced pleasure in tandem with abuse, a very common experience, or gender-diverse people for example, who may receive little support and or positive mirroring around their identities.

Psychedelic integration that welcomes erotic pleasure can first start with the individual: How can I feel pleasure, safely, on my own? What feels good to my body? A hot shower? Self-touch? Massage? During integration we can take the time to go back to the fundamental building blocks of sensuality and discover, maybe for the first time, simply what feels good. These foundational practices can lead to more explicitly erotic self-touch. You can then notice whether your protective parts feel comfortable to engage in more or whether they want you to slow down. Not bypassing your protective inner parts, staying present with pleasure, and going slow are all ways of reengaging eroticism in the process of healing or reconnecting to our sexuality.

Psychedelic Harm Reduction: Engage in Some Heavy Vetting

Make no mistake, at the time of writing, the single most dangerous thing about psychedelics is that they are federally illegal. Although multiple cities and a few states are decriminalizing* the use of psychedelics, federal use remains illegal. This, combined with the associated stigma surrounding so-called "illicit" drug use, creates serious hazards and obstacles to enjoying a successful experience. Since obtaining psychedelic medicines often requires engaging in extralegal transactions, if something goes wrong with a setting or substance, one has little, if any, recourse to address the harm. It also means people wishing to experience psychedelic ceremonies must sometimes travel far from their own

---

*According to the Cornell Law School Legal Information Institute, "decriminalization" means the act would remain illegal, but the legal system would not prosecute a person for the decriminalized act.[6]

systems of support in order to do so, making a successful integration process much more challenging.

Because psychedelics are unregulated and federally illegal, it can be very difficult and at times impossible to know whether the substance you have is what you think it is. For example, there are a number of LSD analogues (such as 25I-NBOMe) that carry radically different risk profiles. While LSD itself generally has a very good safety profile in terms of physical risk, other substances like 25I-NBOMe can carry risk of cardiac arrest or seizure leading to death.[7] The most acute of these issues is the presence of deadly fentanyl in the recreational drug supply. Sometimes, psychedelic users are persuaded to engage in unsafe situations or with unsavory facilitators in an effort to gain access to plant medicines. There are reports from the Amazon of ayahuasca-related deaths, sexual violence, coercion, and other dangerous practices that are not the result of a traditionally prepared ayahuasca brew itself, but due to the introduction of other plants into the mixture that are toxic (like *toé*), that can cause wild hallucinations and disorientation.[8] Matched with predatory facilitators, this makes for an incredibly dangerous experience. Heavily vetting any retreat center, facilitator, or shaman with whom you plan to work is a must.

It is essential to test your substances to know they are safe. You can do this with at-home kits provided by drug education organizations such as Dance Safe* to be sure as you can that your medicine is safe is also essential. As long as we have prohibition, we are all exposed to unnecessary risk from unsafe substances and unsafe people. Because people who have been harmed are understandably reluctant to expose their own substance use, and/or may not even know how or where to seek accountability, compromised people may proliferate (and harmful substances may circulate) without consequences for long periods of time. Chapter five will deal with the specific issue of sexual harm in psychedelic spaces in depth.

Another aspect of harm reduction is managing our expectations for

---

*Dance Safe is a 501(c)3 tax-exempt organization committed to education and risk reduction efforts, providing drug education, information, and harm reduction materials.

a psychedelic experience. While a positive attitude toward psychedelic experience and the intention to enjoy it (hurray for pleasure!) are predictors of positive outcomes, chasing the mystical experience and the presumed gains it brings (that is, focusing too much on a specific outcome) can lead to disappointment and worsening mental health outcomes if it fails to happen.[9] The most psychedelically at-risk clients I see in my therapy practice are the ones who say, "This has to work because I have nothing else left. If this doesn't work I don't know what I'll do." When we place our hopes in a single psychedelic experience to change entrenched behaviors or heal trauma we've been carrying for years, we are hoping for a miracle. This search for a miracle is an understandable pursuit when long-time sufferers see pervasive media reports that portray psychedelics as a magic bullet. But psychedelics are not a miracle, they are a tool. Developing realistic expectations, including that we may see no immediate changes, or even a temporary worsening of symptoms after a psychedelic experience, is helpful. There is a delicate balance between positive expectation, which we know leads to better mental health outcomes,[10] and over-investing in needing a certain experience or medicine to save us. There is simply no such thing as "ten years of therapy in one night" as psychedelics are often promoted. Psychedelics are merely an accelerator on a trajectory that you have already set.

PSYCHEDELIC PREPARATION FOR COUPLES AND POLYCULES

When couples or polycules* contact me for preparation and integration work around psychedelic experiences, it is often because things have gone wrong in the relationship somehow, and they imagine that a shared psychedelic experience might help them repair it. It's true that this is a self-selecting group of psychedelic users who identify the need for support, as there is a long tradition of people in relationships using psychedelics and entactogens successfully for garnering connection, enhancing

---

*A polycule is a group of more than two people who are in a committed, romantic relationship with each other.

communication, and recreation. Psychedelics are allies in pleasure, cultivating genuine presence, and deepening connection. This is a benefit not only to couples or polycules in distress, but to all people aiming to deepen a bond. There is literally nothing like tripping together to bring you closer.

The scientific literature on couples and psychedelics is a developing area of research that has so far mostly focused only on couples in which one (or both) have a mental health diagnosis such as PTSD, and in which the focus of study is how mental illness has impacted the relationship. However, treatment of mental illness in one or more partners is only the tip of a large iceberg of what psychedelics can do for relationship satisfaction and pleasure. It's impossible not to acknowledge the years of successful implementation of MDMA in couple's work in the 1980s prior to it being scheduled by the DEA as a "dangerous drug" around which much controversy and protestation swirled, not the least of which was from therapists who understood MDMA's tremendous potential. Known to the world of therapy—subsequently underground therapy after MDMA was outlawed—as "Adam," a substance that could bring us back to an original state of shame-free innocence, practitioners such as therapist-turned-underground guide, Leo Zeff, continued to offer it to clients long after its use had been restricted.[11]

To understand more about what is possible in psychedelic-assisted couples work, I spoke to someone who is perhaps the field's leading expert on this matter, therapist and researcher Dr. Anne Wagner. Every time I see Anne at a training or conference, it's like the sun is shining a bit brighter. She's smart and highly principled, but carries herself without a hint of pretentiousness. I spoke with Dr. Wagner about the work she's undertaking with couples and MDMA-assisted psychotherapy. Having led the first clinical trials using MDMA with couples when one partner has a diagnosis of PTSD, Anne's work is leading the way in the field of psychedelic-assisted therapy for couples. I asked her about moving past the reduction of symptoms as a basis for healing trauma in relationships. "It feels like reducing symptoms is this much of what it's really about . . ." she said, lifting her fingers to indicate something very tiny, ". . . and the rest of it centers on, how are you relating? How is this living in your relationship? How can the experience increase your intimacy in different ways? How can greater intimacy heal the relationship? How can I help you grow? How can this experience together help you navigate the world differently? When you're in a relationship with another person, you're creating shared realities all the time depending on how each individual sees the world, and then there's the co-constructed reality that you're seeing as well." Anne and also I talked about personal transformation that's possible through this work. "Non-ordinary states can be very powerful shared experiences. Obviously, when symptoms go down, there's more ease that comes into the relationship and the interactions in a couple. Trauma is not taking up as much space, so you're able to focus on other things. MDMA-assisted therapy can help people to feel deep empathy for one another."

Presumably it also provides new ways to see yourself. Many of the best practitioners in the field of psychedelic-assisted therapy are doing the work because psychedelics have made a tremendous impact in their own lives, myself included. Dr. Wagner shared of her own healing journey, "There have been multiple different ways psychedelics have helped me to explore and understand my own identity. For me, psychedelics have helped me around the issue of feeling 'queer enough. . . . '" Anne shared, "I felt uncomfortable taking up space in a world where I want to support and center others. My psychedelic work helped me to connect to the knowledge, 'of course I'm queer enough. Because I'm enough. There's no 'enough,' it's just that I am enough and queerness is part of that."

Our ongoing work in accepting ourselves at the deepest level is actually what's necessary for not only personal transformation and liberation, but for having honest, connected, and loving relationships.

Creating Context for Psychedelic Experiences in a Couple

For better or worse, Western psychotherapy has promoted a model of psychedelic healing that entails a reflective, individual, inner journey where the star of the show is you, clad in eyeshades, in quiet contemplation. When couples come to my practice for preparation work, they often question whether their self-directed psychedelic healing should take a form like this. When preparing for a psychedelic experience as a couple, the first consideration is intention. What do you hope this experience will do for you and for your relationship? The quiet inner journey is certainly not a bad model for healing, but is it the model that will suit your intentions for your relationship? If a couple's intention is to understand their own inner complexities in service to better communication and connection, then co-journeying might be a good start. Couples can have quiet inner experiences side by side, and later share their insights, or choose only to interact when the medicine is wearing off. I've experienced dozens of ayahuasca ceremonies with my partner beside me. While we did not interfere or interact with each other during the journey, after being ripped through a cosmic vortex for six hours, coming home to each other's arms after the ceremony concluded was pure joy.

But the relational model for psychedelic healing is also an alternative. Rather than an interior journey, a couple or polycule can instead decide to be directed toward one another for the duration, or part of, the experience. If this is the model being used, having specific aims can help direct and support your experience. In my integration practice, perhaps the most common reason couples are interested in psychedelic work is to promote connection or resolve conflict in a relationship. In these cases, couples often talk about things being at an impasse, or finding that they so rapidly lose the capacity for compassion that conflict resolution breaks down. Substance choice plays a major role constructing an environment where conflict can be discussed directly. Tryptamines, meaning the "trippy" ones like psilocybin, can be a catalyst for connection to mystical states and perceptual shifts that can support a couple in rising above conflict. Couples report that expanded states of awareness that garner a connection to all beings and phenomena suddenly make our human conflict look small. But the most popular medicines couples generally gravitate to are the ones that promote feelings of compassion, connection, erotic feeling, and softening, like MDMA and 2C-B. These more lucid psychedelics that generally garner deep pleasure and embodiment can be very powerful vehicles to confront relationship difficulties with less defensiveness. But never forget, there are some very important moments in life when just being able to abandon your own bullshit and feel deeply connected to someone you love in bliss is the healing.

The Importance of Self-Knowledge: Preparing for Vulnerability

One of the single most useful awarenesses to have around setting intention as a couple and having an experience with psychedelics that is useful to you and your relationship is to know that psychedelics can rapidly blunt protective parts of yourself that perhaps, for very good reason, keep your partner at a distance. An example of this might be an inner protective part that remains judgmental and angry after infidelity. When a substance rapidly opens up perspective and compassion toward your partner, a few things can happen. First, this could be the best medicine for your relationship; moving past resentment and reconnecting with understanding can transform angry people into connected people. But that's not the only possible outcome. When a relationship seems to be on the line, we can be motivated to take extreme steps to avoid abandonment and loss. When this is the case, psychedelics can create a temporary container for connection and perspective, but a backlash may follow. Feelings of vulnerability or exposure, or even openness and agreeableness, can have a dark side. When the effects of the medicine wear off, individuals in a relationship can be left feeling manipulated or even violated that their inner protectors who have been serving to keep them safe from hurt were banished so rapidly that they now have to reconfigure a state of protection to function in the relationship.

Psychedelic preparation for couples can include several considerations that can help prevent this backlash and lead to increased feelings of connectedness and improved communication. Why are we doing this? Are we ready for this? If your psychedelic experience is designed to be a last-ditch effort to prevent an end to a relationship, that is a lot of pressure to put on a medicine. A way of aligning that goal toward a more achievable aim might be to craft an intention for more openness, curiosity toward each other, or space to resolve the aftermath of specific conflict or problem. Much like some couples enter therapy with the belief that "if this doesn't work, we're done," which rarely leads to successful outcomes, psychedelics similarly can be ineffective or even retraumatizing if that much emphasis is placed on trying to prevent disaster. Similarly, reflecting on whether you are ready for a psychedelic couple's experience might really rely on whether you have worked sufficiently with your protective inner parts so that they are comfortable with you being in a more vulnerable state with your partner. Building trust, or at least a genuine willingness to trust, and attunement beforehand is necessary.

Preparation for journeying as a couple should also consider other important factors, such as whether the experience will be structured or unstructured. If one person needs time to themselves or in quiet reflection, can the other partner or partners be emotionally self-sufficient during that time? What are our sexual boundaries during the experience? Remember, my earlier statement about inner protectors especially applies to sex. If desire or making time for sex is a struggle in the relationship, incorporating physical intimacy into the experience can be healing. However, when sexual connection is conflictual, using psychedelics as a means of overriding inner parts that keep us distant and unavailable for intimacy can elicit the biggest backlash of all. Unwanted sex, even with a committed partner while on a psychedelic, can create major issues afterward. With my clients who struggle with maintaining intimacy in their relationship, I notice that most often it is not that there is a full-on "no" to sex, but rather an inner ambivalence. Part of me wants to feel connected to my partner, doesn't want them to feel rejected or undesirable, and another part really, really wants to stay safe and sex is not on the menu. If this is the case, your intention for your joint experience may not be to *have* sex, but to be able to *talk* about sex and work with these inner conflicts directly. Compassionately witnessing your partner sharing about inner conflicts and then being able to receive your partner's feelings can be tremendous medicine for healing.

Crafting a Life Worth Living
But what about the other delicious reasons you might want to try psychedelics with a partner? Like fun. Like connection. Like erotic plea-

sure or joy. Now we're on to something. Perhaps your relationship is not in distress, but instead you want to deepen the love you already have. Clearly, the medical model is not known for focusing on this, but it is likely the most common reason people in relationships choose to journey together. Because really, when you love someone, who doesn't love to take a journey? The limits of this journey end only at the deepest places in yourself. I've worked with couples for whom psychedelic work together is a tune up for their relationship, a pause from the madness of modern life to enjoy and cherish each other. Imagine a world where this kind of family-based healing (and it *is* family healing) could be safely accessed and discussed? In these cases the preparation intention might not be to fix anything at all, but to use psychedelics as enhancement of connection and appreciation for life and the life you share. These can be the richest journeys of all. What's better than having it good and being in full awareness and gratitude for it?

One of my true passions is to support the creation and design of culturally respectful, legal psychedelic rituals for healing. I believe we suffer a deep and often unseen wound when we have no means to mark rites of passage, or to celebrate and affirm our connection to the Earth, and to community and family. Whereas I would love to see the expansion of community-based psychedelic ritual, there are perhaps other ways to fit psychedelic ritual into our modern families. Dr. Anne Wagner and I discussed how this might look in the context of broader clinical access to psychedelics outside of tightly controlled research settings. "When the safety, tolerability, and efficacy of MDMA work with couples is known and we have the data to support us, therapists will be able to use this in their practices in exciting ways. What if MDMA could be used during periods of life transition such as when parents are facing an empty nest when kids leave home, or marking other significant life events?" It occurred to me in the context of my interview with Dr. Wagner that this too is ritual. Ritual *can* happen in traditional Western psychedelic psychotherapy. This type of living ritual will mean we are using psychedelics in the sacred container of therapy to process transition, loss, or marking significant life events as a couple or family. This is indeed a moving vision for the future.

PSYCHEDELIC INTEGRATION FOR COUPLES OR POLYCULES

Maintaining Change

Psychedelic integration for relationships is parallel to individual integration, but instead we focus on what practices, changes, or communication we need to implement in the relationship, which means it is a two-way street (at least.) All partners need to be invested in maintaining change. As previously mentioned, this is not always easy when we have inner protective parts who want to come raging back into a state of control. But perhaps the most grand challenge is exactly what contributes to sexual dissatisfaction, disconnection, and isolation; that when the psychedelic experience ends, we don't just go back to our ordinary consciousness, we go back to our ordinary lives which can be filled with the demands of kids, jobs, and making money. When all of these demands come rushing in after the happy psychedelic container we have created is over, the same circumstances that created our overwhelm in the first place are there waiting for us.

The hardest reality for any psychedelic work, but especially for couples, is that in order to maintain the connection, insights, or new ways of being we glimpsed in a psychedelic state, we have to change our life. I've seen couples fall apart not because of a lack of love, but because one person was so obsessed with maintaining the role of provider or securing a financial future, for example, they simply weren't present in a manner required to maintain true connection. An aim of integration can be to clarify your shared values as a couple and then make concrete plans of how you intend to live by them. No easy task. If you want real connection and intimacy, that requires not only vulnerability and sacrifice, but also time. Because of its finite nature, time is a precious resource (for some more so than others), but it is a resource worth spending when it comes to working to improve our interpersonal connections. Any time dedicated to connection and relating makes a difference.

Specific integration activities can be dedicating time to having conversations about the state of your connection, but then making time for deep dialogue, recreation, intimacy, and eroticism. These things are usually the first casualties of a busy life. It's helpful to ask yourself whether you are sharing activities together, building a life around shared projects or goals, or are you actually *sharing your lives* with each other, your inner worlds, feelings, and thoughts? Psychedelics have the potential to wake us to the fact that this life is very short. Are you spending your relationship waiting for retirement or when you get that promotion, or are you living aligned with your values right now? What would you do if you lost your partner tomorrow? Would you be happy with how you're living now?

Let's again come back to the concept introduced at the start of this chapter: living ritual. The idea of creating ritual in our lives, or indeed creating a life of ritual, can seem accessible when we are thinking only of ourselves in the context of having the space and time to do so. But this is not how we live our lives, and it is not the reality of our modern relationships. How do we foster a practice of living ritual amidst the chaos, conflicts, and demands of our existence? How do we find a life of grace when we are bombarded with the suffering in the world? Suffering that we ourselves may be experiencing. Deeply.

Living ritual in the context of our relationships can be the practice of incorporating the opposite values of how we are conditioned to function in modern-day Western culture. Instead of multitasking, we can be alive and present in our conversations with the people we love. We can stop what we are doing and truly listen. We can commit ourselves to making connection a priority. We can take the most radically anti-establishment stance there is and embody the practice of experiencing the pleasure our bodies offer as enough. And it is indeed enough, because it is a limitless well. Perhaps we can't afford time off, or a fancy psychedelic retreat. But we can breathe. We can live the ritual of each breath, each sensation, each morning as a gift. This is the ritual of simple awareness, simple gratitude. To return to a metaphor I used earlier in this chapter, having a psychedelic experience can be like standing in a pitch-dark room full of jewels and someone, for a moment, lights a match. It is our job to try to find the jewels again when the match is extinguished, when the ceremony ends. But, honestly, the good news is, they are really not all that hard to find. Our ritual is simply remembering that all the love, all the beauty, it is right there waiting for us.

PREPARATION AND INTEGRATION IN CONTEXT
The Extended Case Study of Valeria

Preparation

Valeria was a 38-year-old woman who reached out to me after being invited to a group ritual using 5-MeO-DMT. She was a therapist herself, specializing in working with clients with obsessive-compulsive disorder. She shared that her work was fine, but she kind of fell into it during a grad school internship. She really didn't feel any particular draw to working with her clients, or the disorder. She was warm, connected, and came to our intake dressed professionally. While everything on the surface seemed fine (Valeria had a good job, a partner, and friends), she described herself as having "a hole inside." "I'm just missing out on joy. Everything is fine, and I just can't feel happy." At first, I considered whether Valeria was just depressed. Her description of herself and her life seemed to point in that direction. But as we began to work together, a deeper understanding of Valeria and her life emerged.

Valeria had only had a few psychedelic experiences in college, "I took mushrooms a few times with friends. I really have a hard time understanding how that experience, like, heals people's depression. It was enjoyable, but it never did anything big for me." She shared that she decided to try 5-MeO-DMT because she really trusts the person who invited her, a friend who had experienced amazing benefits from the medicine. Also, the experience was going to be a group retreat just for women with an experienced facilitator which felt safe. In my mind, I wondered how making the jump between a few low dose mushroom experiences right into the very deep and glimmering water of nature's most powerful psychedelic substances would go for Valeria. But Valeria was prepared; she was seeking expert preparation and integration, she had read up on the substance, and she reported she was taking no medication, no one in her family was psychotic or diagnosed with bipolar disorders, and had never experienced these things herself. I thought,

"My job is to prepare her, not scare her. So let's dig in!" I understood that approaching Valeria with curiosity and respecting the autonomy of her choices was a far better approach than giving her guidance she had not asked for. I gave her more context about the 5-MeO-DMT medicine and shared with her some cautions including that some people experience a "reactivation"* of this particular medicine after the experience is over.

During our first few prep sessions a clearer picture emerged. Valeria's parents divorced when she was ten, but remained collaborative with each other, even celebrating holidays together in an effort to make Valeria feel supported. Neither remarried. She described her mom as "someone who is so smart, but never really lived up to her potential. She always felt like she had to take care of me." Valeria's wise adult inner self recognized this was her mother's decision and not her fault, but she was also in touch with a part of herself that felt guilty whenever she exceeded her mother's life accomplishments. Her PhD felt hollow. Her job was nothing to write home about. Her father had died a few years before, and she was still grieving the loss of his warm presence in her life.

For three sessions, Valeria volunteered little about her romantic relationship. When I asked, she gave straightforward answers with little embellishment. So, all I really knew is she was partnered with a nice guy, a friend from college turned romantic mate, and that he worked in banking. Not a lot to go on. She did not want children. They agreed on that. Valeria was grateful there was little conflict and feared rocking the boat with her partner, even though he had never been argumentative or rejecting when she did address issues with him. Sex? Meh. A few times a month. It was fine. She described her partner as attuned; he made her feel safe, and did not push for sex when she didn't want it. When I asked about her sexual history, she gave me much the same story. Nothing spectacular. Her first time having sex was during her senior year of high school and was "a good experience."

Great. Wonderful to hear she felt safe in her life and her relationship.

---

*There is a deeper discussion of the reactivation phenomenon in chapter six.

But what did Valeria want? For a straight, cisgender* woman with high educational attainment who checked nearly every box of stability and privilege, she was flat.

Valeria moved through her life like an appeased ghost. The more we talked, the more we came to realize that what showed as mild persistent depression on the outside (and could probably be clinically diagnosed as such), was actually a total absence of meaning in her life, a deeper existential problem that antidepressants weren't going to solve. Valeria was careening toward middle age stuck in what psychologist Erik Erikson dubbed the crucial conflict of "generativity versus stagnation." Was Valeria going to create meaning in her life, or would she be stagnant, lost in a world of "fine-ness?"

Finally after a few sessions, I asked her, "If you could come out of this medicine experience you are about to have changed in some way, what would that look like?" This was the first time I ever saw Valeria come to life.

Her eyes gleamed, "I want to feel something! I know the medicine is supposed to, like, blast you through the stratosphere, but I'm not even afraid of that. I think that's what it's going to take to shake something up inside of me. There's a part of me that wants to find a new life direction, but I'd actually really like to start feeling some joy in the life I have."

I was puzzled as to why Valeria had chosen me as a therapist. I mostly work with clients in the queer community, Valeria was straight. I focus on sexuality, but she claimed her sex life was fine and didn't occupy much of her mind. I work with trauma survivors, she claimed no traumatic experiences. Something was lurking in the relational field of our therapy that had not yet been said. Certainly unknown to me, and perhaps to Valeria too. I tried to come around to things in a different way.

"What's your relationship to pleasure?" I asked.

"Like, sex?" she countered.

---

*"Cisgender" is a label people use to identify themselves as someone whose gender identity matches the sex they were assigned at birth.

"Sure, sex but also just pleasure in your life. What feels sensual, what makes you feel good?"

Valeria began to tear up. "I'd really like to feel more pleasure. I would like to be more in my life. I just feel numb," she said.

"When did you start feeling numb?"

She paused, "Well, if I'm really trying to think back, I really had a lot of life in me as a child."

I could see Valeria pondering. I waited. A long moment passed. "You know, I'm just remembering that in my junior year of high school, the theater teacher used to really like me and I got a lot of roles in the plays. My parents were really proud. But it meant staying after school a lot. He was always normal when he saw me, but he used to call my house and pretend he needed something related to school and try to have phone sex with me. I could hear his breathing. I remember thinking, gross, he's touching himself, but I couldn't say or do anything. I would just sit there on the phone and listen. Then I'd go into school and he was totally normal. He never tried to touch me or anything. He just would do the weird phone thing."

It had never occurred to Valeria the impact that this had had on her. She told no one, both ashamed of what was happening and afraid she would be held back from the one area in which she shined: theater. She didn't want to ruin things for anyone else. Although she had had years of psychotherapy during her training, this memory never came up. She could remember it, but she never thought about it anymore. "I just pushed him right out of my mind," she said. Valeria spent her life in a very narrow zone, doing only the safe thing with safe people, part of her trapped in a state of suspension on the phone with her creepy teacher. But something inside her was ready to hang up that phone. She wanted her joy back. Her adult perspective could easily place the blame on him. But some younger part inside her still felt very afraid to feel. That part of her said, "If you stay numb you will never have to feel like this again."

In the session before her 5-MeO-DMT retreat, enough trust had been built between us that Valeria was willing to step outside the box of her cognitive behavioral training she herself used as a therapist in her work with clients. I asked her about the numb feeling. If she closed her eyes and imagined she could see it, how did it show up for her? "Like a brick wall," she said. I asked her if she could try to see over the brick wall. Although this was way outside of Valeria's normal comfort zone, she indulged me.

"Well, I'm there. I'm a teenager and I'm just there by myself."

"Can you talk to her?" I asked.

"Yeah, I think I can."

"Go ahead and try," I prompted.

It was a long while before she said, "She's been stuck there a long time. She'd also like to feel. She wants to come out from behind the wall."

"Fantastic, let's get her out of there. Where would she like to go instead of being behind the wall?"

"With me, I guess." Valeria described taking her teenager self out from behind the wall and going for a walk in a forest together. Valeria liked her younger self. She commented that her body was tingling during the session. "I think you're magic," she said.

I replied back, "I am no more magic than you are. This magic is coming from inside you!"

I asked Valeria to explain to this teenage part of herself that she was going on a retreat in a few days, what was supposed to happen there, and what Valeria wanted from it.

"See if she's ok with that or has any concerns."

"I think she's cool with it," Valeria replied. She ended the session feeling lighter. The next time I would see Valeria would be after her medicine retreat.

Here is a breakdown of some of the areas and questions I assessed with Valeria in her preparation for medicine work. You can consider these domains for yourself, or with a therapist or coach. They are not exhaustive and will be slightly different for everyone.

- What draws you to use psychedelics? What medicine and why?
- What is your previous experience with psychedelics? How might it compare to what you are about to do?

- What is your personal history that might be relevant to your medicine experience? Is there a personal or family history of psychosis or bipolar disorder? Any health conditions that would make it risky for you to use psychedelics (like high blood pressure)? If so, more medical evaluation is necessary.
- Explore the set and setting for psychedelic work. Is it safe? Led by an experienced facilitator?
- Gain insight about your history including previous trauma.
- Assess your current relationship to pleasure and embodiment. Name specific ways the psychedelic experience can enhance your relationship to pleasure and your body.
- Envision outcomes you'd like for yourself.
- Understand your inner system of "parts."*
- Assess your readiness for the experience directly beforehand. Is there anything, or any "part," that would make it difficult or unsafe for you?

Integration

Valeria bounded into my office two days after her retreat ended.

"Well, how was it?" I inquired.

"Literally the most beautiful thing I ever experienced. Also one of the hardest. I cried a lot. I screamed. A lot. I really didn't expect that. I don't think I ever actually screamed in my life. It was held in a circle, and people sat and watched each other have a turn with the medicine. At first I was terrified because I didn't want people to see me look weird, and I was afraid I'd say something stupid. But really once the medicine came on, not only was I not aware of them, but I was in this totally expanded state. When I started to feel like I was coming back to my body I first thought, wow, the other participants must really be bored. I've been occupying too much of the group's time in the center of the circle. But then I thought, you know, I have a right to be here. I'm

---

*My working style is inspired by Internal Family Systems therapy. I have found the IFS approach superior for psychedelic preparation. There are also other ways of understanding parts, including Jungian archetypal work, tarot iconography, animal parts, and protectors, etc. Find what works for you.

going to stay here a while longer. It was that moment when I realized I had a right to take up space. And I have a right to my feelings. I think then I was both crying and laughing at the same time."

If Valeria had taken a longer-acting psychedelic like, say LSD, there might have been a much longer discussion about the actual content of the experience including visions, realizations, and narrative as well as body sensations and emotions. But for shorter-acting medicines, sometimes it is the somatic, emotional, and meta-perceptual experience that is the most important. Valeria continued. "So for my second turn, I thought I'm really going to work with this younger part of myself who has been trapped for so long. Again, the first part, I think it was about ten minutes, was like a giant rush. But then when I started to come back to myself I thought, go find her. See how she's doing. And I could find her. She was cheering me on and told me to remember how good it is to laugh. So I laughed. It was weird because at first I started to make myself laugh. Then I started really laughing. And then I started crying. I asked the women in the group if they could all grab my hands and I reached out and held them. I stayed like that for a long time because it felt so good."

My integration work with Valeria lasted for about six sessions. We identified key areas of her life where she would like to feel more connected and alive. Now that her young part, who was previously numb and traumatized, was in a better place, Valeria felt open to exploring pleasure. Some of the work we did in the actual sessions had to do with remembering sensations she had experienced in the medicine work and anchoring them in her body, we used breath to explore connecting to a feeling of expansion. We also created a storyboard together of all of the emotions, sensations, and ideas she had while she was in the retreat.

Valeria reported she had started taking a dance class, and as requested, was spending more time in nature. After a morning in the woods herself, she exclaimed, "It's so quiet, but also, like, so full of sound." Literally the first time she'd ever really heard a forest! But the sexual part was coming less easily to her. Her partner was supportive but felt like something changed really fast and was thrown off by it. I asked Valeria if she would like to bring him in for a joint integration session. José, her partner, came to my office with her the next time we met for an additional session. José was jovial, but looked a little uncomfortable. He was clearly checking me out and getting a read. I asked how this was going for him.

"Well, I really don't know. I'm a very open-minded guy. But Valeria is very energetic . . . about life, all of a sudden and I'm not sure how I will fit into that."

Valeria thought it would be helpful if I told José what was normal after psychedelic work, so I did. I asked José if he would have liked to have been included in our sessions before Valeria did the medicine. We hadn't invited him previously.

"Nah, it was her thing. I just feel like I'm trying to wrap my head around all this now. Obviously the sexual part is something because Valeria and I . . . I thought we were having a perfectly good sex life, but now she's saying she wants more and I don't know where to start."

First, I asked José what he meant by sex. Was it penetration? Was it something else?

"Penetration, I guess," he said. I asked him if it would be possible to build a bigger container around sex. Wherever he felt comfortable starting, that's where the container could start. Did he like to be naked together and just breathe together? Was there something he was interested in exploring that Valeria didn't know about?

"There are things *I'm* interested in that you don't know about!" Valeria chimed in. While I don't encourage cross talk, we had an opening. Valeria really wanted José to be interested in what made her feel good. She didn't necessarily care if they were having penetrative intercourse more frequently. "Things have just been the same for so long," she said. José could relate to that.

I gave Valeria and José an assignment: to make a list of everything they could possibly think of that would be erotically pleasurable to do together. Things that when they thought about it gave them a little charge. That felt good for them, and they took the assignment home to work on. They agreed to share it with each other a week later. During this session, Valeria realized that her teenage trauma, which she didn't even recognize as a trauma, actually was about a feeling that men would never be interested in her boundaries or emotional needs. With José, things felt so safe, but also so predictable. It was a comfortable box to stay in, to a point. Valeria told José for the first time her experience from high school and shared with him that leaving that behind made her feel free to feel a lot more and she hoped he could be part of that.

I saw Valeria for one more session. She seemed radiant, but said she was getting back to her normal life and felt our work was at completion. I agreed. She reported that she and José had tried six things on their various lists. There was actually a lot of overlap. They weren't having more penetrative sex, but they were spending a lot more time relating to each other's bodies, showering together. She also yelled at José for the first time. That wasn't super pleasant, but we recognized together, that feeling more means, well, feeling more and expressing it. Valeria was in a new place. Alive and well.

Integration approaches in my work with Valeria included:

- Creating narrative: what actually happened in the medicine experience?
- Creating meaning: how is what happened important to your life?
- Somatic Awareness: what sensations do you remember and how can you come back to them?
- Assessing goals: what will change in your life because of your medicine experience?
- Embodied practice: how do you relate to movement, embodiment, and pleasure?
- Sexual healing: what about sex and pleasure would you like to be different for yourself and how do you achieve it? How creative can you be about embracing pleasure?
- Expanding the frame of sex and pleasure: what is it now, and how can it be bigger and more intentional?
- Family/community healing: how is this healing carried over into your relationships, family, and community for support and deeper connection?

Valeria and José, are of course, made up. But I've seen so many clients like this. Stifled in their lives. Not feeling connected. Hampered by trauma that no one has ever given them permission to look at or they had not ever thought of as traumas. Psychedelic integration and preparation is not complete unless it touches explicitly on how your medicine experience can bring you into a deeper connection with the world, with yourself, your body, and pleasure. It's not all about what you think and what happens in your head. Our world, and our deepest healing, is about blending the cognitive with embodied states of joy and pleasure-enhancing life practices. This is how we walk the healing into our lives every day.

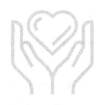

5
HIGH IMPACT

Recovered Memories, Sexual Abuse, and Power Dynamics in Psychedelic Healing

And now the wheels of heaven stop
You feel the devil's riding crop
Get ready for the future
It is murder

"THE FUTURE" BY LEONARD COHEN

WHERE DO YOU TURN when the person who was entrusted to guide you through one of the most vulnerable experiences of your life sexually abuses you? What happens when your attempt to heal sexual trauma retraumatizes you? How do you make sense of psychedelic visions or emerging memories you aren't even sure are memories? What boundaries are needed around strong sexual attraction for a psychedelic guide or medicine person who is neither your therapist nor your friend? These questions represent some of the most troubling and complex realities that surround sexual healing with psychedelics medicines. This chapter will delve into topics that are underrepresented in scientific research and are strongly polarizing among psychedelic practitioners including the emergence of "repressed memories" of sexual trauma or abuse, the horrifying reality of sexual trauma occurring at the hands of people entrusted to guide healing work, and an evaluation of power dynamics in psychedelic spaces. I hope to not only shine a light on these topics, but also to provide blueprints for understanding and healing in their aftermath.

These issues on their own are complex, and many therapists and communities alike are understandably unclear on how to support psychedelic users when phenomena such as recovered memories emerge, or sexual abuse occurs. Developing an approach for how to address these destabilizing events in psychedelic integration work or create appropriate responses to abuse are made all the more difficult by the current psychedelic landscape. While each setting for psychedelic healing has its own unique power dynamics and risks, we can broadly divide these contexts into two categories: regulated (medical, research, and certain retreat contexts) and unregulated ("underground" medicine work, recreational experiences, and some forms of shamanic ritual). Unregulated contexts have the potential to leave the people harmed by it feeling abandoned and alone with little recourse when things go wrong. Psychedelic guides (and even many trained therapists) may be ill-equipped to support people having spontaneous memories of previous sexual trauma. When sexual abuse occurs, survivors fear not only self-incrimination, making law enforcement intervention not feasible, but might find little support in communities either eager to avoid controversy or blame survivors for the abuse. While regulated contexts with oversight might seem like a brilliant remedy for these risks, recent examples of sexual abuse occurring within the context of clinical research have occurred. Institutions can only protect people if the institution is willing to take accountability for harm.

I will illuminate several under-explored areas related to psychedelics and sexuality that lead us to questions as deep as the nature of memory, the power of desire and projection, and what constitutes genuine accountability and healing in psychedelic spaces.

GHOSTS IN THE MEDICINE
Trauma, Memory, and Sexual Abuse

It was perhaps eight or so years ago that I got a call from a young woman named Molly who shared that she hadn't slept in several days after coming home from an ayahuasca retreat near the Peruvian Amazon. She was shaken and exhausted. The first of these ceremonies had been helpful, beautiful even, seeing visions of her ancestors and animals. But as Molly progressed through the program of every-other-night ingestion of ayahuasca medicine, things devolved into terror and confusion. She explained to me that it started as a feeling, a feeling that she had been carrying something unexplained her whole life that made sex feel shameful and difficult. The medicine seemed to guide her toward exploring this sensation of disgust. Then, during her third ayahuasca ceremony, she "remembered" an experience of her father, who was seen in her ayahuasca-induced visions wearing a ceremonial robe with a hood surrounded by other adults who took turns sexually abusing her.

She emerged from the ceremony extremely upset and sought the support of a Western woman who presented herself as an integration coach working at the retreat center. This coach told her that not only were her memories true, but that the medicine was prompting her to confront her father. Her work with ayahuasca would not be complete until she "looked him in the eye" and told him she knew what he had done. The trouble was, Molly had no conscious memory of ever having been sexually abused, much less in a room with several adults wearing ceremonial hoods, and had a loving relationship with her father who was present and involved in her life. On one hand, Molly *did* experience unexplained symptoms of sexual dysfunction that seemed to line up with what she had read about the aftermath of sexual abuse. But the rest of the story didn't fit for her. Molly called my therapy practice after leaving the Amazon confused and frightened. Should she tell her family? Was the integration coach right, that this must be true? Not only was Molly "recovering" memories of possible abuse, but the experience of being alone in the jungle, completely immersed in these terrifying scenes, was traumatic in and of itself.

Molly's story, of course, is a composite, not meant to represent one individual. But it reflects aspects of many clients who have contacted my practice over the years with similar stories that have upended their lives. Cases range from survivors who have clear and distinct yet fragmented memories of sexual abuse that most certainly did occur retrieving more complete memories or heightened somatic sensations related to the experience, to people like Molly who have no memory or belief that they had been sexually abused, and who have positive relationships with the alleged "abuser." Additionally, one of the more common and troubling calls I receive are from family members reaching out on behalf of their children or spouses either alleging sexual abuse or accusing a family member of having abused them. These cases require some of the most clinically complex and delicate integration work.

When journeyers emerge from psychedelic experiences with these visualizations or feelings regarding previous sexual abuse from childhood, several conflicts and ethical dilemmas must be considered. First, the #MeToo movement has given us a vital imperative to "believe survivors." This is a very straightforward value when talking about people who have been sexually harmed, often by those with far greater power than themselves, and have broken their silence around the harm, and survivors with clear knowledge of previous abuse in childhood. But "believing survivors" becomes complex when, say, the survivor themselves may not be sure if the alleged abuse occurred or, the memory was "retrieved" in a form that includes fantasy elements such as highly ritualized or religious scenes of sexual torture, for example. Because psychedelic states make people more susceptible to suggestion while also inducing a *noetic* quality, a term often used to describe transpersonal revelations, but can also point to an inner knowing about personal or psychological narrative and history,[1] we must consider the possibility that the psychedelic user may have been unduly influenced by the therapist, ceremonial facilitator, or guide.

Memory fragmentation is common in the aftermath of sexual trauma, particularly in childhood. Fragmentation means a survivor has only a "flash" or portion of a memory, rather than an intact, chronological memory. The trauma shows up in somatic responses, reactions such as dissociation, and relational issues, rather than concrete scenes in a survivor's mind. Psychedelic experiences can reconsolidate fragmented traumatic memories so all of a sudden they fit into a bigger context. Psychedelic journeyers can also remember traumatic memories that were not repressed, but forgotten or otherwise compartmentalized. It is well documented in the scientific literature on trauma that a person can indeed experience childhood sexual abuse and due to their age at the time, lack the context to understand that it was abuse. Such cases like these often involve an adult close to the child who contextualized abuse around a "special relationship." Young children may not have the framework to understand the nature of the abuse, experiencing it instead as special treatment, or even find themselves sexually stimulated from it. All of these experiences are normal for young survivors. It is not until the adult survivor recontextualizes the memories with an understanding of appropriate boundaries, power, and abuse that they may only come to feel traumatized by the event later. Memories of abuse can be forgotten precisely because the abuse was not experienced as terrifying or traumatic at the time it occurred in childhood.[2]

As a contrast to Molly's story, some survivors experience a reconsolidation of actual memories from childhood that become clear, somatic, and overwhelming after psychedelic use. Raul contacted my practice after several MDMA sessions facilitated by an underground guide. He knew that he had been sexually abused as a child not because he had very clear memories of it, but because his parents discovered that Raul, as well as a neighbor's son, had been abused by a local babysitter. They observed Raul's temperament and play changing. When a neighbor called and stated they had caught Raul's babysitter abusing their child, they contacted police, a therapist, and family doctor immediately. Raul had vague memories, traumatic in their own right, of being questioned by these adults. He also had "flashes" of memory of the abuse itself, in which he remembered playing games that required him to take off his clothes and be touched. Although he had had therapy over the years, Raul's primary complaint was numbness, lack of interest in relationships, and having intense separation anxiety. Even the somatic therapist he saw told him he was OK because his body "didn't seem to be holding onto the abuse," because whenever Raul tried to bring up these fragmented memories he felt nothing.

During his MDMA experience, every sensation, every part of the sequence of traumas from the abuse itself, from keeping the babysitter's secret to the police and doctors further violating his body, came rushing back. He trembled and screamed during his MDMA experience. Afterward, he did actually feel better temporarily. His emotions were "back online" and his body had released something long held. But in the days and weeks after MDMA he felt dysregulated and overwhelmed. Full of memories that felt half processed, he debated taking MDMA by himself because he could not afford another two thousand dollars the sitter was charging. He also had the sense that her capacity to help him was limited by her role as a guide, not a therapist.

Raul's story is the other side of the trauma memory coin. Psychedelics can facilitate the somatic and emotional remembering and reprocessing of abuse that has been either fragmented, suppressed, or not contextualized as trauma at the time. An ethical approach to psychedelic integration around these emerging memories requires a great amount of discernment, knowledge, and care on the part of the survivor and the integration specialist. To understand more about the phenomenon of psychedelic-induced "recovered memories," we first need to understand more about the nature of trauma and memory and the controversies that have swirled around these topics.

The concept of a repressed traumatic memory is controversial and polarizing among trauma specialists with a soft divide seeming to occur between clinicians, many of whom believe that traumatic memories can be repressed to the unconscious only to be unearthed later in therapy, and research scientists who fail to find credible evidence to endorse the belief that a person could experience a terrible trauma only to have no recall of the event.[3] The roots of this controversy extend all the way back to Sigmund Freud and the French physician Jean-Martin Charcot, known as the Napoleon of Neurosis,[4] who first conceptualized that the mind could relegate terrible experiences to the unconscious, and the memories could later be retrieved in treatment. But the real debate around memory and trauma took off in the 1990s during the so-called "Memory Wars" when there was a dramatic increase in reports of childhood sexual abuse and satanic ritual abuse. How were so many people recalling these events when there was no scholarly evidence that such memories could indeed be forgotten at all? Was it due to therapist suggestion? Was it a cultural phenomenon?

While there is little scientific evidence derived from clinical research that a traumatic memory can be repressed to the unconscious, there is ample evidence that false memories can be suggested by a therapist and believed to be true by a client. In clinical research studies, anywhere from zero to seventy percent of subjects were susceptible to false memory implantation (where a psychologist suggests and asks a subject to elaborate on a "memory" of an event that did not occur).[5] One study showed that subjects with a high level of fantasy proneness, dissociation, and absorption appear to be more susceptible to the suggestions of false memories.[6] This information is crucial, as psychedelics are shown to make users even more susceptible to suggestion.

Yet, over ninety percent of participants in a survey of EMDR trauma therapists believed that the mind is capable of blocking out memories and later recalling them.[7] Why? Because it is very likely that they have witnessed spontaneous traumatic memories emerging in treatment. As a trained EMDR therapist myself who uses this evidence-based modality widely in my practice, I have personally witnessed clients "recalling" and processing traumas going back to the first days of life, including birth trauma and penile circumcision-related trauma. What could possibly be happening here? How do we make sense of clients having meaningful and lasting benefit from processing traumas that they believe to have occurred during a time in their life before language acquisition or common memory recall? The science simply doesn't back this up. Yet practitioners in the field of trauma therapy who actually work with clients in a clinical setting (rather than a research setting) seem to witness either the retrieval of repressed memory or preverbal trauma becoming accessible.

This background is helpful in trying to determine an ethical and compassionate approach to the experience of psychedelic-induced repressed memories. I, as a therapist, want my treatment approaches to be driven by scientific evidence. Yet, there is a human side to this controversy. When a client calls a therapist stating they have recovered a memory of sexual abuse during a psychedelic experience, is the therapist to say, "Well, the science really says that can't be true because you should have been able to remember it before. Sorry about that!" Of course not.

So both therapists and psychedelic users need a better framework for understanding these experiences and how to work skillfully with them. It is also worth stating clearly that the science of the brain is in its infancy. Based on my actual clinical work, it is essential to keep an open mind, weighing the current science against the very real possibility that our understanding of the brain may later give us more scientifically observable evidence that unconscious repressed memories may be real and may indeed be directly stimulated by psychedelic use. It is also important to remember that the conditions of a lab are not the conditions of real-life therapy. This may cut both ways, as psychedelics may end up not being such a blockbuster treatment after all when they make their way from research to clinical practice. Likewise, we may also find that unconscious repression of trauma and its subsequent retrieval in psychedelic states may become an even more widely documented occurrence.

It's important to remember that these are real experiences that happen to real people, and our approach to recovered memories needs to be grounded in compassion and curiosity for the experience of the psychedelic journeyer, while also acknowledging that these visions of abuse leave people terribly confused and destabilized. Much like childhood sexual abuse itself, one big trauma can contain multiple traumatic parts. In the case of psychedelic recovered memories, there is the potential childhood trauma, the recall or reexperiencing of the trauma under the influence of a psychedelic medicine which can be traumatic in itself, and the trauma involved in trying to make sense of the experience later, including family response, therapist support or lack thereof, and internal confusion. Some preliminary considerations and questions when trying to make sense of these experience may include:

- What intention did the psychedelic user establish for the experience? Was it related to resolving trauma, somatic, or emotional distress? Or did the abuse vision emerge completely unprompted?
- Did they have any knowledge of being sexually abused prior to the psychedelic experience? Was this entirely new to them, or did they have fragmented memories that became more vivid or linear during the medicine work?

- How does the journeyer feel about the memory? Are they destabilized? Curious? Are they having somatic experiences related to trauma? Or do they feel like something has been processed and resolved during their psychedelic experience?
- What do they want to do with this experience? Do they want to confront family members whom they "saw" perpetrate abuse? Do they want to pursue law enforcement action? Do they just want to heal themselves?
- Did the traumatic vision come in a form that seemed fantastical or incredible to the journeyer, or clear and realistic?

The answers to these questions can support a roadmap to healing for psychedelic users and the people who support them. Therapists and integration professionals hold an extremely high responsibility to be supportive and validating, while not suggesting or endorsing that they can conclusively say any detail previously unknown to the journeyer prior to the psychedelic experience is literally true in the way the person experienced it. This can be very hard. Survivors of sexual trauma deserve to be believed. Indeed, it's crucial to repeat clearly that any person who has experienced sexual abuse or assault and has clear knowledge of it happening, whether or not it was experienced as traumatic at the time, is in need of support, validation, and healing, not disbelief and questioning. But the situation gets far murkier when these visions emerge in psychedelic users who have never previously recalled memories of abuse in their history. Therapists and integration professionals are literally holding the very fate of lives, communities, and families in their hands in how they navigate these situations.

What could possibly be happening during these instances of traumatic psychedelic visions or memories? Drawing upon over a dozen cases from my integration practice, I believe there are several possibilities. First, I do believe that people may repress and later recover a traumatic memory in a psychedelic state. Given my work with survivors who were later able to verify some aspects of their visions, this does seem to be a genuine possibility. I also believe that these visions can be the result of not a literal act of sexual abuse, but rather a consolidation of feeling states from childhood. Remember, psychedelics most often teach us using an interplay of visual imagery and a feeling of inner knowing. I believe in some cases experiences such as emotional abuse, extreme vulnerability, neglect, or even strong sexual feelings toward an adult caretaker can be concretized into visions that present during psychedelic work much like a dream, for the purpose of creating narrative around intense feelings so our minds and bodies can work through them to heal. I also believe it is possible for an unscrupulous or unaware guide or therapist to suggest that a client's current issues might stem from sexual abuse and thus influence the mind to create what is essentially a healing narrative around this. I believe our whole being gravitates toward healing. If you don't know what it is you're healing from, that task can seem impossible. Suggesting that a set of symptoms or issues could stem from sexual abuse can indeed influence someone to "remember" sexual abuse.

A useful approach to making sense of psychedelic recovered memories is to first ask, what needs to be healed? Why did this come up as part of my healing work? How is this trying to help me in my healing? I'll share a personal example that does not have to do specifically with sexual abuse, but illustrates a point. For many years, I had a very specific issue around food. Not restricting or overeating, but rather a neurotic obsession with making sure I would have food accessible to me. By 10 a.m., I would be in my office plotting and worrying about where to buy the best lunch. I would overbuy groceries for fear of running out of food. I also had an intense fear of hunger and not being able to eat. (Imagine all the snacks I would take to an airport. Imagine the distress at plant medicine ceremonies that required fasting!) During an ayahuasca ceremony, I was shown a vision of myself as a child witnessing my parents fighting violently in the kitchen. My child self was cowering in the corner and a plate flew off the kitchen table by itself and smashed on the wall. The medicine was "showing" me that my food issue was based on a childhood fear that my parents would divorce and I would be left alone and hungry with no one to care for me. Some background: my parents are not divorced—they are married to this day, and they certainly would not have left me alone and hungry. I asked them if such a fight happened. It did not. But it was so clear in my vision. I felt completely as if I had remembered it. Is it possible that it did happen and was forgotten by my parents? I suppose, as this alleged fight would have been nearly forty years earlier.

The medicine gave me context for understanding a childhood fear of abandonment that translated to dysfunctional behaviors around food, stitching together these intense emotions in a way that could be directly experienced and felt above and beyond what would be possible in talk-based psychotherapy. The result was immediate relief from my food anxiety that persists to this day. Here we have an example of a "memory" that may or may not have been real that pointed me to a very deep terror my inner-child-self had held for decades: abandonment and starvation. Understanding and releasing that fear changed my adult feelings and behaviors dramatically. How would I have fared if it was extremely important to know my vision was real? My successful resolution of this anxiety was directly related to my willingness to accept that it was a gift from the medicine for my healing, and may or may not have happened. The stakes are astronomically higher when we are talking about a state of uncertainty around sexual abuse, especially when it may have involved an otherwise trustworthy figure.

Successfully working with psychedelic recovered memories may require tolerance for not knowing—not knowing if a vision was "real," if it happened with that person or in that situation. That can be a bitter pill for people desperate for answers. Supporting psychedelic users during integration might be about shifting the question from "Did it happen?" to "Why did this vision emerge; how is it meant to be part of my healing; what do I do with this now?" It is also crucial to remember that integration psychotherapy after psychedelic experiences can help those who recover memories to come to some form of resolution around the memory or vision through a process of inner knowing and meaning-making, rather than outer confirmation of facts. One might ask, "What would it take for me to be at peace with this experience and understand how it emerged to support my healing process," instead of "Did this really happen?" That can be difficult.

The first place we look in supporting the healing process is the body. Body-based trauma therapies such as EMDR, Somatic Experiencing, and Internal Family Systems, all of which use elements of visualization and somatic awareness and processing, are excellent modalities to support the integration process. After a psychedelic experience that reveals traumatic visions, integration work can center the body's process. Does this "memory" induce a charge or sensation in my body? Where are those sensations felt? What are they trying to tell me? Is the *memory* traumatic, or was the *experience of remembering* traumatic? I have worked successfully with many survivors in integration psychotherapy by adhering to two core principles: to connect with openness and curiosity about the experience, and to let the body lead the way to healing. Remember, if this vision came up, it came up for the purpose of your healing.

Working with the body requires openness on the part of the client to center the integration process on working with somatic experience, rather than an insight-oriented approach common in psychotherapy that seeks to understand and make meaning of the trauma memory itself. Therapists can unwittingly become complicit in affirming a "memory" that is simply untrue otherwise. I may ask a survivor to recall a traumatic image from the ceremony (whether they believe it to be true or not). We then notice the feelings, emotions, and sensations the body holds related to that image. This provides a jumping off point where therapists skilled in EMDR can use that tool for moving the client through a somatically driven process. Likewise, sensorimotor psychotherapy and Somatic Experiencing both help the body to develop internal resources, and move through the sensations of trauma. The work is done not when the client has conclusive evidence or resolution about the memory, but rather when the body is no longer reactive. In other words, when the feelings associated both with the memory and with the trauma of *remembering* are safely placed in the past.

Those seeking integration support should proceed with caution around any provider who suggests confrontation of family or an alleged perpetrator is essential for healing, or insistence that a memory is in fact real because it occurred in a psychedelic state. Moreover, beware of therapists who simply cite "the science" and are unwilling to consider that more might be going on simply because psychedelics were involved.

Remember, it is possible to resolve trauma being held in the body without knowing the facts of what happened. It is possible to embrace different ways of believing. We can believe survivors when they tell us they were sexually abused, we can believe that the body has a deep healing capacity that can be accessed through psychedelics, and we can believe in the promise of healing even without specific details of abuse.

Distinct from the emergence of memories or visions that had been previously unknown to a journeyer, another common experience in psychedelic healing is the reexperiencing of traumatic memories. Reexperiencing is an affective and somatic immersion in a traumatic past event about which the journeyer *was* previously aware during a psychedelic experience. A recent paper explored the prevalence, therapeutic value, and ethical considerations related to traumatic remembering occasioned by ayahuasca in a retreat context.*

A study on traumatic memory and psychedelic states found that women who were sexually assaulted and people who had self-reported a lifetime diagnosis of PTSD were most likely to reexperience trauma during an ayahuasca ceremony. In fact, of all adverse life experiences, sexual assault carried the highest reexperiencing rate, with women respondents reexperiencing it in psychedelic states more frequently than male survivors. However, they also found that this reexperiencing, though uncomfortable and difficult, held therapeutic value and catalyzed healing, with those reexperiencing trauma being the most likely participants to enjoy a reduction in neuroticism immediately after the ceremony as well as at a three-month follow-up. The researchers explain that through a psychoanalytic lens, ayahuasca may reduce defenses that normally impede the emergence of traumatic memories. They also describe that psychedelic experience may "assist in activating and modifying trauma memory structures through exposure" to memories with

---

*In my clinical practice, ayahuasca is the medicine I see most commonly associated with both the emergence or reexperiencing of traumatic memories, though it is possible with any psychedelic or even non-psychedelic altered states, Holotropic Breathwork most prominently.

which we may prefer not to engage in normal life. Psychedelics may also help us to reevaluate self-blame for our trauma, and instill that trauma can be remembered without us being harmed. A robust informed consent practice must include explaining to trauma survivors that these memories can be reactivated during psychedelic experiences, as well as making specific plans for support during integration.[8]

A popular psychedelic adage is that there are no bad trips, just difficult ones. I disagree. It can be truly traumatic to enter a ceremony space to pursue healing and be confronted with hours of visions and sensations of sexual abuse, especially if it was completely unexpected and journeyers are left with limited support. Psychedelic users who experience this type of trauma have been gaslighted by those who refuse to admit that psychedelics can be unpredictable and challenge people in startling ways, causing lasting impact including putting self or others in harm's way during the experience, behaving aggressively, or enduring psychological damage.[9] However, with support, most psychedelic experiences can be used to generate healing through introspection, meaning-making, and reimagining personal narratives. Even very challenging psychedelic experiences often hold the exact ingredients for the personal transformation we seek and the healing container to face our worst moments and biggest fears.

It is also worth noting that psychedelics don't just promote negative autobiographical memory, they also are known to prompt beautiful memories and experiences as well. These medicines help us remember back to the moments when we have been loved or experienced great joy. They can reconnect us with those we've lost, with our ancestors, or with a direct relationship to a Higher Power. Adverse life experiences can create a black hole within us that draws every other positive or loving memory toward it, distorting and obscuring them. Psychedelics can and do help us to access the bigger picture to see that our adverse experiences do not define us. A pleasure-centered approach to psychedelic integration places priority on situating ourselves in our beautiful bodies (and they are all beautiful, yes, yours too), here, now. Finding our way back to pleasure often means walking through the valley of darkness, through the darkest shadow of our psyche, until we find the light.

IN THE VALLEY OF SHADOWS
Sexual Harm in Psychedelic Spaces

Healing from sexual abuse often means that the individual survivor must engage in a re-narration of the story of their trauma. Many survivors' internal stories about abuse contain some element of self-blame: "If I hadn't worn that, if I had protested, if I hadn't gone on that trip . . ." Or even the profoundly confusing reality that pleasure or attraction coexisted with abuse. It is essential for the healing and wholeness of survivors that they receive support in shifting self-blame and telling a new story about themselves, a story in which they weren't at fault. Accepting that abuse is not our fault often requires confronting the horror that we are not always in control. We have been powerless, and someone took grave advantage of the opportunity to harm us. Sexual abuse and assault is never the fault of the person harmed. There is no cause, familial, religious, or psychedelic, that is more important than a survivor being able to speak their truth and take their power back. No survivor deserves to be left in the shadows alone with their story.

Over the past number of years, the psychedelic community has been polarized over reports of prominent people, often (but certainly not always) men, who have used their influence, status, power, and access to vulnerable people to perpetrate sexual abuse. There are a number of excellent journalistic resources that illuminate these wrongs and share the stories of individuals who have been sexually abused in psychedelic spaces. These stories of sexual trauma (like most stories of sexual trauma) have multiple traumatic parts: the abuse that occurred, the aftermath for the survivor, and the response to the survivor's disclosure of the harm. Cultural movements that have created space for survivors to tell their stories and growing awareness of the prevalence of sexual harm broadly in society are helping to transform our views about sexual abuse and assault, and about the nature of power and harm. But the fact that we have a bifurcated psychedelic landscape consisting of the realms of clinical research on one hand and unregulated or ceremonial work on the other, presents tremendous complications for survivors and for meaningful community response to sexual harm when it occurs during or after psychedelic healing work.

In conventional psychotherapy, sexual feelings between therapists and clients is a common occurrence. Sexual contact, however, should never occur. It's a core tenant of the profession. When psychedelics are added to the mix, intense feelings of closeness between the client and guide or therapist can take hold, clients can hold idealized views of their guide, or psychedelic facilitators can get caught in a web of their own narcissistic needs or erotic feelings for their clients. Moreover, intense somatic sensations can be a common feature of a psychedelic experience. The mix of strong sexual sensations in the body and exaggerated sense of closeness, attunement, and connection with a psychedelic facilitator can create a mirage of meaning where a client can easily mistake these feelings for wanted sexual contact. The relational matrix of adoration, sexual feeling, projection, and narcissism can prove a disastrous mix. And then there are predatory therapists and guides who simply use the opportunity afforded by clients in an extremely vulnerable and suggestive state to knowingly and intentionally sexually harm them.

Reporting sexual harm perpetrated by a person sanctioned to provide psychedelics by the medical establishment means combatting institutions eager to maintain pristine reputations while catapulting psychedelics away from their reputation as dangerous drugs to a place of respectability (not to mention liability-oriented lawyers and institutional boards). These cases are often passed off as the "bad apple" scenario where one offending person may or may not be cast out of practice, shamed, while the institution itself soldiers on with little change.* When sexual harm occurs in shamanic, underground, or community contexts, survivors have been told that they will hurt the movement, break up the community, or that they are actually not enlightened enough to see that unwanted sexual contact was for their

---

*For those familiar with some of these abuse cases, I'm not referencing a single organization, but rather that sexual harm has occurred, to my knowledge, in clinical research, around psychedelic educational and training organizations, and by therapists trained by these institutions but acting outside of their official capacity.

healing. Even worse, survivors harmed in these contexts may feel they simply have nowhere to turn when a retreat center is far away, a "shaman" comes to town and disappears into the ether, or when disclosing means incriminating themselves. I have had conversations even with respected women in the psychedelic community that hold beliefs such as "What did she think was going to happen when she was invited to stay overnight with that facilitator?" or the like. It certainly doesn't make a survivor confident they will receive support after disclosing abuse.

I will attempt to unpack the complex issue of sexual abuse in psychedelic spaces by looking at the profiles of sexually transgressing therapists and guides; exploring the interpersonal and relational dynamics in psychedelic work that lead to sexual harm occurring; and trying to grapple with the troubling question of individual, professional, and community responses to sexual abuse. In my psychotherapy practice, I have worked with a number of individuals who have experienced sexual harm at the hands of a therapist or guide during or after psychedelic work. I have also worked with transgressing psychedelic facilitators. Similar to many therapists, it is easy to access compassion for the survivors, but truthfully, it has been my work with perpetrators that has taught me the most about the complex reasons these violations occur. As a sexual violence survivor myself, what does it mean to sit and try to understand the inner world of someone who has done horrible things? It requires perspective and discernment. Many therapists believe that perpetrators cannot be redeemed and inherently have personality disorders such as narcissism or psychopathy and manipulate therapists, making therapy ultimately unhelpful for them. That may be true for a percentage of sexual transgressors. That's where clinical discernment comes in. But working with perpetrators has also given me a palpable sense that sexual abuse occurs in a cascade that often starts with the perpetrator's own unhealed trauma.

Sexual abuse and assault is an epidemic unfolding around us. No one can deny its pervasiveness in our culture. But we respond differently when sexual abuse is perpetrated by someone who represents an idea or institution that not only are we supposed to trust, but are discouraged from questioning. In chapter two, I mentioned my experience around sexual harm in Buddhist communities, but this surely applies to the Catholic Church and other religious organizations, and conventional psychotherapy as well. Over fifty percent of lawsuits against conventional psychotherapists involve sexual misconduct.* One study described that in the United States, four to seven percent of mental health professionals admitted to sexual contact with client (by anonymous survey—the number is almost certainly far higher), and perpetrators are most often senior members of their profession with power.[10]

It says something positive about the psychedelic community that these issues are getting so much attention, and genuine attempts at creating accountability structures are underway. It is also helpful to remember this is not a uniquely psychedelic problem, it is a human problem. However, there remains a lack of sophisticated analysis around why sexual harm occurs and what can be done about it. The key to preventing sexual harm exists in creating meaningful ways for survivors to report abuse and receive accountability, vet facilitators for previous reports of misconduct, and enhance institutional responses to this problem that extend beyond rooting out single perpetrators and declaring the job done. One way we can provide the education people need to have safe containers for psychedelic healings is to normalize the confusing and intense feelings that can flow in both directions when power, trauma, emotion, and medicine come together. Having a working understanding of these dynamics can ultimately lead to more meaningful responses when sexual abuse occurs that can genuinely offer healing to survivors, but also address the harm caused by perpetrators in more sophisticated ways than simply exiling them. The most essential ingredient to crafting impactful ways of responding to sexual abuse in psychedelic spaces is to decriminalize psychedelics. When survivors have recourse and do not fear legal jeopardy themselves, the space will emerge to create more robust systems of accountability.

---

*A mental health attorney I know once put this into one pithy description: *gross*.

UNDERSTANDING AND PREVENTING PSYCHEDELIC SEXUAL ABUSE

Monster, sociopath, narcissist. These are some of the most common tropes that swirl around people alleged to have sexually transgressed with clients. What does the clinical literature actually say? How can understanding perpetrators help us to craft a substantive response to sexual harm in psychedelic spaces? Andrea Celenza and Glen Gabbard, both experts in the field of therapist sexual abuse, dispel several of these myths. Based on over 150 cases of in-depth assessment of therapists and pastoral counselors who have participated in illicit sexual relationships with their clients, they name three common beliefs about who exactly these perpetrators are: they are probably psychopathic (meaning they are manipulative and have a pathological lack of empathy); they have exploited more than one patient; and they are not amenable to rehabilitation.[11] But in fact, these seem to be truths in a minority of cases evaluated by these professionals. Celenza and Gabbard found about twenty-five percent of the therapists they assessed were psychopathic or severely narcissistic predators.[12] Not a small number! Certainly, these cases are the ones often described in the media since they represent the most repugnant and salacious scenarios, a repeat predator in our midst manipulating and harming multiple survivors.

There is an important caveat to the work of Celenza and Gabbard. They work with therapists who admit to sexual boundary transgressions and want to take accountability. In fact, these therapists willingly participate in three to four years of extensive rehabilitative psychotherapy after a transgression and submit to ongoing supervision and accountability to the survivor and professional bodies. It is very unlikely that the most pathological offenders pursue this type of voluntary rehabilitation, so their sample statistics are drawn from the therapists most open to introspection and who have genuine remorse. The reality is that the majority of therapists who sexually transgress are not pathological, but the majority of survivors are harmed by the smaller number of serial predators who are indeed pathologically narcissistic or psychopathic.

Let's try to understand the percentage of therapists who are not serial predators and may be good candidates for accountability. How do we relate to them? Our desire to see all people who get involved in inappropriate sexual relationships or even enact more overt abuse as monsters may stem from a disowning of our own shadow. After all, if these are "normal" people who inflict this type of harm, then what does it mean about us? We see a massive boundary violation and recoil, first, because it is shocking—how could this person do such a thing? Not only that, but how could they betray our cause? How could they sully our psychedelic mission? The reality is that *any* person who has been involved in practicing psychotherapy or has consistent experience as a psychedelic guide can name instances of regret, misjudgment, or porous boundaries most often done in the name of benefitting the client. As Celenza and Gabbard point out, "The profile of the one-time transgressor, at least on the surface, is too much like you and me."[13]

What leads these therapists, the ones who are not narcissists or sociopaths, to violate boundaries and what can be done about it? A study of therapist trainees who have been involved in sexual boundary violations provides a fascinating discussion of reasons why abuse might occur. Looking at therapist trainees or inexperienced therapists is especially helpful because psychedelic guides may be mentored rather than psychologically trained, may have limited oversight, or trained therapists who engage in "underground" psychedelic work may be doing so enmeshed in a curious web of professional ethics and stature, while also actively engaging in illicit behavior that must be kept secret by the therapist and their clients. The authors of this study of therapist trainees argue that under-trained therapists are likely to misinterpret a client's attraction to them as personal rather than relating to their professional role, and may even believe that sexual boundary violations are good for the client.[14]

How could any therapist believe such a thing? A consistent theme throughout the literature on sexually offending therapists is that loneliness, working in isolation, and personal crisis are correlated with boundary transgression. I would vigorously add therapists' own unprocessed sexual and relational abuse histories to the mix. These therapists (and by extension guides) enact with their clients complex relationships that include a belief they are saving the client, while using the therapeutic relationship to meet their own emotional needs.[15] The interplay of sexual feelings that can flow between therapist/guide and client are called erotic transference and countertransference. Put simply, erotic transference and countertransference are concepts derived from psychoanalysis; erotic transference refers to a client's overt sexual feelings for a therapist and also the latent reasons that that attraction might be occurring having to do with past relationships, traumas, or fantasy, while countertransference refers to sexual feelings a therapist might feel for a client which are wrapped up in their own unmet needs, unresolved past trauma, and an inner desire for a client to adore them.

Lay therapist and psychedelic visionary Ann Shulgin articulated her thoughts about sexual contact in psychedelic work clearly in her guidelines for psychedelic therapy: *All sexual feelings are allowable; they can and should be discussed, but they will not be physically acted out here.*[16] But a complex relational field is created when sexual attraction occurs during psychedelic work. Whereas the rule of no sexual contact seems direct enough, we also need more basis to understand how to manage the erotic feelings that can occur between facilitators and clients. While appropriate boundaries and avoiding sexual harm are covered in virtually all psychedelic therapy and guide training programs, they most often don't deliver sophisticated education about erotic transference and countertransference. In fact, psychodynamic therapies such as relational, interpersonal, or psychoanalytic therapies, are the only forms of therapy that have strong theoretical concepts around sexual feelings between therapists and clients. As these relational therapies get sidelined in the medical psychedelic model in favor of cognitive-behavioral approaches, which focus only on challenging the thoughts and beliefs of the client, therapists will simply not be equipped to navigate and understand the minefield of sexual feelings, both overt and latent, that can occur in psychedelic work if they are never trained in the more relational theoretical frameworks. It is not enough simply to train therapists or guides to avoid sexual contact with clients. It is equally necessary for the therapist or guide to be able to understand and discuss these feelings with clients who may be acting out past trauma, or fantasizing that the guide can be an ideal sexual partner for healing, while being aware of and acknowledging a guide's own feelings.

One study suggests that both training programs and clinical supervisors can normalize discussion of a therapist's (or guide's) sexual feelings toward their clients, and provide therapists with the tools for discussing the sexual feelings of their clients toward them. A sex-positive approach to psychedelic therapy is one where facilitators are equipped to manage a client's sexual feelings towards them, and also have access to nonjudgmental instructors and supervisors who can normalize their own experiences of navigating the intense emotions, attraction, and idealization can arise in psychedelic work. In a field where the prevailing instructions therapists receive can be as blunt as "don't fuck your clients," psychedelic practitioners can be discouraged from even admitting and exploring sexual feelings for fear of being labeled problematic, rather than as humans having normal human emotions. The authors state, "The most fundamental misconception is that good, well-adjusted therapists can avoid, control, or contain sexual feelings without the need for supervision . . . if they have to discuss their feelings they must be weak or otherwise maladjusted."[17]

All psychedelic training models for guides and therapists teach that therapists should refrain from engaging in nonsexual, supportive touching of the client if sexual feelings are disclosed.* The practice of withholding touch after attraction is acknowledged is a best practice for psychedelic therapy. But clients are not stupid. If a client displays sexual attraction to a therapist and the therapist follows the guidelines of eliminating supportive touch to the client, but without equal skill at discussing the client's feelings, their own feelings, and having time to discuss explicitly why they are not available for hand holding or other nonsexual gestures, this can be deeply retraumatizing of a client who may have experienced abandonment or harbor feelings that

---

*In most psychedelic-assisted therapy models there is another co-therapist in the room, a factor that in and of itself might discourage verbal disclosure of erotic feelings. I mean, imagine admitting to your therapist you have sexual feelings for them with a second therapist sitting there staring at you. Because of this, such a "disclosure" is often not verbal, but rather the client showing preference or flirtation toward one therapist over another.

their sexuality is too much or bad, and lead to further acting out. It is perfectly wonderful to follow guidelines to the letter that help prevent sexual abuse in psychedelic spaces. But without the support, education, supervision, and time to fully explore these dynamics between guide/therapist and client, both parties are deprived of a richer, more human, and more emotionally sustainable dimension of the work. Just wait until managed care eventually comes to psychedelic medicine, and the therapeutic interaction is lopped to a minimum. The results could be disastrous.

The majority of psychedelic-assisted therapists and underground guides I've known in my professional life have had at least one situation arise where a client exposed their genitalia to the therapist during a psychedelic experience, asked for sexual contact, or, even more, insisted sexual contact was necessary for their healing. In the most extreme cases, I have heard of clients threatening to expose the guide if they did not comply with their desire for sexual contact. It is always, without any exception, the responsibility of the guide or therapist to maintain the ethical boundaries in a healing relationship—even if the client gets really, really mad. But if we aren't training providers to know how to work with these issues, and we don't have nonjudgmental networks of support for clinicians and guides, how do you know what to do?

On a sunny, humid afternoon I sat down in a bustling New York City coffee shop with Dr. Bill Brennan, an expert in this area. I met Bill during a training for the EMBARK model of psychedelic therapy, a modality he pioneered with Dr. Alex Belser who contributed the foreword of this book.* Dr. Brennan is warm, mild-mannered, and thoughtful, and relates to this issue through both an academic as well as personal lens, having done research on the topic of relational issues between psychedelic facilitators and their clients, as well as having been involved in community response to sexual harm. I started our conversation by mentioning my concern that as psychedelic therapy is moving into the medical model, it is very likely that the therapy itself will be truncated due to cost, resulting in diminished opportunities to build

---

*I served as a clinical supervisor for the EMBARK program.

meaningful and deep relationships between therapists and clients and minimizing robust conversation about consent. This, combined with a lack of preparation and meaningful relationship-building before psychedelic therapy sessions and therapists taking more liberty to use touch with clients, could all lead to increased risk of sexual harm. He chimed in, "Yes, that's exactly right. I can see that happening."

I discussed with Dr. Brennan that in conventional psychotherapy, I feel very well equipped to talk with clients about erotic feelings that might arise. Most clients come to traditional psychotherapy with an idea of how the relationship is supposed to be. Therapists are trained to know how to address and tolerate both a client's sexual feelings toward them as well as their own sexual feelings without having sexual contact. I expressed that I have felt fear in psychedelic sessions when a client's sexual feelings are amplified, and they may request contact with me I am unwilling and unable to provide. He responded:

> You used the word "fear," and that really resonates with me. When we are sitting in our chairs in traditional therapy and sexual feelings come up, that feels manageable. But when someone is writhing on the ground asking to be touched in a way that I'm not going to do, it's harder for me to respond in a way that's not rejecting. We can't just get up into our chairs and say "Let's talk about these feelings, let's talk about your transference." The less verbal nature of the client's altered state makes it harder to do the kind of dialoguing toward a shared understanding that could take the sting out of a "no." Instead, I would probably manage it in a way that would feel less satisfying for the client, like saying, "I want you to have all of your feelings within your experience, but I'm not going to participate, even though your feelings are good and I still care about you." That's maybe the best way we can deal with it in a medicine session, and the rest needs to be addressed in integration.

But knowing how to address sexual feelings while minimizing actions that could be perceived as rejection by our client takes extraordinary skill.

I asked Dr. Brennan about the trope of the "seductive client;" in other words, a client who acts out sexually toward a therapist to draw them into a transgression. I shared, "It feels really straightforward to me. The therapist is always responsible for preventing sexual contact with a client." He nodded, "Of course they will sometimes try to seduce you and of course it's your responsibility to not be seduced."

Together, we tried to hash out other complexities surrounding this issue. I shared my concerns that as relational models (meaning, an approach to psychotherapy that centers on a complex understanding of the relationship between therapist and client) fall out of favor with psychedelic-assisted treatments, therapists are not going to have the support and knowledge to navigate intense feelings that can arise. Bill reflected:

> It's a major misstep to think that cognitive behavioral therapies are going to be the best fit for psychedelic therapy. Just because they're held up as the evidentiary gold standard in traditional psychotherapy does not mean they're best suited for the kind of experiences we're supporting. These modalities really don't have much to say to the profoundly relational nature of psychedelic therapy. There are so many rich, complex relational dynamics that come up in and around a psychedelic session that we are asked to navigate skillfully. We will not be well-served by models that uncritically graft these nonrelational modalities onto psychedelic therapy because of their reputation as the gold standard in other treatment contexts. We need to move toward models that are more responsive to the relationality of the psychedelic experience. But, as we continue to move toward minimizing the importance of the therapeutic framework, at least within the corporatized, medicalized psychedelic industry, there is a growing laziness around the therapy component, with many clinicians copying and pasting what others did in prior studies. And what's being copied and pasted originates from academic researchers who get really enamored by approaches that have gotten the most research attention but who are not clinicians out there working in the field, and probably not people who did psychedelic work before they started studying it within the frame they decided to put it in.

SYMPATHY FOR THE DEVIL?

The Problem of Predators in Psychedelic Spaces

One of my professional activities is providing education and training around psychedelics to therapists, a job I really enjoy. In the context of these seminars, I have mentioned a Brazilian organization that has conducted religious ayahuasca ceremonies with incarcerated people to help them heal, reduce recidivism, and garner empathy for their victims.[18] I generally get nods of approval at this open-minded approach from students who are often more liberal-leaning and are critical of justice systems. But then I present the next slide which asks the question: "Can psychedelics be used to treat perpetrators of sexual harm in psychedelic spaces? Can we effectively design psychedelic treatments for survivors of sexual harm, but also to address offending therapists, guides, or sex offenders?" The energy palpably shifts. I don't suggest I have an answer to the question, but even asking it almost always results in discomfort. Do transgressors deserve psychedelic healing too? More importantly, how can the psychedelic community itself create systems of protection and reporting that might safeguard users in the context of drug prohibition?

Let me be clear: with regard to the abusers who are indeed psychopaths, narcissists, or serial abusers, the priority is stopping them to the best of our ability from causing further harm. This may take the form of barring them from community events, publicizing their abuse, and creating reliable systems and bodies to which sexual harm can be reported. But abusers who have been exiled have been known to pop up in other communities in new locations where they have access to vulnerable people and do the same thing over again. For a community that is as avoidant of traditional carceral systems of justice as the psychedelic community, both in terms of values but also a reluctance to involve law enforcement for fear of exposing other extralegal activity, what is a community to do with these predators? As noted, despite the fact that the majority of therapists and guides who sexually harm clients are *not* serial predators, the majority of people sexually harmed during psychedelic experiences are harmed by narcissistic predators who abuse many individuals. What do we do with repeat offenders who lack empathy, are poor candidates for rehabilitative work, and seek to evade attempts at accountability to continue to use their power to abuse vulnerable people?

Dr. Brennan suggested that client-driven reputation management is a possible solution. He explained that this would entail a voluntary database with psychedelic therapists and guides and note any accusations that have been made against them. In this database, a guide or therapist can also clearly explain their approach to holding space for psychedelic work. Maybe they use more touch and body-oriented techniques, or maybe more traditional psychotherapy where they will hold your hand in a hard moment. After a guide or therapist and client agree to do a session and concrete consent and boundaries have been discussed, the client can then circle back and review whether that guide followed the consent agreement or acted harmfully. Dr. Brennan elaborated:

> And it's done so in a way so that it's not Google reviews. Instead of reflecting a global assessment of the session, it focuses on how well prior consent agreements were upheld and whether relational harm occurred. This kind of client-driven service feels helpful because it can be flexible around what kind of psychedelic work is happening. There are professional organizations currently trying to come up with universal guidelines for practitioner interventions, and I think they are going to be so broad that they don't really help anything. Or, they're going to be so restrictive that they're only going to favor the medical model. So, we need to have something that is tailored to specific client-practitioner relationships. Reputation management services that can respect the diversity of ways you can work with psychedelic medicines could be a useful approach.

Psychedelic communities have turned to transformative or restorative justice models to address abuse with mixed results. Restorative justice is a method of creating dialogue between people who have been harmed and the people who have harmed them that results in co-created accountability that can include psychotherapy and submitting to supervision for the perpetrator of harm, and apology, financial restitution, and other accountability measures to the harmed person. As wonderful an approach as this is, I believe these methods utilized within the psychedelic community have sometimes fallen short for a number of reasons. Serial perpetrators who become the focus of highly publicized restorative justice processes may be more concerned with holding on to their power and status than genuine rehabilitation, inspired to participate in these processes more to avoid being "canceled" than a genuine desire for introspection. Likewise, the psychedelic community is not a monolithic community that shares accountability and mutual concern for its members. It is a collection of disparate groups of people who all like psychedelics. Love and genuine commitment to one another needs to be at the foundation of any meaningful process of accountability. The fact is, it's likely that restorative justice *will* work very well in small cohorts of people who care deeply for one another as a means of dealing with harm caused by a facilitator capable of empathy and self-reflection. However, when the ingredients of community care and empathy are not present, such processes create emotional drain on those harmed, instead focusing attention on the narcissistic abusers for whom rehabilitation is unlikely.

CROSSED LINES, BLURRED BOUNDARIES
Power, Desire, and Sexuality in Psychedelic Healing

We'd like to believe that power is absolute. That he who holds it is easily identified and can follow a set of standards to responsibly use that power. Those who transgress these rules can be extracted, isolated, and punished. But power is instead a complex matrix of identity, economic realities, and situational truths that constantly shift and morph. To understand power dynamics in psychedelic healing work requires a continual willingness to look at oneself and the subtle relational oscillations that can occur between all parties in these vulnerable states and relationships. Power comes from many places, not the least of which are institutions, social status, and access. Examples of this might include the authoritative power held by medical professionals or researchers, or broader forces such as supremacist movements, unearned social power based on race, gender or other immutable characteristics, or the power held by having access to financial capital. Understanding power on this gross social level is necessary to bring greater equity to psychedelic healing.

There are many in the psychedelic field that can speak to intersectional power dynamics far better than I. There is also a growing awareness both in medical psychedelics and elsewhere that there is a desperate need for more therapists and facilitators of diverse identities and backgrounds who can safely hold spaces where power differentials are reduced (but never eliminated) between members of traditionally marginalized groups. But here I will focus on more subtle types of power exchange in psychedelic healing that center on sexuality, desire, boundaries, and trauma. Exploring power through this lens opens possibilities for a more meaningful evaluation of how sexual harm can be prevented in psychedelic spaces.

The emotional environment in which psychedelic healing occurs is paradoxical. Many approaches to psychedelic-assisted therapy or guiding encourages us to trust a journeyer's inner healing wisdom to unfold organically to promote healing, but we've just read about confusing "recovered" memories that can arise in psychedelic experiences that require discernment, wisdom, and guidance from a trained facilitator or therapist to effectively integrate. Therapists and guides are told that they must maintain professional boundaries with clients, and yet many psychedelic guides describe a need for extensions of care such as texting or contacting a client after a psychedelic session, touching them during psychedelic work, or disclosing personal experience that would be anathema to traditional psychotherapy but feels necessary in psychedelic healing. People in pursuit of a psychedelic guide are told to be wary of anyone who says they, personally, can heal you, yet many are drawn to shamanic contexts precisely because they are told that a shaman does indeed work with the spirit world on your behalf to do exactly that—heal you!

An illuminating study led by Dr. Brennan explored the unique facets of psychedelic work that present relational and ethical challenges for clients and facilitators alike. The study highlights multiple descriptive themes, including guides feeling compelled to: be more authentic and flexible than traditional psychotherapists, utilize supportive touch during sessions, and be more broadly available to the client (accepting texts or calls after the session). There may also be deep feelings of intimacy and connection as well as a need for more self-disclosure on the part of the guide. Clients may be more vulnerable, more sensitive to the therapist's needs, and may experience an impulse for nudity and sexual expression. Additionally, many contexts in which psychedelic healing occurs promote dual relationships. Facilitators and journeyers may be in the same communities, and the line between professional relationships and friendship can be blurry.[19] These themes point to a need for an expanded and sophisticated analysis of power dynamics between journeyers and psychedelic guides, but clearly, we are operating in a sea of complex realities where the rules are less clear.

While there is a need for standards of practice, perhaps what we need to be focusing on even more are values. Rules tell us clearly what to do and what not to do (remember "don't fuck your clients"?). Values such as respect, autonomy, and non-hierarchy are more vague, but may be fundamental to developing a flexible and sophisticated relationship to interpersonal power dynamics in psychedelic work. The most important value is respecting the wisdom and autonomy of the client, while holding fast to professional boundaries. The facilitator most likely to transgress with a client is the one who believes they know what the client needs, rather than responding to what the client says they need. Believing your client needs to be cuddled right now to deal directly with their fear of intimacy is very different from your client extending a hand for support in a difficult moment.

The truth is, as much as we might try to have a values-driven relationship to psychedelic healing work, we are attracted to power. We desire others who radiate power. Power is an aphrodisiac. We are enraptured when someone seems more wise, experienced, and confident. We are seduced by the fantasy of being saved, of feeling cared for in deep ways, of feeling that someone can help us, and being specially chosen for that attention. We also want power. We love feeling that we are in some way in possession of special knowledge or medicines shrouded in secret that we can offer to others. We are the holders of something very special. Guides and clients alike, even those who are self-aware, can slide into these projections and archetypes because they are sexy, exciting, and deeply human. Even between two people that would otherwise not feel attraction, power can be an intoxicant.

It is very easy to sit on the outside of this and either judge, or think, "I would never be susceptible to getting caught up like this." However, until you've worked with a person under the influence of a psychedelic medicine who is telling you they feel seen and loved by you in a way no one ever has before—you are a goddess, or a wise sage, you are adored and revered—you don't know the intense gravity of such a projection. A projection so strong it can warp values and bend standards, especially when there is no one else there to offer perspective and grounding. Likewise, vulnerable, suggestible journeyers can be convinced that being close to this powerful person in various ways is the only thing that can heal their wounds. When there is cross-cultural exchange between participants from the Global North attending Indigenous healing rituals with a shaman, such as the case as with ayahuasca ceremonies, intense romanticism and veneration of Indigenous healers can occur so that they are believed to be gurus or all-powerful healers.[20] These intense idealizations can lead to harm both for participants who are not aware of possibilities for exploitation, and for Indigenous people who, in being seen as more than human, are actually not seen as truly human at all.

It's been reiterated throughout this text that therapists, facilitators, and guides always hold the responsibility of maintaining all boundaries with clients, sexual and otherwise. But it is also necessary to look at ways clients can hold power and why expressions of this power can lead to harm. This occurs more predominantly in "underground" or extralegal healing contexts. Make no mistake, the central issue the psychedelic community must focus on is stopping guides or facilitators from sexually abusing clients. But much less often named, are the situations where participants engage in trauma reenactments, sexual fantasies, or pursue relationships with facilitators. When these situations occur outside of clinical contexts, facilitators can fear legal exposure resulting in arrest, or professional censure for providing extralegal services on top of the violation of sexual boundaries.

In the aftermath of sexual trauma, some trauma survivors can be unconsciously drawn to recreating situations similar to their trauma for their healing. I have worked with innumerable survivors who share in therapy their shame at seeking out porn, kink play, or other fantasy enactments of their trauma. When fantasy enactment occurs in this way, in the realm of fantasy between consenting peers, it can be a deeply powerful vehicle for healing. However, extralegal psychedelic work often takes place in the context of secrecy because of drug prohibition. Having an intense relational experience in the context of secrecy may parallel sexual abuse for many survivors. Enactments can include intense idealization of a guide, requests for sexual contact in the service of healing, believing only the guide can give them a safe sexual experience, and other fantasies to which a guide needs to be completely steadfast in denying sexual advances while simultaneously not shaming the client for their desires.

I have worked with a number of survivors of psychedelic sexual abuse in my psychotherapy practice who discussed having not only initiated but heavily pursued sexual relationships or fantasy enactments with guides or facilitators. When they finally achieved what the traumatized part of them wanted—sexual contact with the facilitator—the bubble of fantasy burst, and they realized that they had been abused. Or perhaps the guide cuts off the relationship for fear of further engaging in a transgression leading to the client feeling abandoned. This decision on the part of the guide can feel unilateral and compound the client's trauma. Guides who engage in sexual transgressions initiated by the client often find a multitude of reasons for denying or covering up their behavior for fear not only of judgment and social shaming, but also because they simply can't reconcile their inability to hold their own stated boundaries.

So, is there ever a time when a sexual relationship can be nonexploitive between a facilitator and a participant in psychedelic work? This question commonly arises in psychedelic community healing spaces where a group of peers hold psychedelic ceremonies together. In this context it will be essential for communities to develop common norms and guidelines around relationships. To say that *no* sexual relationship can be healthy if it includes unequal power, would mean *all* are unhealthy because all sexual relationships include multiple, complex intersections of power-over and different agendas, needs, and desires. The standards of behavior commonly accepted between psychedelic guides and therapists in "underground" or community contexts are informed by Western medical approaches to healing that seek to avoid dual relationships between facilitators and clients. A more holistic view of healing work acknowledges that people can hold multiple roles together in community, if indeed we are committed to psychedelic healing being fostered in community. This may require a much more rigorous and values-driven evaluation of the ethics of sexual relationships because it must respect that people operating in a community can hold different roles that carry different types of power simultaneously. If we assert that a client can never have a relationship with someone who has held a position of power, or that their feelings are always a projection of fantasy, we are actually disrespecting the autonomy and, by extension, a belief in the innate wisdom of that person.

However (and it's a big *however*), as much as we may yearn for such a community, utopian models for decommodified healing (a healing modality free from the confines of a for-profit medicalized system), held for and by members of a community invested in each other, we are still limited by the fact that we are socialized with certain norms. When clients bring the expectations of Western psychotherapy to community healing models, they can be harmed by sexual relationships, because when someone holds space for our healing, something intrinsically changes in that relationship. Many people who, for example, ask a friend to sit for their psychedelic work find that the friendship is forever changed in some way. In order to have safe community healing rituals, we may have to also move toward communal values and community accountability. If we want to accept that in certain cases sexual relationships can be ethical in community contexts, we need large networks to provide introspection, feedback, and support. Most importantly, community-based healing might have to abandon the expectations set by Western psychotherapy that someone is there holding our specific, individual healing process. Instead, we might imagine community-held rituals that are aimed at garnering togetherness, joy, pleasure, and that center the experience itself.

All this may mean that if the aim of our psychedelic journey is a psychotherapeutic outcome like healing trauma or treating depression, it may best be held within the boundaries of Western psychotherapy or consciously guided work. But it is also possible to cultivate non-hierarchical psychedelic rituals for the purpose of sharing the experience itself together in a group that can minimize the complex dynamics that lead to power-based abuses by uplifting pleasure as the intention for the journey.

6
IN THE GARDEN OF EARTHLY DELIGHTS

Psychedelic Medicines for Sexual Healing

Who are you, who are we, what are we doing here?
Are we here to make war, or are we here to make love?
                                    NICK SAND, LSD PIONEER

SOME PEOPLE AND CULTURES relate to psychedelic substances with an animist worldview, that each medicine has a spirit yearning to be in close relationship with us, a guide in our healing. Research science and psychedelic therapy models take a more materialist view: that each medicine interacts with our body, brain chemistry, and consciousness in ways that generate distinct experiences that unfold along a semi-predictable trajectory, depending on the set, setting, and intention for our journey. Perhaps a middle ground would be to describe psychedelics as each having a unique personality. And like people, not every personality is exactly who we want to be in a relationship with, and some personalities light us up and bring out the very best in who we are. This harmony between the right medicine and the well-prepared journeyer can create positive change that can fundamentally affect how we view ourselves, our relationships, and our sexuality.

This chapter will explore several individual psychedelic medicines—

some created by science and others that are plant or animal-derived—that present with unique attributes that can support sexual healing and connection with pleasure. For each medicine I will describe a core theme specific to pleasure-centered integration. We have more information about psychedelics, their use, and safety (and more unique psychedelic medicines widely available) than any time in human history. But what often goes unmentioned are the various relationship configurations between people and psychedelics, and how the relationship varies depending on the way the medicine is used. Psychedelic therapy and "guided experience" models rely on a relationship between the journeyer and the trusted guide or therapist. In this case, the medicine is most often seen as an aid in relational, therapeutic, and intrapsychic healing. But ritual use, as well as naturalistic use of psychedelics, is often far more about the relationship between the journeyer and the medicine itself, a direct and intimate connection between the personality of the sacrament and the recipient. This is the relationship that will be the focus of this chapter. What happens when we turn our focus to that relationship, the intimacy between person and medicine for the enhancement of personal erotic health, or how psychedelics can aid couples in reaching deeper levels of connection, sexual pleasure, and joy, acting as an intimate "third" in the relationship?

In the sea of existing literature on psychedelics, the impact of these medicines on our sexual satisfaction comes perhaps second only to pleasure itself as an underrepresented topic. One person is working to change that, to ask the questions within a scientific context that have tremendous potential for healing the wounds we carry around our sexuality, and perhaps even mold the future of psychedelic-assisted couples therapy. Tommaso Barba is a PhD candidate at Imperial College in London. I had the honor of talking with him on the very day his and his team's research was published in the prestigious journal *Nature Scientific Reports*, marking the first scientific contribution to the field on the topic of psychedelics and sexual satisfaction. Tommaso is a rising psychedelic star, animated and full of vitality as he talks about his work. With a background in both neuroscience and psychoanalysis, Tommaso is opening the door to scientific inquiry about how exactly psychedelics can benefit not only people with depression or other mental health disorders, but well people interested in growth, deeper relational connection, and optimizing their lived experience (including in the sexual arena), and doing so in a deeply humanistic way.

Barba and his team conducted two comparative studies, one looking at the impact of psychedelics on sexual satisfaction and well-being in 261 healthy volunteers outside of a clinical context who took psychedelics in medicine ceremonies, or in other naturalistic settings. In the second part of their inquiry, the team administered a validated questionnaire to participants with clinical depression in a research study comparing the efficacy of the commonly prescribed SSRI antidepressant drug escitalopram with psilocybin as a treatment.[1] As noted earlier, a shockingly pervasive side effect of SSRIs is loss of libido. In fact, many people cite this loss of interest in sex as a main reason they choose to discontinue SSRIs which, despite their spotty efficacy, remain the first-line pharmacological intervention for depression. It's important to note both branches of this study were looking at the post-acute effects of psychedelics on sexuality, meaning the impact on the participant *after* taking a psychedelic medicine, not the effects of psychedelics *during* a sexual experience. Tommaso explained:

> This research was inspired by trying to understand what happened in the 1960s and '70s. Even if people are not familiar with psychedelics, they tend to be familiar with the hippie, "Make love not war" ideology that became very popular then. Psychedelics became associated with hippie subculture and sexually liberal values, but the question is, was this synergy merely a cultural byproduct of the time? Or could psychedelics actually induce a form of sexual flourishing? In our study of naturalistic psychedelic users, participants answered questions about their sex life before they took a psychedelic, and up to six months after the psychedelic experience. We wanted to see if there was any impact. We did find that after these big psychedelic experiences, people reported improvements in sexual communication, sexual pleasure, satisfaction with their partner, they also were more satisfied with their appearance and bodies, and were open to try new things in their sex life. Another interesting finding was that

people perceived sex to be more of a spiritual experience compared to how they thought of it prior to their psychedelic experience. We were not really sure what to make of that, but I think it has to do with connection. When the word spiritual comes up, people highlight tantra and New Age ideas. But I think what this finding might mean is that people put more attention around the connection and the psychological experience of sex. Or maybe they are more likely to surrender, to go into the experience, and maybe they end up experiencing feelings they thought they were incapable of.

Tommaso continued to outline the second arm of the study:

We wanted to see if these results extended to depressed people, especially given that SSRIs are a major cause of sexual dysfunction. We were interested in whether there were differences in sexual satisfaction in people treated with SSRIs or psilocybin. We found that people receiving psilocybin tended to report improvements in sexual arousal, sexual interest, and satisfaction with their partner, and decreases in the anxiety associated with sex. People treated with SSRIs tended to report decreases in sexual arousal and sexual interest. *And* these drugs were quite comparable in treating the negative depression symptoms—the sadness—so to speak. I think this adds to the body of evidence that says psychedelics might be beneficial for enhancing well-being and positive valence systems of our mood beyond merely alleviating negative depression symptoms such as sadness. Despite the fact that psilocybin and SSRIs might be equally effective in reducing sadness, SSRIs end up reducing your entire emotional spectrum so that you could end up numbed. That doesn't mean that SSRIs can't be beneficial, because they can be great for a lot of people. But sometimes you end up losing depression, but also not gaining anything in your ability to feel positive emotions. Patients really care about this.

As our conversation continued, it became clear to me that Tommaso and I were not only aligned in our interests and vision for psychedelic sexual healing, but also found strikingly similar areas to be the most interesting ones for further clinical exploration. He shared:

> Then there's the question of *how* psychedelics can improve our sex lives long after the effects of the drugs vanish from our bodies. It's something we don't have data on yet, but by doing research on psychedelics and research on sexual function and dysfunction, a key common aspect is mindfulness. We know that psychedelics boost mindfulness capacities for months after the experience. The ability to be in the present moment or focusing on sensations is mindfulness. There is evidence that mindfulness interventions improve sexual functioning in both men and women. So if you put this together, it appears that maybe psychedelics can improve sexual functioning through this route. The other area to explore is around empathy and connection with your partner. If you increase empathy, then it can have downstream positive effects on sexual satisfaction.

It felt thrilling to hear Tommaso speculating about new lines of research around the exact same mechanisms presented in chapter two of this book as perhaps the most rich in potential: the tremendous power of being connected to sensation in your body in the present moment and the deepening of empathy for one's partner bolstered by psychedelic experiences.

I expressed to Tommaso that I carried a sense of skepticism about how the conventional medical world views sexual dysfunction; namely, that a systemic etiology is rarely considered. Remember, the medical world can emphasize the presence of a physical problem, and focus less on the social and emotional sources of sexual issues. I mused on the pleasure gap between men and women (mentioned in chapter three) and the complex social, physical, and emotional reasons for this, many having to do with socially reinforced ideas about women's sexuality and pleasure. Tommaso laughed and shared this perspective: "When we think about sexual dysfunction, given that everything is so centered around men, it's possible that in straight relationships women might be thinking they have sexual dysfunction and they don't know how to achieve sexual pleasure. But *maybe* the guy is just really bad at sex. It doesn't come into the mind of guys that they can just be really average, if not below average, in making women experience pleasure." He continued:

> There was another study that I read a while ago that was looking at men's attitudes towards household chores and sexual satisfaction in women. It shows that if men were more helpful and communicative in helping their partners at home, women were also more sexually satisfied and open to having sex with their partner. I think this really speaks to the fact that sexual satisfaction doesn't come from sex itself, but as a process that is built up step-by-step around connection and communication. It happens in everyday life. A lot of women aren't even aware of that because we are living in such a medicalized space in which if something isn't right, then it must be your body's fault. Gay men experience much more sexual dysfunction than straight men, for example, and I don't think it's because they have a biological variance. It's because they carry more shame, they end up knowing less about how to have sex. They end up having more casual sex with people. This contributes to a higher level of anxiety that in turn, contributes to dysfunction.

Tommaso added thoughtfully:

> Another interesting point is that in our research, psychedelics did not increase the subjective importance of sex in the everyday life of participants compared to baseline. It shows that psychedelics are not making people hyper-aroused or sexually disinhibited. So psychedelics don't increase sexual arousal in the traditional sense, but I think by improving how people feel in their own bodies, and creating this deeper sense of connection and intimacy, they can. The impact that psychedelics have in sexual functioning is not really physiological, like a lot of drugs that are marketed towards this. They offer a path to satisfaction that is more rooted in emotional and psychological well-being. People don't end up thinking about sex all the time, but they change their perception and the attitudes that they have towards it.

If this is the new generation of psychedelic researchers coming to the fore, I'm optimistic we are in good hands.

Remember, this research looked at psychedelic users in both clinical settings and naturalistic settings, but all were taking full doses of psychedelics. What about microdosing? Microdosing is the practice of taking very small, sub-perceptual doses of psychedelics for general wellbeing, depression or anxiety, or enhanced creativity. A small study from the United Kingdom looked at couples in therapy who were microdosing psychedelics and examined the impact on their relationships. The four couples enrolled in the study noted reduced levels of stress and performance anxiety which facilitated deeper emotional connection. Couples also discussed increased relationship satisfaction, sexual self-confidence, and willingness to explore sexually. While the study was extremely limited by small sample size consisting of white participants hailing from the United Kingdom, Europe, and America, the authors noted that microdosing can lead to "greater feelings of intimacy and enable a sexually satisfying relationship."[2]

Another novel piece of research was conducted by Leah Moyle, Alex Dymock, Alexandra Aldridge, and Ben Mechen. This team sought to reconceptualize users' motivations for mixing sex and drugs via qualitative interviews. The authors note that the topic of using drugs for sexual enhancement is most often explored in the context of what is known as *chemsex*. Chemsex is a pathologized practice of combining drugs such as methamphetamine or GHB (gamma-hydroxybutyrate) for sexual enhancement or pleasure, usually by men who have sex with men. In fact, the LGBTQIA+ community has often been the locus of research looking into "unhealthy" or harmful practices of combining drugs and sex.[3] These researchers found something quite different. They found that people of *all* sexual orientations were quite interested in combining drugs and sex for the purpose of increased enhancement and excitement, disinhibition, and in fact, therapeutic goals such as reducing anxiety, overcoming body image issues, and ameliorating the impact of previous difficult sexual experiences. People who used psychedelics such as MDMA in this way were predominantly women reluctant to frame their experiences purely around pleasure. The authors propose a new term, *pharmacosex*, and describe that the "therapeutic dimensions of drug-taking . . . cannot be neatly distinguished from purely hedonic motivations."[4]

What follows is not an endorsement of illicit substance use and is meant to garner perspective, provide education, and spark inquiry. My hope is to shed new light on medicines that have been either pigeonholed by the parameters of specific research goals, are under-discussed in the context of sexual healing, and contribute to an evolving dialogue about the many ways of understanding psychedelic medicines. My emphasis will be on the post-acute effects of these medicines for sexual transformation and erotic growth.

MDMA, *THE ORIGINAL LOVER*
Integration Theme: Embodiment

Of all the medicines on this list, MDMA, the Original Lover, had to come first by virtue of its tremendous capacity to connect us to pleasure, embodiment, and closeness with ourselves and others. MDMA (3,4-methylenedioxy-methamphetamine) has masqueraded by many different names including Ecstasy (a name allegedly not endorsed by its modern chemical godfather, Alexander "Sasha" Shulgin) or Molly (short for molecular).* It is not, strictly speaking, a psychedelic at all but commonly referred to as an entactogen or empathogen, meaning a substance that can induce enhanced interpersonal bonding, connection to self, or feelings of oneness. MDMA is also the medicine most studied for healing PTSD in ongoing clinical trials. While this use of MDMA should certainly not be overlooked, the healing of PTSD is only one facet of a gleaming gem that also shines in its ability to induce euphoria, relatedness, melt the user into a sacred fusion of bliss

---

*Although the two terms are often used interchangeably, "molly" and "ecstasy" are slightly different. "Ecstasy" refers to the pressed pill version of the drug, which, in addition to MDMA, often contains other substances. "Molly" (which comes from the word "molecular") refers to pure MDMA, often in the form of crystals or powder.[5]

with their loved one, and deeper levels of connecting with self. Few medicines truly live up to their epithets, but "Ecstasy" just may do exactly that.

MDMA has a fascinating story that illuminates the innovations in use, secret history, and administrative catastrophes that occur around substance use and regulation in the United States. (The story of MDMA's ban is described in chapter one.) MDMA was first synthesized in a Merck lab in 1912, and was resynthesized by chemist Alexander Shulgin in the 1970s (along with a veritable treasure trove of other substances). MDMA was preceded by a widely available chemical relative with comparable effects, MDA, that was outlawed in 1970. All it took was adding a little N-methyl group to create a new substance, a legal, *designer* substance that would itself experience wide use by therapists, a recreational golden age, only to suffer a ban that led those seeking its healing potential or capacity to induce connection to be driven underground.

In the early days after MDMA's resynthesis, Shulgin quietly shared it with friends, including the therapist Leo Zeff, who was dazzled by its potential, utilized it (and other psychedelics) with clients, and in turn trained hundreds of other therapists to do so as well. Couples therapy seemed to be highly benefited by the addition of MDMA. There was no way a medicine as powerful as MDMA would ever be restricted to psychotherapy. Like all of these medicines, therapy is a fabulous place for them, but to limit them only to a therapist's office dishonors both their power and discounts the massive human will to experience altered states of consciousness in a variety of settings. MDMA was always destined for bigger things, and it still is.

MDMA is the Original Lover because he has the power to bring us back to states of openness, connection with our bodies unburdened by shame, and to see others as well as ourselves with fresh eyes free from the hard edges of our defenses. After all, the first code name for MDMA was Adam, a moniker that implies a state of primordial innocence that looks upon the world as if it is the first day of creation. It is worth noting that lab-created psychedelic substances are rarely discussed in gendered pronouns as is common with certain sacred plant medicines (ayahuasca is a "she," whereas huachuma is a "he"). Relate to these medicines anyway you wish. But in my mind's eye, MDMA is the disco star Sylvester, a fabulous gay man in flowing robes glittering in gold trim, singing disco like it's a church revival.

There are many sources of information on the clinical trials with MDMA and its scientific applications. Allow me to introduce you to some of the other research that is less well-known about MDMA. In 1986, researchers John Buffum and Charles Moser conducted a small study with MDMA users in the San Francisco area exploring MDMA and human sexual functioning. Their research described the sexual experiences and perspectives of seventy-six MDMA users having self-directed (rather than therapeutic) experiences. A key takeaway from the work of Buffum and Moser is consistent with my opinion, that MDMA is indeed a drug of *sensuality* rather than *sexuality*. MDMA users were largely not inspired to take part in sexual activity that was outside of their pattern, and their receptivity to being sexual during the MDMA experience was middling, with thirty-four percent of women and forty-six percent of men likely to initiate sexual activity while on MDMA.[6]

But what *did* happen? MDMA, unsurprisingly, increased feelings of emotional closeness, and helped people come to terms with their sexual identity, decrease jealousy, and release trauma from the body. The real joys of this article rest in the details. MDMA users report the subjective experience, "Salad oil session—no holds barred," ". . . fantasies with real desire to act them out. I want to make sexual love with several of my close friends, including threesomes and foursomes. Seems to be a large emotional component to it."[7] One important conclusion we can draw from these scintillating descriptors, is that MDMA does not overwhelm one's capacity to control their behavior, but may open one up to increased novelty and exploring sexual feelings related to self and others. A later study concluded that MDMA moderately to profoundly increased sexual desire and satisfaction, but impaired sexual performance while on the medicine.[8]

Why would it be that MDMA would make people feel more sexual desire and greater connection but not necessarily prompt people to have sex while on it? MDMA users will make jokes to the effect of "I don't necessarily want to have sex, but I do want to cuddle and tell you that I love you so much!" What could be happening here? Yet another study of MDMA and human sexuality noted that what users report as sexual receptivity is actually emotional closeness. Here's where things get really interesting. A whole cascade of neurohormonal changes occur in the body both during MDMA consumption and during and after sexual activity. One of the hormones affected by both is prolactin. Prolactin is known to increase after orgasm and stay elevated for an hour or more. Prolactin is thought to contribute to feelings of sexual satiation. MDMA also increases prolactin. The authors of this study hypothesize that MDMA's capacity to induce the release of prolactin basically delivers you into a state that is the equivalent of orgasmic afterglow. People aren't craving sex *per se*, and experience inhibited sexual functioning, because the body is already bathed in an endogenous chemical elixir of post-sex good feeling![9]

MDMA can be a seductive substance, and the desire to feel good can override our good judgment unless we closely follow the rules of responsible substance use. There are several practices that are imperative to harm reduction with MDMA. First, you *must* test it. Any substance purchased extralegally that comes in the form of powder (and especially in the case of an Ecstasy "pressie," which—as noted earlier—is a pre-pressed pill that often contains multiple substances) should be treated as if it's adulterated until you conclusively know differently. Testing kits are available from several reputable sources online that allow you to test MDMA for purity. You must also test every single dose separately for the presence of fentanyl as fentanyl can be lethal in even small doses and is not evenly distributed throughout the sample. Known as the "chocolate chip cookie effect" small amounts of fentanyl "chips," if you will, might be found throughout an otherwise clean sample, so each and every dose must be tested.

MDMA is also a substance that must be taken in measured doses. No eyeballing it. Pure MDMA is safe for most people with healthy cardiovascular systems. But the difference between a standard dose of around 60 to 125 mg and a dose that can cause physical harm is very easy to mistake in a social setting, poor lighting, or a festival environment. It should not be mixed with alcohol. Additionally, MDMA can, in some users, cause a depressive dip one to two days later due to serotonin depletion. Although, at least one study debunked the myth of the "blue Monday," as no depression was observed post-MDMA in clinical trials, leading researchers to conclude that it was actually impure substances, poly drug use, alcohol use, and sleep deprivation that were the real culprit.[10] Anecdotally, some users claim there is a "sweet spot" when it comes to MDMA dosing, and that ingesting a higher-than-necessary dose (whether in the form of a single dose or multiple re-dosings called "booster doses"), is more likely to result in deleterious effects. Moreover, multiple re-dosings in a single MDMA experience or chronic use can also cause health complications. One way of mitigating all of these risks would be full drug decriminalization that would allow users access to safe substances, abundant testing supplies, harm reduction education, and safe environments in which to experience the effects.

MDMA Integration
Core Theme: Embodiment

MDMA is often touted as a gateway to psychedelic experiences, as its very core mechanism for healing is pleasure and embodied good feeling. Let me first start with some cautions about MDMA important to integration that extend beyond the physical and substance-related risks. MDMA can bring about good feeling, but it can also loosen the mind's protective barrier that holds traumatic memories at bay. I have worked with a number of integration clients who assumed their MDMA experience would be a pleasure tour, and instead, what they got was a flood of associations, fragments of traumatic memory, and body sensations related to unprocessed trauma. The challenge in integration was as much the experience itself, as the unexpected nature of these trauma-related phenomena. In fact, I once heard a seasoned MDMA researcher hypothesize the psychodynamic interpretation that the depressive drop some users experience after MDMA could in fact be related to users repressing emotion in recreational settings that would otherwise be expressed and felt in a clinical setting.

Another facet of the MDMA experience that rarely gets discussed is that before MDMA becomes euphoric, it can be very, very activating. The first "wave" of MDMA at the onset of effect is often highly stimulating and can be anxiety-provoking in some users. MDMA users ingest the substance prepared to sink into a state of bliss, but may instead be met with sensations that mimic the intense activation that occurs in the body during a traumatic experience. In fact, I have heard from a number of integration clients that the onset of MDMA launched them somatically right back into a traumatized state. Later, as the brain is bathed in serotonin and other neurotransmitters, the qualities of peace, perspective, and warmth take hold. But at first, it can be an amphetamenic rough ride, and the body can be triggered back into traumatic memories and body states.

Another concern is that the increased trust, agreeableness, and feelings of love MDMA fosters can—depending on context—actually cause trouble. I was surprised to hear couples in my practice mention, "We took MDMA together and the experience was great, but I never would have agreed to *that* if I were sober." *That* might be non-monogamy, different sexual acts, or shifting relationship agreements. I'll again echo, be careful with whom you take substances. MDMA might be a fantastic tool to increase communication and empathy between a couple, but those conversations need to be revisited once our protective inner parts that are fearful of change are back online. In the worst cases, MDMA can be used to manipulate a partner into feeling open to something they truly do not want. Ethics and the willingness to create ongoing space for discussion are essential to the MDMA integration process.

What about when things go right? Integration of an MDMA experience is about insight and perspective, but it is also about embodiment. Many times, journeyers report *never* having felt so good. Let's say your intention for your MDMA experience is not to heal trauma or confront difficult feelings, but it is simply to feel pleasure. You'll never find this in any research paper, but feeling good is a fantastic intention. More good-feeling people make a happier world. But perhaps even in the context of a relational medicine experience centered on joy there are deeper levels of experience to probe. One question to ask might be, can feeling this good actually facilitate transformation? During an MDMA experience, users can take note of the experience of being directly embodied. Where is your mind when your body feels good? Is it relaxed, happy, peaceful? Notice tactile sensations. Do you want to be hugged, touched, embraced? Are you with someone safe to offer that touch? How is it to explore solo sensual touch? Noting these qualities during an MDMA experience opens up the ability to work with them afterward.

Integration practices after MDMA can include listening to music and mindfully moving your body. I highly recommend collective, sober ecstatic dance practices and breathwork for MDMA integration as both root us solidly in the body. Integration can also be sensual explorations of your own body that may or may not be sexual. How does it feel to take extended time with your body, simply breathing, running your fingers along your skin? If you have a trusted partner, extended embraces can bring us back to a place of peaceful connection. I found at least one study that referred to MDMA as a "hug drug." But guess what: hugs are great even without drugs!

While the thoughts and feelings experienced on MDMA are helpful to work with in integration, I find what often is overlooked is anchoring the body in feelings of bliss, peace, and connection. It is especially helpful to take note of what is *not* happening during an MDMA experience, for example the presence of trauma triggers or stress. For people who are using MDMA for trauma work, it is especially important not to over-intellectualize the integration process. What does it feel like to be without tension, anxiety, or activation? Integration can be the process of helping the body return to this state of bliss. Remember back to the best sensations of the experience. Let your mind rest in that space of openness, even if you can only access it for a moment. The process of returning back again and again to good feeling is showing your body that you can willingly return to a blissful state without any substances. Coming back to our bodies in pleasure is the way we heal.

AYAHUASCA, *THE QUEEN OF HEALING*
Integration Theme: Discernment

It's curious to situate ayahuasca into a pleasure paradigm. She is profound, powerful, and sometimes wrathful. She is none other than the Queen of Healing, the Mother of the Jungle. Ayahuasca experiences can be overwhelming, confusing, and physically challenging, but they can also be the most vast, astonishingly beautiful experience one can ever have. I recall very early on during my experience sitting with ayahuasca being shown the creation of the universe *from the inside*. I was there while stars were being born, the universe expanding and exploding. I thought I was special to have seen such a thing. A few weeks later, the ceremonial leader prepped the group by saying, "You might even get to see the birth of the universe. Many people new to ayahuasca experience that." What? *Many* people get to see the birth of the universe? If that's true, that means that ayahuasca is both generous and reliable with extending her mystical insights. In fact, ayahuasca users with no shared cultural background, in different contexts, with different facilitators who are not in any way predisposed to do so, consistently see the same visions: the serpent and the jaguar. Visitations from ayahuasca herself.

Before we go any further, it is vital to place ayahuasca in context. Just a few decades ago, ayahuasca was largely inaccessible in the Western world. People who had worked with her were often the intrepid or privileged enough to afford travel to Peru, Bolivia, or Ecuador to visit communities with ayahuasca healing traditions. The scene is very different now, with ayahuasca ceremonies proliferating around the United States and Europe. In some cases these ceremonies are held by Indigenous lineage holders seeking either to share their ancestral wisdom with seekers or bring financial sustainability to their communities and families (often it's both). But in this era of ayahuasca globalization, many times these ceremonies are held by Western practitioners, some of whom have proper training and authorization by Indigenous teachers to serve medicine. There are many however who don't. I am not a trained *ayahuascero* (a traditionally trained ayahuasca facilitator). But I do know for certain if it takes at least a decade of training, initiation, and discipline to serve ayahuasca in Indigenous community settings, it certainly takes more than drinking the medicine a few times, acquiring the necessary plants, and watching a YouTube video for some dude from Brooklyn to safely serve her.

Indigenous activist Daiara Tukano describes in an essay that the "global context in which ayahuasca is currently more accessed by white and economically privileged non-Indigenous people than by Indigenous people, in which academics, scientists, and religious leaders widely discuss the expansion, legalization, democratization, commodification, medicalization, syncretization of medicine, it is necessary to question the importance of the representation and autonomy of Indigenous peoples in the midst of these discussions." Tukano also notes there are over 160 Indigenous ayahuasca drinking groups in the Global South each with distinct practices, preparations, and names for the medicine.[11] The original keepers of the wisdom of this medicine are Indigenous.

To give a contemporary example of the different ways ayahuasca is used, a recent news story covered around the world detailed the plight of four children, the youngest of whom was only eleven-months-old and the oldest thirteen years old, who were lost in the Colombian Amazon after their small plane carrying the children and three adults crashed. The bodies of the three perished adults were recovered, but the children had vanished into the rainforest in territory riddled with venomous snakes and dangerous animals. A major search and rescue operation took place led by the Colombian army and Indigenous volunteers. The party searched for thirty-nine days for the missing children to no avail. On the thirty-ninth day, the Indigenous members of the search team drank ayahuasca. On the fortieth day, an Indigenous elder drank more ayahuasca and emerged from his visions certain the children would be found that very day. And indeed they were, only sixty-six feet away from where the group had previously searched. The children's father was reported as crediting ayahuasca for the return of the children. Ayahuasca's power is not only about emotional healing. She has been used for physical healing and divination to this day.[12]

Unique to all plant medicines, ayahuasca is an admixture of two plants—the *Banisteriopsis caapi vine*, a monoamine oxidase inhibitor (MAOI), and a DMT-containing plant such as *Psychotria viridis*, otherwise known as *chacruna*. The MAOI allows DMT, which is not normally orally active, to be processed slowly in the body creating an extended psychedelic effect.[13] Ayahuasca brews are heavily proprietary from community-to-community and shaman-to-shaman, and may contain other psychoactive and non-psychoactive plants. Imagine the spiritual attunement and breathtaking knowledge needed to know that two plants completely unalike (one is a leaf, and one a woody vine) should be boiled for hours into a tea that has the capacity to heal so deeply? Any notion that Western science has a more sophisticated understanding of plant medicine than Indigenous wisdom holders do is laughable.

The subjective experience of ayahuasca encompasses all things. It can be highly visual or completely emotional. It can be terrifying or beautiful or terrifyingly beautiful. It can induce the experience of speaking directly to ancestors or guides, of seeing the past or future. One can have visitations from aliens, cosmic serpents, or jungle cats. You can also be pulled through cartoon fantasyland space-time and spit back out the other side. One can experience death over and over until one agrees to face it head on. A common requirement for ayahuasca preparation is a restrictive diet that eliminates pork and some other meats, heavy spice and salt, caffeine and alcohol, among other things. A nearly universal prohibition is sex, either with a partner or with yourself, for several weeks before and after ingesting the ayahuasca brew. It has been described to me that sex is powerful medicine and orgasm diminishes your vital life force. Our life force needs to be fully intact for the ayahuasca ceremony. The female plant spirit ayahuasca is also described as a "jealous" spirit that likes to bond monogamously with those who drink her in. She does not want the energetic presence of anyone else in the vessel of your body. Anthropologist Daniela Peluso describes how very experienced ayahuasca shamans may meet and get to know an entity in their ayahuasca visions who is to become their sexual partner and spouse in the spirit world. She notes her source, a Shipibo-trained shaman, also stated rules that this spirit sexual relationship must not interfere with the shaman's earthly life or produce spirit children.[14]

While the content of an ayahuasca experience may include aspects of eroticism, the drinking of ayahuasca medicine itself is most certainly erotic. What could be more powerful than taking a spirit within your body and allowing her to overtake you entirely, to possess you? She is in charge, and you can do nothing but submit to her. For that experience to be safe, you must trust not only her, but also the facilitator. All the more important that ayahuasca ceremonies be held with the utmost care and ethical practices. Dr. Yalila Espinoza studied the spiritual and erotic awakenings of women who worked with Amazonian plant teachers such as ayahuasca. She identified eight core themes that emerged with the women she interviewed after ayahuasca ceremonies held in the Shipibo Peruvian tradition: purification and support for reproductive health; increased sensory awareness; transformation of the relationship with self; empowered decision making; enhanced intimacy with others; increased cognitive awareness; connecting with subtle energies; and connecting with God. She writes that "physical and emotional purification and as well as cognitive and behavioral realignments" are necessary for sexual and spiritual healing. All of the women interviewed for the study described a reconnection with their bodies, and facilitated a "reprogramming" of their nervous systems that increased sensitivity and allowed energy to flow freely through the body, facilitating healing. These women also described increased awareness of their intimate relationship to God.[15]

Clearly, sexuality and the erotic are deeply entwined with ayahuasca and what may be experienced during a ceremony. However, during my work supporting people after ayahuasca ceremonies, I have found that another shift relating to sexuality might occur. Ayahuasca drinkers can also experience a loss of interest in the way they have traditionally approached sex. Users report decreased desire for sex, decreased interest in pornography, or realignments in their sexual interests. In my therapy practice, I've encountered many people confused and frightened by these shifts. But when we dig further, it becomes clear that after ayahuasca, it is not so much their sex drive that is diminished, but that they no longer feel a pull towards sexual activities they normally used for high stimulation, self-soothing, or in ways that constitute harmful or disruptive compulsive behaviors.

It is not that ayahuasca dampens our erotic potential. What ayahuasca might do is break the hold of patterns that ensnare people in a web of pursuing sex that they later regret, spending time or resources they do not wish to spend on pornography, or engaging in other sexually compulsive behaviors. After ayahuasca, they come to therapy stating they lost their sex drive, when in fact what they have often lost is not their sex drive but their compulsivity. This opens up the opportunity to rediscover a new way of relating to sex and pleasure free from traumatic reenactments or out-of-control sexual behaviors. But even though the change might be a positive one, tearing away behaviors we have historically relied on for stimulation or soothing can be destabilizing, and support is often needed to imagine new ways of being.

Ayahuasca is our ally in healing. Thus, she helps us change things that need healing, and accept the things we might want to change but in fact do not need healing. Clancy Cavnar's work looked at gay and lesbian participants in ayahuasca ceremonies to explore the relationship between ayahuasca and sexual identity and self-acceptance. Themes of self-acceptance and seeing the self as connected to part of everything, or part of God, emerged. All ayahuasca drinkers reported feeling their identity was affirmed and their lives were enhanced by their ayahuasca use.[16] Gay and lesbian sexuality is not a pathology to be healed, but powerful (and magical).

As noted earlier, psychedelics have been used, sometimes by very powerful and beloved figures in psychedelic history, as tools of conversion therapy. One cannot change their sexuality or sexual orientation by any type of therapy including psychedelic therapy. Homosexuality is not a disorder. What needs fixing is a broken society that insists on regulating, oppressing, and discriminating against LGBTQIA+ people. Psychedelics can be powerful agents to help us all move toward self-acceptance and self-love. Ayahuasca, or any plant medicine, cannot fix what is not broken. She is here for all of us to find what is best in us and cherish it, every bit of it. It is my entirely personal opinion that ayahuasca helps us to see the true diversity and beauty in us and among us, to embrace the parts of ourselves that are unexplored or disowned, reconnecting to them in love.

Ayahuasca Integration
Core Theme: Discernment
Ayahuasca is one of the most consistently challenging medicines to integrate precisely because the intensity and vastness of the experience can be confusing and overwhelming. Ayahuasca can also show us depictions

of things that are not "real" memories. She may speak to us in symbols that are difficult to understand. Some say she can be deceitful. In my early days of my interest in shamanic practices, like many people, I read Michael Harner's *Way of the Shaman*, a book that now feels quite different to me given that it is written by a white man accessing and benefitting from Indigenous traditions. But one story always stands out to me. Harner describes being given ayahuasca to drink by an Indigenous person in the village in which he was working as an anthropologist. In his visions, he encounters reptilian creatures that claim to have created life on earth and were the true masters of humanity. Harner was told by these creatures he was dying and thus safe to receive the revelations. After his ceremony concluded, still very much alive, he consulted multiple people about his experience including Christian missionaries who likened it to the Book of Revelation. Were the serpents the true masters of humanity? Harner found his way to a blind shaman, a source of great wisdom, who waved him off, stating: "Oh, they're always saying that. They are only the Masters of the Outer Darkness."[17]

This classic story illustrates that ayahuasca is not always what she seems, and thus the main focus of integration must be discernment. How do we know what in an ayahuasca experience are the true gems and what is not at first what it seems to be? There is no easy answer to that question, and ayahuasca requires that we sit with her teachings, sometimes for many months, before we act on them. The previous chapter outlines the slippery experience of confusing "memories" of abuse that seem to occur more often with ayahuasca than any other medicine. But ayahuasca can also help us confront fears, often the fear of death or illness, and she can also bring us directly back to experiences of trauma with the ability to either reprocess, navigate, or rescue our still-suffering former selves from these experiences.

If an experience with ayahuasca has clearly helped you to process a previous trauma to completion in a way that feels like healing for you, trust it. However, if you walk away with a kaleidoscopic experience of confusing biographical material, spiritual symbols, and personal gnosis, it requires further exploratory work to sort through. Professional integration help may be necessary in these cases. But should you not have access to that, I recommend taking things very slowly. Journaling everything you remember about your ayahuasca journey chronologically is a first step. This can also be done pictorially by making a "storyboard" of the experience. While journaling is a fairly common and innocuous assignment for psychotherapy, the practice of psychedelic integration journaling engages the unconscious mind as you seek to take something experienced in symbols and images and convert it to words. Often associations and interpretations previously unknown to you will emerge.

Reckoning back to Yalila Espinoza's work, ayahuasca integration practices can also act as a purification practice. I use this word "purification" very hesitantly, as we are most acquainted with it through the lens of oppressive purity culture that seeks to control our relationship to sexuality, especially women. In the case of ayahuasca, purification takes on other dimensions. Ayahuasca integration can be about purifying ourselves from practices and habits that are not supportive of our erotic growth, or tending to our body in new ways. It can be as simple as spending time in nature and taking conscious deep breaths of fresh air. We take in what is pure and release what is no longer needed. It might mean trying old things in new ways. For example, if you typically masturbate mindlessly watching pornography, try erotic self-touch relying only on the fantasy in your mind. Only you can decide what "pure" means to you. Perhaps it's feeding your body food that makes you feel good, or engaging in sex mindfully.

Ayahuasca also facilitates a deeper relationship to the divine. What does it mean to you to connect your sexuality to the divine? Practices can be as overt as creating an altar space in your bedroom, or ritualizing erotic experiences with candles, music, and flowers. But the deeper practice of connecting our sexuality to the divine needs no accoutrements. It is an inner inquiry about the role our sexuality plays in our true divine nature. Integration work with ayahuasca challenges us to see that all that we are, sexuality included, is holy. You can ask yourself, what would be different about the way I relate to sex, relationships, and pleasure if at every moment I remember that I am indeed holy?

PSILOCYBIN MUSHROOMS, *THE SECRET CHILDREN*
Integration Theme: Surrender

The "magic" mushroom has worn many proverbial hats: Indigenous sacred medicine, instrument of divination and healing, clinical agent of combatting depression, and recreational substance enjoyed on college campuses near and far. Mushrooms enjoy a reputation as the safest psychedelic with little to no risk of physical injury consumed in virtually any amount. One source claims you would have to eat your body weight in mushrooms to take a lethal dose.[18] Other sources contend it's more like a few pounds of dried mushrooms. The mystery will likely persist since literally no one is eating pounds of psychedelic mushrooms. The psychological risks of psilocybin, especially at high doses, is a different story altogether. It's for this very reason that I believe psilocybin mushrooms, ushered into a new era of enjoying a decriminalized status in many places whilst simultaneously co-opted into Western medicine, might be one of the most difficult psychedelic medicines to truly understand. They are, in some ways, tricksters. They can bring about laughter and joy, but they can also power cosmic journeys beyond this world that can transform our relationship to ourselves and the divine. They can heal depression through their power to promote mystical experience, but they have also enabled shamans to cure the sick and fuel divination practices. It's hard to reconcile their versatility and many faces. What they can do for you is very much dependent on how you approach them. The history of their use is a dramatic one that encompasses secret cults, lies, betrayal, appropriation, and redemption. It's a story of heroes and villains, although who belongs in each category is dependent upon who you ask.

While widespread use of psilocybin mushrooms is supported by the existence of species known to be endemic to America, Africa, and Europe,[19] our only recorded history of their use extends to ancient rituals among the Maya and Aztec (Nahuatl) people. In his book *Psilocybin Mushrooms of the World*, our contemporary emperor of all things mushroom, Paul Stamets, points out the irony that a priest, Bernardino de Sahagún, from a conquering nation that supported the *planned* destruction of a subculture that engaged in the ritualistic use of mushrooms, is the single best source of information we have about psilocybin mushroom use in Aztec culture.[20] So important was the psilocybin mushroom to Aztec ritual that it was referred to as "teonanacatl," or the Flesh of the Gods. Sahagún, accompanying the murderous Hernando Cortez, is said to have created a text with full color illustrations of the blue-tinted Flesh of the Gods, the *Codex Magliabechiano*, around 1570.[21] But the violent suppression of Indigenous spirituality and the eradication of texts created a vacuum of knowledge that still exists about the ritual use of sacred mushrooms in this time and region of the world. Michael Pollan rightly asserts, "The Roman Catholic Church might have been the first institution to fully recognize the threat to its authority posed by a psychedelic plant, but it certainly wouldn't be the last."[22] Throughout history, if you want to find the villains, look for the burning piles of books, and there they are.

It is worth noting a disconcerting parallel between the actions of the Catholic Church during the Spanish conquest of the New World and the current situation in which many people interested in accessing psychedelic experiences find themselves today. The repression of the use of sacred mushrooms (and cacti) in the New World was motivated by a desire to position an intercessor, specifically a priest or religious figure empowered by the institution of the Catholic Church, as a gatekeeper between a person and an experience of the divine, an experience which had previously been directly facilitated by the use of sacred plants. The Church and its authority figures now became that intercessor between God and humans.

The Western medicalization of psychedelics does much the same, turning psychedelic seekers into patients who must rely on an institution, in this case the Western health care system, manned by doctors and therapists, to access a psychedelic experience of the divine for healing, self-exploration, or sacred connection. The problems inherent in the medicalization of psychedelics might be unique to this moment due to the influence of psychedelic start-ups seeking profit, insurance companies interested in reducing the cost of mental health treatment, Big Pharma, and bias in the health care system. But the story? That's very, very old.

The mushroom-using cults that survived the forced Christian colonization in Mesoamerica were situated in the high mountains in the North of Oaxaca among the Mazatec where the mushrooms were known as "little one who springs forth."[23] And it is from here that the modern history of the sacred mushroom and its journey to North America takes shape. Make no mistake, all of the research, science, truffle retreats, and psilocybin treatments poised to make billions of dollars, can all be traced back to a single Woman of Color. Her name was Maria Sabina, and it's from her power and goodness from which this all grew. To be clear, Maria Sabina's ceremonies with the "little children" or "little saints," were not psychedelic explorations, but instead were primarily cures for the sick, but also conducted to find lost objects and people.[24]

Maria Sabina is a person cloaked in tragedy and mystery. After being deceived into sharing the ritual, or *velada*, with Western people, her life became ruinous. As a direct result of the deception of R. Gordon Wasson, she was exiled from her community, her house burned down, and was jailed, Sabina died in poverty in 1985.[25] She never got to see what became of her "little children" in the 21st century nor did she benefit from the counterculture fame that has sprung up around her.[26] I found myself curious about Sabina when a meme began circulating on the internet with an image of her weathered and wise face next to a poem that concludes, "You are the medicine." While I'm no Maria Sabina expert, all the visionary poetry and songs I've seen of hers include a lot of Jesus and certainly didn't seem like the flowery poem that extols you to "put love in tea instead of sugar, and take it looking at the stars." Turns out after a bit of online sleuthing, that I was not the only one who was skeptical. Authors Eden Woodruff and Tom Hatsis wrote an excellent article debunking this meme and describe the whitewashing of Maria Sabina's culture and identity. They explain that the poem is unlike anything known to have been written by Maria Sabina, and that things like "looking at the world with your forehead" which some believe refers to the "third eye," a trope from Eastern philosophies, she was unlikely to have known.[27] In the history of making Maria Sabina who we wish her to be rather than seeing who she actually was, using her for our purposes, the proliferation of inaccurate memes is the least of the offenses. Somehow, despite the fact that Maria Sabina gave everything, we still need this Indigenous woman to be more.

This brings us to how the mushrooms came to North America. I will only briefly touch on the treachery of R. Gordon Wasson, an investment banker and mycology enthusiast credited as "the man who pulled the trigger and fired the first round in the psychedelic revolution."[28] Wasson, a prolific author of psychedelic books, was searching for the psychedelic roots of religion. He located Maria Sabina and convinced her to conduct a mushroom ceremony for him by telling her he was concerned for his missing son. Locating missing people and objects was one of the uses for the mushroom in Mazatec culture, and Maria Sabina acquiesced under the pressure of a local politician whom Wasson had persuaded.[29] Wasson, thrilled that he was to be the first man to "discover" the elusive mushroom, made audio and photographic recordings of her ceremony which ended up in none other than *Life* magazine in 1957. Although Wasson attempted to mask her identity, it was only a matter of time before this disclosure brought massive unwanted attention to Maria Sabina and her town, which was soon inundated by people seeking the magic mushroom, resulting in disaster for her and her family.[30] It was not only curious seekers who wanted the mushroom. Notably, another interested party was the CIA, who immediately took a shine to psychedelics for the purpose of mind control. This interest grew into the notorious project MK-ULTRA.[31]

Contemporary Western research focusing on psilocybin mushrooms for the purpose of mental health treatment is vast and growing. Companies race to patent their proprietary versions of synthetic psilocybin for therapeutic use. Some in the psychedelic community applaud this, while others consider it a dishonor to the medicine. My feeling is you can't put toothpaste back in the tube. Here we are. We can only do everything in our power to act ethically given the current circumstances. It sent a shiver down my spine however when I began to see the first articles published about just how "cost-effective" psilocybin therapy will be. Trust me, the will to medicalize psychedelics like psilocybin will likely come with paring the therapeutic container down to a bare minimum, and completely overlook the deeply sacred roots of the medicine itself.

As alluded to earlier, because psychedelic treatment within the medicalized model requires close supervision (and aftercare including integration, if done properly) the profit-driven model of Western health care views the "tripping" aspect of psychedelics as burdensome and expensive. Many companies therefore, seeking to increase the "efficiency" of treatment, are working to tweak psychedelic substances either to reduce the psychedelic experience[32] or redesign them completely, to extinguish *all* psychedelic effects.[33]

It is also true the psilocybin mushrooms are the most commonly used psychedelic in the United States *outside* of clinical contexts, with over eight million adults surveyed having used psilocybin for either microdosing or full psychedelic experiences in 2023.[34] But not only is mushroom *use* increasing, the mushrooms *themselves* are getting stronger. A recent article in *Wired* that captured my attention explained, "Cultivators are using genetic sequencing and are hybridizing cultivars from ever more distant lineages (of distinct mushroom strains) to hunt for improvements plus sheer aesthetic novelty." Why is that significant? These super mushrooms are now far more psilocybin-dense then their fungal ancestors of just a few years ago, meaning 1.5 grams of these mushrooms (normally a low-moderate dose) infiltrating the underground supply stream, might have the subjective effects of a much, much higher dose.[35] Since an at-home user cannot easily test a mushroom purchased extra-legally for density of psilocybin, that leaves users in the position of getting way more than they bargained for. My recommendation is to carefully follow the old psychedelic adage, "start low and go slow," meaning until you conclusively know how strong a batch of psilocybin is, take very small amounts and wait to see the full effect before taking more. Otherwise your microdosing day might turn out to be a tripping day.

Let's instead look at psilocybin mushrooms a different way. Given their accessibility and availability, what role might the magic mushroom play in the healing and wholeness of our sexuality? First, I want to disabuse you of the notion that psilocybin is an accessible and friendly psychedelic. It can be. However, subjective experiences seems to be highly dependent on dose; some users may also encounter nonhuman entities and fantastical and confusing scenes, not to mention past traumas and overwhelming body sensations. These experiences can be intense and scary. A respected mushroom ceremonial facilitator I know calls it "going into the hinterlands." In fact, some users report that ingesting a high or "heroic" dose (five grams or more) of mushrooms resulted in an out-of-body experience akin to ones experienced on DMT.[36] The casual mass media depiction of the therapeutic use of psilocybin can harm inexperienced journeyers who may believe it will be a user-friendly superhighway to good feeling or that using it independently will yield the "miracle" results seen in clinical trials. Match this with the proliferation of retreat centers that charge thousands of dollars for mushroom experiences, claiming to deliver the same transformative results attained in the highly curated and controlled container of clinical trials without the same accountability. James Rucker and Allan Young, both psychedelic researchers, caution that "there is no convincing, substantive evidence that providing psilocybin in a retreat center is more safe or more supportive than standard harm reduction advice." They name sensible precautions such as using psilocybin in known quantities in the presence of a sober sitter as a good approach for naturalistic psilocybin use.[37] Indeed, it is in nature, with friends, or in community that the vast number of psilocybin users experience this medicine.

In chapter two, I discussed several features of psilocybin experience observed in research settings that map onto sexual wellbeing: increased mindfulness, openness, as well as the impact of the mystical experience. What about nonclinical settings? One study of psilocybin users consuming truffles (a type of psilocybin-containing fungi legal in the Netherlands and elsewhere) found that anxiety decreased directly after psilocybin consumption, and the trait of non-judgment increased. Users experienced higher traits of agreeableness and lower neuroticism. Journeyers rated the experience as personally meaningful, spiritually significant, and insight-enhancing. These findings mirror studies of psilocybin use both in and outside research.[38] Another study conducted at a legal psilocybin retreat found an increase in divergent thinking (the ability to engage creativity to think of multiple solutions) and increased empathy after participants took psilocybin.[39]

Let's pull all of this together and see how it relates to sexuality. Some of the core difficulties I see in clients seeking either couples or individual sex and trauma-focused therapy include rigid sexual narratives about themselves or their relationship, neurotic fixation on the appearance of the body and sexual performance, and difficulties with empathy and connection. Research of psilocybin use both in clinical and natural settings seems to speak to each of these issues. One can't truly be present with pleasure if you are fixated on body imperfections. Likewise, if your story about yourself and your previous experiences is entrenched, that story can hijack moments of pleasure that are destined to affirm that old narrative. A consistent theme throughout many of the studies on psilocybin is that all of these factors—increases in mindfulness, openness, creativity, and decreases in anxiety, neuroticism, and cognitive rigidity—relate to one meditating factor: ego dissolution. Ego dissolution is the temporary loss of (or loosening of) the concept of "I." This dissolution of boundaries is perhaps what enables us to enter into such a profound feeling of "one-ness" or connection with other beings and our environment. Despite its bad rap, the ego is what gives us a sense of separation between "you" and "I," and as such, is necessary for our both our psychological safety (the ability to create psychological boundaries), as well as ensuring our physical survival (the ability to detect and defend ourselves from external physical threats). The temporary dissolution of the ego afforded by the use of psychedelics affords us temporary distance between our stories, traumas, and attachment to our physical body, rendering us more capable to see ourselves with perspective.

Imagine trying to see Earth (a planet that is undoubtedly round despite what some people would have you think) and conceptualize its shape from standing on its terrain. Now see it from outer space. There she is, a beautiful floating globe of green and blue. Seen from far enough away, the individual features disappear and it becomes a beautiful, unified whole. Mushrooms can be that way. Psilocybin-induced ego dissolution can temporarily get us far enough away from all of the little stories, problems, and imperfections that we can get a sense that the beautiful whole is not so bad. Sometimes solving a problem truly does mean not fixating on it. Sex is one of the prime areas where we develop negative self-referencing beliefs that are internal attempts to keep us safe. We absorb information for our whole lives about what our body is supposed to look like, who is desirable and who is not, and whether who we are as a sexual person is acceptable. The experience of ego dissolution may afford us a temporary lens through which to experience the world outside the confines of a self that has adopted stories that don't serve us. Imagine just simply being able to drop all that? Sometimes, this must happen through the slow process of understanding and working with each of our aspects of self who have a story about us designed to shield against judgment and rejection. But sometimes, the psychedelic experience catapults us into higher consciousness and we temporarily, but indelibly, get a look at the whole bigger picture. You just can't unsee that.

Psilocybin Integration
Core Theme: Surrender

The integration theme of psilocybin work is surrender. We are called to surrender to the experience of the medicine itself. But after the acute effects of the medicine are over, there is an opportunity to surrender our sexual narratives, bias, and the barriers we hold that prevent true intimacy. Why do we hold onto things that clearly prevent us from being fulfilled and present with sexual and sensual pleasure? To again use the lens of inner parts from Internal Family Systems, by living through moments big and small that give us information about the right way (or safe way) for us to be, or generalizing the cruelty of one person into the behavior of all people, we develop a system of inner protectors that can show up with paradoxical messages. A voice inside us that constantly says, *she's wondering why you're even talking to her because you're fat*, or even, *being raped makes you unlovable*, can at first seem like inner tormentors. But if we look deeper, those parts of us that say terrible things are simply conspiring to prevent future harm from happening to us. If we don't talk to the person we are interested in, they can't reject us. If we believe we are unlovable, we don't risk seeing that in someone else's eyes or exposing ourselves to further harm. Psilocybin integration work means moving into a space of willingness to surrender these stories. It can help these protective parts of yourself to stand down, at least long enough to work with them and understand their protective mission.

One of the most difficult patterns I routinely see in couples therapy is some version of, "I need to feel close to you to have sex," versus "I need sex to feel close to you." This dynamic can destroy couples as one person feels the constant pressure to be more sexual while craving emotional connection and safety, and the other yearns for affirmation and closeness through sex. These dynamics occur for various reasons, whether it is the influence of a toxic commercial culture that encourages people to believe their worth is in their sexual desirability, or something as simple as a lack of empathy. The person in the relationship who pursues sex at any cost may experience a disconnect from their ability to feel empathy for the emotional needs of their partner, while the person craving emotional closeness often cannot see that their partner's desire for sex is about feeling chosen, desirable, and wanted. I've seen couples get so close to emotional breakthroughs, when the whole thing crumbles as the partner pursuing sex turns around and says, "Sure, this is great, but when am I going to get more sex?" What could it mean to stay with your own feelings of discomfort a little longer so something new can grow? The cosmic perspective that psilocybin offers, matched with increases in empathy, make it uniquely helpful for couples hoping to solve what may otherwise seem like intractable issues.

Some concrete ways of approaching psilocybin integration for sexual healing include creating a list of beliefs about yourself, your body, and your relationships that you can emotionally relate to as true after your medicine experience, all for the purpose of surrendering dysfunctional beliefs and stories about ourselves. Beliefs might shift from "I'm too fat," to "This is the vessel that houses my spirit, and it's fine the way it is! My body shape will not hold me back from pursuing what I want." Sexual trauma survivors might experience a shift from beliefs such as "This trauma defines me," to "I don't have to have wanted this trauma to know it has made me compassionate toward myself and others."

Using the window of decreased reactivity and cognitive flexibility and neuroplasticity afforded by psilocybin can help us to not only *see* things in a new way, but *feel* them in a new way.

The aftermath of psilocybin experiences is also a wonderful time to expand sexual scripts. Sexual scripts are simply the generally unconscious pattern we follow in our approach to sex. Embracing empathy and creativity opens up the possibility of changing that script. Are there new things you'd like to try? Do you rush through sexual experiences, rather than savoring them? Can you slow down, making time to connect to your body or your partner's body? Take stock of your normal approach to sex and ask yourself: what might a sexual experience feel like if I expand it, slow it down, or do it in a new way? We limit our sexual satisfaction by approaching sex as routine or goal-oriented, or when we disconnect sex from our spiritual selves. Applying the cosmic consciousness of psilocybin to sexuality marries the corporeal body with the spiritual body in an act that supports us in surrendering a rote experience of sex to make way for something much, much greater.

MESCALINE, *THE GREAT FATHER*
Integration Theme: Connection

Mescaline is a medicine very close to my heart. Every time I have been lucky enough to sit with Father Huachuma, a mescaline-containing cactus native to the Andes mountains in ceremonial settings in Peru, at some point during the journey I think, "This is the best day of my life." Because it always is. My story of healing through the pleasure of presence with huachuma medicine is one I've been sharing for a while in different articles and public talks. Funnily enough, it's not just one story. I've written about different experiences with huachuma, during different moments in my healing process, because they always lead me to the same place: deep self-love, connection with the Earth, authentic presence, and unbridled joy. Not too shabby. Of course, plant medicine works differently in everyone, and I don't mean to imply that that my experience will resemble all experiences. But Father Huachuma is widely regarded as a great healer of the heart. He is known for his tremendous capacity to get us out of the head and into our body, connected to the Earth. He is also said to carry healing capacity for physical illness as well as emotional strife.

Mescaline (3,4,5-trimethoxyphenethylamine) is a psychoactive substance that can be created synthetically, although very hard to come by for various reasons. I've heard it said that because synthetic mescaline must be taken in much higher volume than other synthetic medicines to achieve a psychedelic effect, underground chemists find it unwieldy to produce and distribute. It is also contained in certain sacred cacti. As mentioned earlier in the book, most famous mescaline-containing plant is peyote, a cactus with a deep sacred history to Native Americans. Peyote sits in a unique position in the plant medicine world. His habitat in the Southern United States and Mexico is horribly endangered, making it increasingly difficult to access. He is also part of a tradition of healing and resistance to Native Americans. Native Americans in South Texas used peyote as early as 1716. But it was Quanah Parker, the great Comanche leader, who was responsible for a resurgence of peyote use in the twentieth century that was to evolve into what is known as the Native American Church, an organization that helped Native Americans achieve spiritual grounding in the years that followed the forced violent relocation from their native homes into reservations. He is quoted as saying, "the white man goes into his church and talks *about* Jesus, but the Indian goes into his tipi and talks *to* Jesus."[40] Much like we see in the repression of sacred mushrooms in Mesoamerica, the Indigenous use of peyote threatened Western religious power systems that insisted on installing itself as an intercessor to God. Both the sacred mushroom and cacti were attacked and suppressed because of their deeply threatening ability to connect users directly to the divine with no need for a priest to absolve or meditate anything. It is a radical act of resistance to insist that your connection to divinity is personal and does not need to fit into an establishment power structure.

Peyote has generally been excluded from the vast movement toward decriminalizing naturally occurring psychedelics throughout the United States due to its the relationship with sacred Native practices and habitat endangerment. It's curious that peyote, a tiny button of a cactus, gets so much attention, when his cousin, the towering San Pedro cactus (from which huachuma medicine comes) has every bit as much power to teach us. The environments in which San Pedro/huachuma is able to grow are more abundant and less endangered, and the ancient traditions that surround him come from a number of places such as Ecuador, Peru, and Colombia. It is incumbent upon non-Indigenous users to ask critical questions about their use, such as whether they engage with San Pedro in a way that is respectful, minimizing harm to the environment and surrounding communities.

I have already touched on how the Indigenous history of huachuma, and the prohibition of peyote was linked to moral panic and sexual repression in chapter one. The history of mescaline is ancient, vast, and storied. Research into its use confirms that the use of mescaline-containing cacti for visionary purposes extends back 5,700 years in South America,[41] and later into the 19th and 20th century in the United States and Europe where the then-unregulated peyote is consumed by artists, intellectuals, and scientists. In 1888, the chemist Arthur Heffter was given dried peyote samples by famed scientist Louis Lewin. It was Heffter who later isolated the alkaloid responsible for the psychedelic effects of the cactus. He called it mescaline, and thus bestowed us a word so mellifluous it is nearly as beautiful as the experience itself. The author Mike Jay, an expert on the history of mescaline, describes how the first scientific trial of any major psychedelic occurred at what is now George Washington University back in 1895. A twenty-year-old man, under observation, consumed several peyote buttons that originated from Quanah Parker. The subject described "delightful visions such as no human has ever enjoyed under normal conditions . . . an ever-changing panorama of infinite beauty and grandeur, of infinite variety of color and form, hurried before me."[42]

Perhaps the most enduring and famous account of mescaline consumption in the West comes from Aldous Huxley's 1954 book, *The Doors of Perception*, in which Huxley describes his encounters with music, art, and the beauty of common objects.[43] The book was successful yet polarizing; intellectuals of the day battled over the persistent question as to whether psychedelic experience is a true mystical or religious experience.* In fact, Jay notes that Huxley's mescaline experience catapulted him into an immediate conversion from someone who viewed self-transcendence with drugs as "an illusion," to believing mescaline offered "a gratuitous grace," and was a vehicle for mystical experience.[44] Huxley inspired many psychonauts in ages to come, with the rock band The Doors deriving its name from Huxley's famous account. In fact, it was Huxley's correspondence with psychiatrist Humphry Osmond after a mescaline journey in 1953 that birthed another famous term: the word "psychedelic."[45]

So, in this vast explosion of contemporary psychedelic research some would go as far as to call a renaissance, where *is* mescaline? If its use is so vast and ancient, and roots so entwined with Western intellectuals and artists from W.B. Yeats to the likes of Aleister Crowley, why did mescaline virtually disappear from the modern psychedelic science? Well, it must first be said that it did not disappear from the world. While synthetic mescaline is hard to find, San Pedro retreats and ceremonies proliferate in Peru and other South American countries, and the collective peyote ceremonies within the Native American Church continue on. It is also important to remember that mescaline is the chemical ancestor to MDMA and other novel phenethylamines. In fact, it was Alexander Shulgin's experience with mescaline that kicked off his inquiry into other related compounds such as MDMA, which he thought to be less unwieldy.[46]

This doesn't really answer the question as to why the clinical research into mescaline has been a trickle whereas, for say, psilocybin, it has been a flood. The very things that make mescaline an exceptional healer and vehicle for embodied pleasure are the things that make it unappealing to psychedelic therapy. Mescaline experiences are long, often twelve hours. Mescaline also takes a considerable amount of time before the user registers any subjective effects, sometimes taking up to two hours for the journey to begin. The embodied effects of mescaline

---

*As I can attest from my brief stint studying at the C.J. Jung Institute in New York City many years ago as a young therapist, this question is still very much alive and well amid its dusty halls.

can range from total orgasmic euphoria to a feeling of heaviness and nausea. Drawing upon my experiences working with huachuma in Peru, the medicine is a gentle healer whose spirit is described by many as speaking directly to you in simple and straightforward ways. There is a heightened sense of color and some visual distortion, but the cactus produces a shift in perception distinct from the kind one experiences on tryptamines like psilocybin mushrooms or ayahuasca. Mescaline-containing cacti have a long history of traditional use in community or in nature, not the normal settings for modern psychedelic research.

Most clinical psychedelic research occurring today is motivated by a desire to monetize the medicine. In other words, how to create a saleable treatment. I'm not being a cynic. The reality is that any research not motivated purely by academic inquiry (and nonprofit research in psychedelics is being eclipsed by pharmaceutical companies) you must be able to standardize and sell the treatment. Mescaline just does not fit well into this paradigm. How are you going to price a fifteen-hour therapy session? Yet, he thrives in ceremonial use in many settings. And it's in that container that I believe his power shines, helping us connect with others and the Earth, allowing the quality of embodiment and sensuality blossom.

I will speak again of my direct experiences of healing with huachuma medicine. As discussed earlier in this book, this plant spirit brought healing to my life in a totally unique way. It brought me into a directly felt state of bliss, a palpable connection to the Earth, and gave me a sense of being free (if not nauseous) in my own body. Speaking of nausea, a real fear for many curious seekers resistant to physical discomfort, the most recent time I was in Peru working with huachuma medicine, I purged each time I drank. And with each purge, something I was carrying that I did not need was removed. The final ceremony was conducted around a campfire at night. In the back of my mind I was scouting around for a place for the inevitable vomit I knew was coming, hopefully far enough away to not bother anyone. You know what happened? I did not vomit. Father Huachuma told me clearly, "Relax. I got everything out of you that needed to go the last few times you drank me. Enjoy the night."

Mescaline offers us not only the possibility of awe and wonder at our world, but the opportunity to fall in love with yourself. He offers the potential to simply be free of the pain we carry, even if only temporarily. Imagine if you could press pause on thoughts of trauma, of fears—what would you do with that space? This is what healing can look like on an individual level. But mescaline-containing cacti have always also been agents of community healing. Sitting in group ceremonies with huachuma makes your individual experiences and thoughts very, very small compared to the collective power and consciousness of the group. It is he who shows us that we can heal our sexuality by connecting directly with the sensuality of the world. Sexual trauma may make us feel isolated and small, but in reality, we never stop being part of something unbelievably big and heartbreakingly beautiful. Huachuma's gift is his reminder that we are his child, beloved, perhaps for the first time. A Great Father who silently walks with us to the heart of healing.

Mescaline Integration
Core Theme: Connection

The integration of mescaline experiences with particular focus on healing sexual trauma and erotic embodiment rely on cultivating space for pleasure and wonder in our lives. His theme is connection. Connection is what is most lost when we experience sexual trauma. When we are disconnected, we are alone in our suffering, and subsequently seek to numb ourselves to block out the pain. Mescaline's spirit coaxes us to come back online and behold all that is beautiful in the world. Often, after sexual trauma has occurred, sexual activity is not the best place to start when we are seeking a reconnection with our emotions. Starting with relating to our body through breath, direct contact with nature, and in a welcoming community can be safer. Let your body experience what it is to simply *be*. To feel good again. To feel safe. Such an experience is often readily available to us during mescaline experiences, and during integration we can try to remain open to that spaciousness.

A seasoned ceremonial facilitator once reflected to me that mescaline is a slow medicine, and thus his integration unfolds more slowly than any other psychedelic. He requires coming back, again and again, to the feelings and sensation he offers to really feel his full wisdom. We can also pay attention to the feelings and sensations we are not feeling. The absence of trauma. During integration, you can find ways of coming back to this space, this nest of healing. But it may require a lot of you. Just as the medicine unfolds over a long arc, you can try sitting in nature not just for a short walk, but several hours. Feel yourself among the trees, in quiet, for an extended time. Notice what arises. Tune into every sensory experience you can, the sun on your face, the sounds of birds, the wind in the trees. Every moment of direct experience with pleasure and beauty is a moment of healing.

As I write this, I'm noticing a nagging voice in me that I should be giving you something more explicitly sexual. More racy. But this is it. And it's the biggest thing I have to offer. The culmination of all erotic healing exists in your ability to be alive, in the world, in your body, connected to love in this very moment. For the erotic is not only the sexual, but it is also the sensual, there for us in everyday life. Audre Lorde, in her seminal essay "Uses of the Erotic, The Erotic as Power" writes, "The erotic is a measure between the beginnings of our sense of self and the chaos of our strongest feelings. It is an internal sense of satisfaction to which, once we have experienced it, we know we can aspire. For having experienced the fullness of this depth of feeling and recognizing its power, in honor and self-respect we can require no less of ourselves."[47]

5-MEO-DMT, *THE GENDERLESS GOD*

Integration Theme: Expansion

Widely considered the most powerful psychedelic substance known to humankind, 5-MeO-DMT is the active substance found in varieties of plants, created synthetically, or unique in the psychedelic pharmacopia, derived from the dried secretions of the endangered Sonoran Desert toad indigenous to the southern United States and part of Mexico. It is distinct from DMT (N,N-Dimethyltryptamine). While both are part of the tryptamine family of psychedelics that operate on the serotonin system, the subjective effects of 5-MeO-DMT are quite different from

DMT.* Known as the "god molecule," 5-MeO-DMT produces a near instantaneous expansion to a shimmering spirit realm, while DMT, colloquially known as the "business man's trip" and christened the "spirit molecule" can transport users to a liminal space occupied by the likes of aliens and "machine elves."[48] While admittedly beside the point since we are focusing on 5-MeO-DMT, I can't help but comment on the sobriquet "the business man's trip," referencing DMT. Only Americans could come across an extremely powerful psychedelic of short duration and immediately have the thought, "I can fit this into my lunch break, and then go back to work!" It's worth mentioning if only to point out how different a medicine can be depending on the container that is created around it, and our ability to normalize the shoehorning of psychedelics into our overscheduled lives rather than taking the time to create sacred space for them. Currently, there is much interest in developing psychedelic-assisted mental health treatments with 5-MeO-DMT, not only because of its profound power but for its short duration of action. Imagine having the most powerful mind-expanding experience on Earth, with a therapist who may have never used the medicine personally and then stumbling out into a parking lot two hours later? I don't think that's good medicine at all.

Within moments of inhaling the smoked medicine vapors, one dissolves into a white, crystalline, boundaryless expanded state that can encompass a profoundly felt state of bliss and peace or wild vibrational somatic experience (and nearly everything in between). The experience lasts anywhere from twenty minutes to an hour based on the dose. I once heard 5-MeO-DMT described as the star at the top of the psychedelic Christmas tree. The supreme psychedelic experience. The

---

*Like 5-MeO-DMT, N,N-Dimethyltryptamine (extracted from various plants to create a freebase powder) can also be smoked or vaped. The onset of effects from inhaled DMT occur rapidly, and dissipate within 30 minutes. Some users orally ingest plant material containing an MAOI prior to ingesting DMT (a combination sometimes referred to by users as "pharmahuasca"), which prolongs both the onset and duration of psychedelic effects. Some users infuse plant matter containing an MAOI with freebase DMT to create what is known as "changa," (also smoked) with an onset and duration of effects similar to that of "pharmahuasca."[49]

gateway to heaven. It can be all of these things. But the intensity of the experience and reports of shockingly dangerous facilitation practices, some even resulting in death, make 5-MeO-DMT a substance to be approached with reverence and discernment. When held in a sacred way, the rapid dissolution of a sense of self combined with the medicine's unique capacity to enable the body to process and directly release emotions can be magnificently healing. Simply put, it can be the most beautiful experience of your entire life. It may also be difficult; users report uncontrollable shaking, screaming, and involuntary physical movement. This might sound scary, but when held in the glimmering chrysalis of the medicine, journeyers emerge with the feeling that they have released trauma so deeply held in their nervous system they could not have processed it in any other way. The result is often rapid and sustained reductions in harmful substance and alcohol use, alleviation of depression, and substantial shifts in PTSD symptoms.

But medicines of this extraordinary power, especially ones with no specific practice lineages associated with them to oversee and initiate guides, can attract people seeking to be the holder of the most powerful thing on Earth, rather than to be in service to the medicine and the people whom they are serving. The psychedelic world swirled with controversy when a well-known 5-MeO-DMT facilitator allegedly vomited on clients, shoved his thumbs in their mouth, and reportedly touched clients' genitals, all based on his impression of what they needed for their healing.[50] Other shocking reports discuss a different well-known facilitator engaging in not only irresponsible facilitation, but even physical violence, including what amounts to waterboarding clients during their 5-MeO-DMT journeys.[51] I'd like to impress upon you that while under the influence of this medicine, during its peak, you may be entirely unaware of your surroundings with no sense of being anchored in a body. You are certainly not in a position to negotiate consent or even stop what is happening to you if you tried. My intention is not to give you the worst and most shocking practices that have been reported around this medicine, nor engage in psychedelic sensationalism. I'm writing about these terrible wrongs to convey how important it is to seriously vet any facilitator and environment in which you might choose to experience this medicine.

Conversely, clinical trials with 5-MeO-DMT are taking off. Unfortunately, as is the case with all clinical trials, federal drug prohibition makes it nearly impossible for study therapists to experience the medicine themselves in a clinical context. Supporting an experience with 5-MeO-DMT without ever having done it is like the old parable of the blind men and the elephant. There is no possible way to get the bigger picture of this medicine in any way other than direct, first-hand experience. The scenarios I highlighted represent two terrifying extremes. Underground facilitation by wannabe psychedelic gurus abusing clients, or well-intentioned but inexperienced psychedelic therapists administering the most powerful substance on Earth with no conceivable way of having the slightest idea of how incredibly big the 5-MeO-DMT experience is. I would personally never, under any circumstances receive medicine from a facilitator who had not had extensive personal experience with it themselves. So, should you wish to pursue work with this medicine, finding safe, responsible settings with facilitators highly trained and experienced in the use of this medicine is imperative.

The very origins of this medicine are shaded in mystery and deception. What is conclusive is that plants containing low concentrations of 5-MeO-DMT have been used by Indigenous people in South America for thousands of years, but in the form of a snuff which is a fine powder made from ground medicinal plants.[52] It is still sometimes included in snuff preparations with other proprietary blends of plants and forcefully blown into the nose for physical and emotional clearing. But by far, the most common contemporary use of this medicine is smoking it either in the form of a synthetic preparation, or the secretions of the *Bufo Alvarius*, a Sonoran toad that is captured, milked, and the secretions dried. Even some of those who advocate for medicines derived from natural sources, condemn the toad-smoking in favor of the synthetic version because, well, obtaining toad secretions involves the capture and molestation of a now-endangered amphibian. Others swear that sourcing it from the toad is a superior form of the medicine that has unique healing and subjective properties.

Let us pause and imagine that someone, sometime during the later twentieth century, was the first person to venture to dry toad secretions and smoke them, proving that human beings are curious creatures. This original toad smoker was very likely the man behind one of psychedelia's most enduring underground publications. The introduction of the use of smoked *Bufo Alvarius* venom (a practice sometimes known as "smoking toad"), can be traced back to a single pamphlet published in 1984, simply titled *Bufo Alvarius: The Psychedelic Toad of the Sonoran Desert*, written under the pseudonym Albert Most. The booklet detailed exactly how one goes about identifying, milking, and smoking the toad.[53] There has been much speculation by archeologists and anthropologists as to the potential use of the toad in ancient ritual, with images of toads showing up in the art of Olmec and Mayan cultures. Andrew Weil and Wade Davis, both celebrity scientists in their own right, published a much-maligned paper in a small journal (no larger journal would take it) seeking to unravel the mystery of ancient psychedelic toad smoking. The *Bufo Marinus* toad, indigenous to the Mayan communities where the toad art is found, contains cardiotoxic properties. Weil and Davis hypothesized that trade routes between Sonora and the Mayan regions may suggest that it was in fact the secretions of the *Bufo Alvarius* toad that were traded and used in ritual.[54]

The paper was not maligned for its conclusion, but rather that Davis and Weil, armed with Albert Most's pamphlet, found the toad and smoked it themselves, proving it was indeed psychoactive. The story is outlined in Mike Jay's captivating book, *Psychonauts: Drugs and the Making of the Modern Mind*. Jay's work demonstrates that whereas self-experimentation was once a common practice with novel substances from Albert Hofmann to Sigmund Freud, there is no place for it in respectable modern scientific inquiry.[55] Modern practitioners also seem to have perpetuated a constructed history of the use of *Bufo Alvarius* by the Seri people that is unsubstantiated. It seems, after all, that smoking the toad is a totally modern phenomenon despite the fact that toad enthusiasts seem desperate to frame it as an ancient connection. I myself find it quite beautiful that a medicine this powerful emerged in our era.

After all that, why include in this book a medicine so fraught with controversy? It actually makes sense to me that a medicine this expansive and penetrating, and in some ways unknowable, would attract confusion. Anything this powerful, capable of actualizing the deepest healing, is bound to magnetize people operating from their own shadow-seeking power. The 5-MeO-DMT experience is like looking in the face of God. A shaman once told me that when you see non-human entities such as tree spirits or elemental spirits they will often appear in human-like (or humanoid) forms because that is the only way the human mind can perceive them. The human form is our point of reference. 5-MeO-DMT can offer users—no longer rooted in a physical body subject to chronological time—the opportunity to stare into the face of the formless, genderless God. The experience is fleeting, and yet once experienced, can change you forever. I call 5-MeO-DMT the "genderless God" because this medicine is beyond all binary, it is the genderless holy. 5-MeO-DMT represents the possibility of mind without boundary. Of course, boundaries are known to dissolve on many different psychedelic medicines such as psilocybin mushrooms at high doses. But the 5-MeO-DMT experience delivers this state of "mind without boundary" with astonishing consistency. As an integration client once said to me after a 5-MeO-DMT experience, "I never knew how to be in a body, until I experienced being out of one."

The 5-MeO-DMT experience itself can be highly erotic for some users. Vibrations and intense sensations may shoot through the body, a sensation some journeyers find orgasmic—another reason a safe container for this medicine is essential. Another unique aspect of 5-MeO-DMT I'd like to focus on is its potential to occasion massive somatic release. During the peak of the journey, users can experience uncontrolled somatic expression. Unlike more "lucid" psychedelics like MDMA that might create space for intense expression of emotion, during a 5-MeO-DMT experience the body might spasm, the user might vocalize, and emotions can shift rapidly from elation to intense grief. I've worked with a number of integration clients who experience this as a raw emotional release capable of ridding the nervous system of stored emotional residue, without any conscious narrative about what is being released.

The last feature of the 5-MeO-DMT experience that relates to sexual healing is its capacity to break us out of our body and far outside the binary. We all live with the burden of socialized gender roles which serve to limit how we might express our gender presentation, dictate what forms of sexual experience are acceptable, and even tell us what emotions we are allowed to express. The 5-MeO-DMT experience can bring us to a directly felt experience of existing not only out of a body, but out of a binary. This can be intensely healing, especially for people who feel constrained and limited by the experience of their bodies.

5-MeO-DMT Integration
Core Theme: Expansion

Understandably, a 5-MeO-DMT experience can be challenging to integrate. Prior to elaborating on the psycho-spiritual aspects useful to integration, it is first wise to describe a phenomenon associated with 5-MeO-DMT use known as reactivation. Reactivation is a reexperiencing of aspects of the psychedelic effect after the medicine has worn off. The term harkens back to the fear of "flashbacks" which fueled drug hysteria in the 1970s. In one study, of those who experienced reactivation after taking 5-MeO-DMT, up to ninety-six percent described it as positive or neutral (rather than scary or overwhelming). Predictors of reactivation were surprising. The more a user prepared appropriately for the medicine experience (such as abstaining from other substances and setting psychological or spiritual intentions), the greater the mystical experience or experience of non-duality, and the context (specifically neo-shamanic or other structured settings) in which the medicine was administered all seemed to predict a higher likelihood of reactivation. Lastly, the biggest predictor of reactivation was being *female*.[56] While not indicated in the research, in my work with integration clients I have noticed that reactivation can be triggered by transition states such between sleeping and waking, or consuming even mild intoxicants like alcohol or cannabis after 5-MeO-DMT use. Clearly, integration professionals must prepare people for this possibility so that they can be aware of what might be happening.

In the integration process, what do you make of a totally ineffable experience? With clients, I've found art making to be an incredibly useful tool. Creating visual imagery that relates to your experience can be a way of going back and trying to piece together the sensations, revelations, and emotions without trying to formulate them into language. It also encourages you to remember and imprint as much of the experience as you can. Much like a dream, the experience itself can fade quickly, while the emotional and psychological benefits may be long-lasting.

5-MeO-DMT also presents us with an opportunity to explore two dimensions useful to pleasure-centered healing: how did it feel to be disconnected from your normal identity and how did it feel to lose control of your body while still remaining safe? The answers to these questions have massive implications not only for the healing of sexual trauma, but can go a long way towards the dismantling of identity markers that do not serve our full erotic potential. When administered in a group, as it often is, 5-MeO-DMT users are witnessed by an entire group of people watching this free and unrestrained release of emotions and movement. For many survivors, particularly of childhood sexual abuse, who may have spent a lifetime dissociating, repressing, and controlling uncontrollable feelings, the very meta-experience of being witnessed whilst experiencing an explosion of emotion can itself be the healing. Integration work can center on slowly trying to bring more emotion back online in your daily life in safe ways.

There is also a deeply existential aspect to 5-MeO-DMT integration work. During an integration process centered on sexual healing, journeyers can be prompted to examine identity-based notions of who they believe they are allowed to be, how they experience pleasure, and how they relate to emotion. I hereby invite you to spend some time exploring your gender and sexual identity. If 5-MeO-DMT can, in an instant, transport you from the normal confines of a body and connect you to a universal consciousness or occasion a total loss of personal reference point, how can that benefit you in your life? I suggest that the experience of egolessness can be a disruptor to all identity-based preconceptions that hold us back from maximum pleasure. The integration theme of 5-MeO-DMT is expansion. Expansion occurs not just during the medicine experience, but in challenging ourselves to expand our boundaries of love, and expand our conception of ourselves afterward. Perhaps, after we are wherever we are when we are not connecting directly to our corporeal form, we can return back to the Earth, back to the body with renewed appreciation for our physical form as the container for our spirit, the brilliant vessel that enables us to feel so good.

OTHER EROTICALLY SIGNIFICANT PSYCHEDELICS

The psychedelics mentioned above are far from the only ones that have the potential to enhance pleasure, encourage embodiment, or support the healing of sexual trauma. In fact, some of the psychedelics I've highlighted are actually *not* the ones most associated with pleasure and sexuality. The detailed descriptions of MDMA, ayahuasca, psilocybin, mescaline, and 5-MeO-DMT are intended to show that our journey towards pleasure, healing, and good feeling can happen in paradoxical ways. Some of the medicines that allow us to experience pleasure are pleasurable when taken and our present moment awareness of pleasure can be healing, while others help us create a much-needed space for pleasure in our daily lives *after* what can be the uncomfortable process of helping us clear a path through traumas and negative self-referencing beliefs. However, I'd be remiss not to mention two substances that are widely acknowledged to have high erotic potential and have deep historical roots entwined with sexuality, **LSD** and **2C-B**, and one that has emerged as the most common quasi-psychedelic to be integrated into wide clinical use and is enjoying broad applications in couples therapy for its transformative potential, **ketamine.**

Some psychedelics have ancient origins and long lineages of traditional use, while some are being created in clandestine labs as we speak. But there is only one that carries the weight of having fueled a sexual and political revolution in the United States, with varied outcomes. Reviled as a disruptor of the social order, and the substance that buttressed political, medical, and social change from its use in psychiatric institutes for the treatment of alcoholism, as an instrument of torture by the CIA, to the glory of the Woodstock music festival, **LSD** (lysergic acid diethylamide) was birthed into the world by scientist Albert Hofmann right around the same time Robert Oppenheimer invented the atomic bomb. Both of these inventions affected cultural perceptions about society and humanity in profound ways.

When we think about LSD, the most common image conjured up is of free-loving hippies and Timothy Leary adorned with flowers in his hair declaring a new paradigm for the youth of America, free from the constraints of marriage or obligation to comply with participation in unjust war described in chapter one.

LSD had early applications in the area of psychosexual inquiry and treatment as well. In 1962, a woman writing under the pseudonym Constance Newland published her account of 23 therapeutic LSD experiences. Titled *My Self and I: The intimate and completely frank record of one woman's courageous experience with psychiatry's newest drug, LSD-25*, Newland described how LSD cured her specific neurosis, sexual frigidity.[57] Newland was, in reality, an actress, writer, and perhaps most fascinating, a parapsychologist who became known for aura photography, named Thelma Moss.[58] Her account of treatment with LSD became a prurient best seller. Who could not be entranced by a book that boasts chapters such as "The Closed Up Clam," "The Battle of the Sphincters," and a personally relatable favorite, "The Return of the Full Bladder?"[59]

A case report from 1965 entitled "The Treatment of Frigidity with LSD and Ritalin" gives us another look into the history of LSD-assisted psychotherapy for sexual disorders. The report details the treatment of a sexually "frigid" woman, a condition marked by lack of orgasm and low desire or avoidance of sex, considered at the time to be a neurosis with a deep psychological genesis in early childhood. The authors suggest that traditional psychotherapy could be "time-consuming and frequently unrewarding," but that LSD could lead to a "speedy release of the unconscious material and alleviation of its associated sexual and other manifestations."[60] The report details how the female client under the influence of LSD (and Ritalin which is a non-psychedelic stimulant) was able to access, identify, and metabolize psychic material related to sexual feelings and events from childhood resulting in improvement in her sex life with her husband.[61]

I do think that psychedelics can be powerful tools to help people recognize, process, and release intrapsychic material that may block healthy sexual functioning, and chapters two and four of this book detail exactly how I think that might look in the modern practice of psychedelic-assisted sex therapy, a field that is yet to evolve to maturity. I'd like to pause for a moment and think about the undergirding of this treatment described in the aforementioned report, a treatment that appears to have been successful, and the concept of "sexual frigidity" in women.

Leslie Margolin critiques the historical concept of frigidity (now rolled into the contemporary diagnosis Female Sexual Arousal Disorder). Drawing upon medical and popular texts from the 1930s to 1960s, she observes that these texts describe "normal" women as welcoming, joyous, and worshipful, while the sexually frigid woman is bitter and resentful "reaching its apotheosis during the man's attempts to engage them intercourse."[62] While I am truly excited by the prospects of psychedelic-assisted sex therapy treatment, we must also acknowledge that women's sexuality has been pathologized and medicalized for a very long time with little consideration for social and relational reasons she might not crave sex. Even in this case report of LSD-enhanced psychotherapy for frigidity the implied goal is that the female subject achieve "vaginal orgasm."

You might be wondering what the hell that even is? In short, Sigmund Freud—who, in truth, I deeply respect and admire in many ways, but was also full of ideas about women later considered to be misogynistic—believed that orgasms achieved by clitoral stimulation were "immature" orgasms, but that women must graduate to *vaginal* orgasms (or an orgasm originating inside the vagina) to be fully mature sexual beings.[63] It is exceptionally well-documented that the clitoris is the primary locus of pleasure for people with vaginas and the vast majority of clitoris owners achieve sexual pleasure and orgasm from the stimulation of *this* organ, not the vagina per se.[64] And yet the founder of psychoanalysis promoted the idea that that tiny pearl of pleasure was the *wrong* way for women to experience stimulation and orgasm. The early psychedelic psychotherapy movement was deeply entwined with psychoanalysis. So while these analysts were enlisting LSD to enhance many different types of mental health treatments, when it came to women and sexuality, the use of LSD was also wrapped up in unrealistic and unscientific ideas about women's sexuality.

When we think of LSD and sex today, it is certainly not in the context Newland's book or clinic treatments for frigidity. LSD has been, and remains, a sex drug par excellence, paving the way for many to sexual satisfaction and erotic liberation. Some users of LSD report intense feelings of embodiment, unity, and increased desire and energy. Certainly, its storied associations with free love and sexual freedom has earned LSD a solid place in the sexual psychedelic cannon.

However, it is also worth mentioning another drug, one that boasts similar qualities of sexual enhancement, **2C-B** (4-bromo-2,5-dimethoxyphenethylamine). 2C-B is not a classic psychedelic like LSD, but rather sits in the same chemical family as MDMA. Whereas LSD's effects can be felt for a whopping twelve hours, 2C-B is a sensual joyride of five or so hours that users may experience as physically arousing, and, rather than heady and intellectual, induces waves of embodied pleasure. Described by Shulgin as a substance that "heightens all of the senses. You'll enjoy food, smells, colors, and textures. The texture of skin . . . and other aspects of eroticism are thoroughly enjoyable."[65] Dr. Friederike Mickel Fischer, a Swiss psychiatrist briefly jailed for offering psychedelic underground therapy, described the plateau phase of 2C-B as "a mixture of LSD and MDMA."[66] Surely, a wonderful chemical love child for curious pleasure seekers.

This brings us to **ketamine**. The spirit of ketamine has always shown herself to me as a white wolf, mysterious and beautiful, full of power with the potential for danger. This substance has the capacity to rapidly relieve depressive symptoms,[67] instill insight, and lull users into a relaxing silken haze. At psychedelic doses, her gentle fingers might draw you into a dream-like world that can extend back through time and space to events of your past; to other worlds filled with creatures, animals, or symbols; or deep into the earth on subterranean voyages. Often described as a "dissociative anesthetic" (a descriptor coined by the wife of the first scientist to publish research on ketamine as useful medicine for low-risk anesthesia), it can be administered in both surgical and emergency contexts without the risk of respiratory depression or other complications. Because of this, ketamine quickly became a popular anesthetic for use in the battlefield, and continues to be used in military conflict today.[68]

What became clear over time was that ketamine at lower, non-anesthetic doses could help users shift suicidal thoughts, unblock stuck patterns of thought, and quickly dissolve the heavy blanket of depression via both the substance's pharmacological effect on the brain as well as the resulting benefits from a psychedelic-like experience. Given that ketamine's medical utility as an anesthetic was unquestionable, it never suffered the same fate as other psychedelic substances, all of which were quickly burdened by restrictions on their research and use soon after their appearance. Ketamine quietly existed, and still lives today, on the United States federal government's Schedule III as a controlled substance prescribed for anesthetic purposes. The flexibility that this status imbues is exactly what has enabled the ongoing research and clinical use of ketamine in diverse settings for mental health treatment. This is in spite of the fact that generic ketamine for the treatment of mental health issues is currently not FDA-approved, and therefore, its use for such purposes is considered "off-label."

In some ways it's peculiar that ketamine has really led the charge in creating the model for what psychedelic therapy could look like when it's more broadly integrated into the health care system. Now, there are ketamine retreats: companies that will send orally active ketamine to your home in curated boxes with designer eye masks and playlists; therapists offering ketamine to their clients in the privacy of their practices; and most alarmingly (to me) infusion centers with no trained therapeutic staff hooking clients up to intravenous ketamine drips, shooting them into the stratosphere, and then sending them home without support. I name ketamine's cultural positioning as peculiar because this substance boasts an incredible profile for both safety and efficacy with few adverse effects, but also risks that are distinctly more pronounced than the risks most psychedelic plant medicines carry, namely bladder cystitis as a result of prolonged use, and addictive potential. And ketamine addiction is not a pretty thing. I've sadly witnessed how ketamine addiction can sway misusers toward the very opposite of its intended transformational qualities, instead engendering a sense of disconnection, spiritual narcissism, and compulsive attachment to her watery twilight realm.

Taking all of this into account, I was skeptical the first time I acted as a co-facilitator in a room full of couples, all cuddled in their own "nests" of blankets and pillows, on the floor of a retreat center for a ketamine-assisted couples therapy retreat. How could this dreamy, psychedelic-like substance create embodiment, connection, and love in couples when ketamine is certainly not a reliably heart-joining substance like MDMA, or even a more physically grounding substance like mescaline? But what happened over the course of that retreat, and the number of other retreats I've guided since then, was quite powerful. When it comes to couples and intimacy, it would certainly seem that ketamine's magic functions in unique ways. At higher, "psychedelic" doses, couples journeyed next to one another, emerging together to share deep inner visions, grateful to be close to each other, with a deeper capacity for empathy. Reactivity was lowered, making connection easier and painful topics more accessible for discussion. At lower, more lucid doses, recently coined a "relational dose,"[69] couples fell into relaxed states where the normal somatic responses that erroneously trigger danger signals in the body were turned down so soft intimacy could take hold.

As a practicing ketamine-assisted psychotherapist, I have now guided hundreds of hours of ketamine journeys in my office, all safely held with medical oversight. I've worked with couples looking to resolve unmanageable conflict. I've worked with sexual trauma survivors who experience so much physicalized fear they can't even talk about their trauma. I've worked with people who have caused relational harm whose narcissistic defenses otherwise don't allow them introspection into their own behavior. Hundreds of hours, dozens and dozens of people, and for nearly all, ketamine opened up space to heal their sexual wounding, open up to deeper intimacy, or achieve a deeper connection with their body. How is it that this short-acting "dissociative anesthetic," the Pluto of the psychedelic solar system—in the mix but not regarded by science as the genuine article—help people achieve this?

In my experience, ketamine's healing power in therapeutic settings comes from a particular alchemy of the medicine's somatic and psychological effects in different dose ranges, the transpersonal experience of the journeyer, and the psychopharmacological impact of the medicine itself. While the psychotherapy I provide in a ketamine session to, say, a couple in distress is going to look very different from that of a sexual trauma survivor, I'm relying on the same ingredients to support healing. There are hundreds of popular media accounts of ketamine therapy describing it as both a life-saving miracle *and* a scary or destabilizing experience. And of course, once you release a transformative substance into the therapeutic wild, the results and quality of care are going to vary.*

But when it comes to the core theme of this book, pleasure and sexual healing, there are some features of the therapeutic ketamine experience that consistently support a return to embodied pleasure. When ketamine is given in a therapeutic setting, the likely first effect is a quality of floating, disconnection from the room and one's body, and the emergence of a dream state of visions and messages. While these visions and messages can be crucial material for good therapeutic integration, it is what happens with the body that is just as important. As the journeyer emerges from the more visionary part of the experience, they become more verbal, related, and thoughtful. However, as thoughts come back online, as the *personality* comes back online, the body remains in a calm, deactivated state. Topics about sexuality, memories of trauma, difficulties in relationships that could not be tolerated in a normal state of consciousness are suddenly accessible in this relaxed, spacious state. Our protective parts take a backseat from running the show. I've worked very effectively with clients who saw their bodies as disgusting, their traumas deeply denied, or their very ability to exist in a body compromised. The lessening of somatic activation after ketamine can be an anchor for how to be, and how to feel, without being completely overwhelmed by painful sensations. Not to mention that in the

---

*There are still active discussions on a popular ketamine listserv for practitioners about whether therapists working with the substance should have had personal experience with it. This is where we still are, so screen your potential therapist very wisely if you pursue this treatment.

days after ketamine administration, my clients often report a profound space from their habitual anxious or dark thoughts.

I've come to see ketamine as less of an "antidepressant" as we traditionally think of them, and more as a layer of insulation from our body's deeply held fear and our mind's habitual negative thoughts, all without the dampening of feelings overall that accompany SSRI use. And wouldn't you know it, when most of my clients experience this distancing from the tight bindings of their own unmanageable thoughts and body sensations without an overall dulling of feeling, pleasure is right there waiting for them. My integration work often centers on rebuilding connection to nature, to touch, to opening up to the curiosity of your own mind when not battered by difficult thoughts and memories. Turns out, pleasure shows up quite naturally when there is space for it. Not only space in your life, but space in your heart. Ketamine, that majestic white wolf, works her healing in subtle and mysterious ways.

This chapter offers a look at various psychedelic medicines in terms of their forgotten histories and unique properties relating to sexual wholeness, healing, and pleasure. Since we are living in an era in which the medical industrial complex is actively hijacking psychedelics and selling us the story that they—the startups, pharma companies, and doctors—are the only safe purveyors of psychedelic experience (a story echoing the efforts of Catholic Church to ban Indigenous use of mushrooms in order to instill itself as the only legitimate purveyor of the divine experience), a refreshing end to our inquiry of psychedelic medicines can be found in a recent research study that examined increased intimacy in couples who used psychedelics together in naturalistic settings. Researchers Jonas Neubert, Katie Anderson, and Natasha Mason explored how shared psychedelic experiences with substances including psilocybin mushrooms, LSD, DMT, 5-MeO-DMT, and mescaline (in other words, the classic psychedelics, which excludes MDMA) could shift relationship dynamics and impact relational intimacy.

The researchers noted three central themes that emerged in psychedelic-using couples: Navigating Anxiety, Reshaping Practices, and Encountering Bliss. Most couples discussed their psychedelic experiences as carefully planned rather than undertaken spontaneously, including cleaning and preparing their shared space together, creating playlists, and making other intentional arrangements relating to the cocreation of an agreeable setting. All study participants described experiencing their partner as a calming presence who ameliorated anxiety about the trip ahead. Couples reported the ability to communicate directly and engage in intensive discussions, including improving how to relate to each other.[70]

But most luminous was the thematic category of Encountering Bliss. Every couple interviewed for this study recounted shared moments of joy. This joy was derived from leaving behind everyday tasks and responsibilities to connect and experience the non-ordinary together. Couples described encountering the unexpected and appreciating the beauty of the phenomenal world as powerful relational experiences. One couple commented, "no amount of research would have explained what to expect." The authors note both the act of willingly putting yourself in a vulnerable state with a partner and committing undivided attention to the present moment as powerful vehicles for intimacy. The study authors conclude that the distinct phenomenological quality of the psychedelic experience including increases in trust, openness, connectedness, mindfulness, and empathy actually point to a distinct way of connecting supported by shared altered states they call *psychedelic intimacy*.[71]

The beautiful thing about psychedelic intimacy is that it can actually stretch much farther than what these researchers studied. Yes, psychedelic work in couples can encourage a unique experience of deepened intimacy, but psychedelics can also expand our awareness of ourselves, our sexuality, and our erotic shadows, leading to an intimate knowing of the self. At best, these medicines help us to appreciate every part of ourselves, so we can be truly available to connect to others and the world. The psychedelic experience can also garner intimacy between ourselves and the divine, removing barriers to the somatic experience of feeling spirit move through us and with us, noticing the way the sacred is in our lives at every moment. And lastly, by increasing our capacity to experience and witness the phenomenal world in new ways, psychedelics enhance our intimacy with nature. They seduce us to fall in love with the planet so we might be inspired to save her. These feelings of intimacy and connection to others and the world are not just for our own benefit—they are imperative to ensure a more just, equitable, and loving collective future. Perhaps this is really how these medicines love us back. They give us bliss, so that we may joyfully accept the responsibility of cultivating love in the world.

7
Stories of Transformation

Personal Narratives of Psychedelic Sexual Flourishing

Love's vast sea cannot be emptied
And springs of grace flow easily everywhere
Where is nirvana?
Nirvana is here, nine times out of ten.

HÔ XUÂN HUON

IN THIS CHAPTER you will read first person accounts and interviews with people of diverse identities, ages, and sexualities, all of whom experienced sexual healing or deeper connection to pleasure through the use of psychedelic medicines. Some use their real identity, others, in order to protect themselves in an ongoing era of psychedelic prohibition, requested pseudonyms, and are noted as such with an asterisk. All of them are courageous beings and have my undying gratitude for sharing their experiences with me and the readers. The opinions and perspectives in their narratives represent their own unique experiences. Here are their stories.

Eve*

Eve, 40, is a visual artist, pianist, and sacred musician who emigrated from Asia to the United States as a child. She verbally shared with me the story of her first ayahuasca experience which helped her heal from sexual trauma she experienced during her childhood. Every part of the narrative she shared, originally over an hour long, was deeply moving. We have curated this excerpt in collaboration for this book. Here is her story:

> *This is the story of my first time sitting with ayahuasca. The experience was a pivot point in my life. As a seeker I felt very drawn to ayahuasca, and for a year she was making appearances in my consciousness, through friends, and coming up in things I was reading. You know how she does that! I'd already started dabbling and being interested in psilocybin and LSD in recreational settings. I was having very powerful experiences in nature already with these medicines. I was at a juncture where I needed to do something else to help myself and I became very interested to explore ayahuasca. The first time I sat with ayahuasca, it was with a healer I really trusted, but it wasn't in a great setting. It was an old dojo in Brooklyn. I was like, "OK, this is gonna be my first time. It's not gonna be in Peru, or, you know, something amazing like that. It's going to be this!"*
>
> *Leading up to the ceremony, I was pretty fastidious about following the ayahuasca diet, abstaining from other substances, sugar, salt. I was feeling pretty raw, and totally nervous. But I also went in with a lot of reverence. I remember writing a letter to the ayahuasca before the ceremony on the advice of a friend. To her spirit, her presence. I didn't know what she was, so I treated her like a spirit who I could communicate with. In my letter I thought about what I really wanted to address, what I hoped and prayed for. I was very specific. At that point in my life, I had one traumatic memory that I felt in my being. I just could not quite get over it with therapy, medication. I had tried everything. There was just a part of me that could not let go of this trauma—it was so violating. It was a memory that I had with my*

father growing up. When I was very little, I must have been four or five years old. At this point in my life, I was living in Asia with my parents, my father and my mother, and also my brother. There was a lot of violence in my family that was initiated by my father.

There were also things about my father . . . moments of sexual discomfort. Even children have a nascent sexuality, and I knew when something was uncomfortable. When I would sit in my grandfather's lap it felt safe, but I was not quite comfortable in my father's lap. One thing I really did love was driving in the car with my father. He had a fancy car, and I loved to go out in it. Even though he was abusive, he was still my father and there were things I loved doing with him. Despite my fear of him, I really loved him too. One night we went out driving. I was in the passenger seat, and he was in the driver seat and the sun was setting. It was getting dark. We were talking and he leaned over and started grabbing at my thigh in a way that was clearly crossing a line. It was beyond affection. It was uncomfortable. The first time he did it, I swatted him away but I didn't say anything. Then he did it a second and third time. This time I clearly said, "No!" very loudly and pushed his hand away. Then he grabbed my hand and said, "I can do whatever I want to you. I am your father." He was livid and raising his voice. At that point he was so mad about my swatting his hand away, exerting autonomy over my body, and me not wanting to be molested, that he stopped the car and reached over me and opened the door. He told me to get out. I remember it was really dark outside by this point. I didn't know where we were. I just remember we were on some road, like a deserted highway. He told me to get out, and then he closed the door and he drove off. He left me on the side of the road. I remember watching the car go away, breaking into tears. That was a decisive moment in my life. It was the first time I felt my life was in danger. I was in utter fear. I thought I was going to die. My father eventually came back for me. It could have been five minutes later or twenty minutes later. It was hard to tell, because I was afraid of being punished for not wanting to be violated. We drove home like nothing happened.

This memory stayed with me. I pushed it down, but it would

resurface in various parts of my life. I remember going off to college, which is the first time in your life you aren't governed by your parents. I was having sex, and I was very interested in sex. But the one part of me no one could ever touch was my thigh. If someone touched me there I felt this rage, this burning, and then the memory would come back. No matter what I did or how much I talked about it, I just could not get over it. As I got older, I got over the fear of my father, and I came to some level of forgiveness toward him. But my body did not heed that change. So this was the memory I wrote about to the ayahuasca spirit before my first sitting. I was like, "Dear Ayahuasca," and I asked for some insight or some way of being able to move past this because my body could not. My body was in shock about it. I'm sure it was affecting me in other ways. Because of this experience, somewhere inside myself I believed that if I stand up for myself, I'm going to be abandoned. I'm going to get hurt. That it was not ok to have autonomy over your body or you'll be punished. I was asking for help, for insight.

I go to the ceremony in this old dojo and there are like forty or fifty people there, and it's kind of chaotic. They served us the medicine. And of course, ask anyone who's ever drank ayahuasca: you remember that taste forever! I can taste it right now while I'm talking. The facilitator led us through a series of breathing exercises because everyone's starting to freak out. I remember how the medicine started out with sparkles, like little plays of light. But then it went full visual. It felt like there was reality, then someone took an Exacto knife and slit it open. It opened other portals, other worlds started opening up. I was sitting there, and I was just like, "This is a lot." I remember very distinctly looking down and thinking, "I don't see the floor right now." The floor is opening up into something. I was trying not to freak out. I also very badly needed to purge in like the most epic way. I remember someone told me if you need to purge, purge like you're a lion. Get on your knees, get on all fours, and just let go. So, that's exactly what I did. I remember there were things that were coming out of me that I was letting go of. I was physically releasing something I was holding onto. That was also an incredible experience that made me feel even more open.

After I purged, all of these dimensions were opening up in fractals. I started to get scared and panicked so I reached out my hand for the assistant to say I needed help. He tried having me sit in a different way and blew smoke around me to calm me down. So I put myself in a cross legged meditation pose, and when I looked up to the upper right hand corner of the room, suddenly I saw these figures up in the corner, like six or eight of them. They were like black smoke with white faces and white hands. I made eye contact with them, and when they saw me see them, they started flying towards me. I thought, "This is just not going well. Nothing is making sense, it's all fucking terrifying." I put my hands up to my face, and the assistant suggested I put on my eyeshades and lay down on my right side. Kind of like in a fetal position. I was like, whatever. I'll try anything. The moment I did that, a giant dark portal opened up in front of me, and the periphery of it was moving. The tunnel was moving and at the end was a very faint light. Suddenly I said aloud, "I'm coming for you." Don't know why I said that, but I was like, "OK. I guess I'm going looking for something."

I decide I'm going to crawl through this tunnel. On the walls were scenes from my childhood, memories of family, and some really weird scary stuff too. Violent imagery mixed in with my own memories. I thought, "Whatever this is, I have to get out of this thing." I was crawling and crawling through this tunnel of chaos and violence. I started to make it to the end, and the light grew brighter and brighter. I started to see a figure of a person. As I came closer to the figure I could see it was myself as a child, the moment my father left me on the side of the road. I remember seeing the outline of her hair, I had long hair and bangs, and what she was wearing. She turned around and looked at me. She was crying, so scared. I remember feeling just so overwhelmed by the sense of incredible tenderness for this child who's me but not me. I went to her and grabbed her and looked in her face and said, "Do you know how perfect you are? Do you know how much I love you?" I remember feeling how smooth her face was and how sweet she was. I remember telling her, "I'm not going to leave you. You're going to be OK. I'm here." I wiped away her tears, and her whole disposition just changed from being hurt and abandoned to calm. Eventually she started smiling. I told her, "You're perfect and I'm here for you." At this point she felt complete joy, and she smiled and I smiled back at her. She jumped up on me and wrapped her legs around me and hugged me. It was the best entheogenic moment in my life. We just held each other—there was no me or her. My chest opened with light, and the light turned into a rainbow. That's what white light is, all colors. I should not even use the word "we." We were one. Here I am a woman at the time in my 30s after living with this traumatic experience, and we finally became one. At this point in the journey I was just laughing and smiling. Ayahuasca became like a connector. I was able to go back and rescue that part of me that was stuck in the past and finally heal. It was ecstasy.

Malena AND Øistein

Deep in the woods of the Catskill Mountains, I met and worked with Malena and Øistein at a ketamine-assisted therapy retreat for couples focusing on sexual healing. Married fourteen years, they are both professionals in their forties and have two children. Ketamine work helped them find deeper connection with each other and address long-standing issues around intimacy in their relationship. Here is their story.

> **Malena:** *I'm a fifth-generation Argentinean woman of Jewish descent. I emigrated to the U.S. when I was twenty. My sexuality can be described broadly as queer. I use the term bisexual as well, though perhaps I am more of a pansexual person since I'm attracted to gender-fluid and gender queer people too. But as Margaret Cho says, "I like 'bisexual' because it's kind of '70s." When I met Øistein, I wasn't looking for a partner at all. I was disillusioned with people and relationships, and not entirely sure whether I could even be in a monogamous partnership. Meeting Øistein, however, was like a breath of fresh air. He was unlike any man or woman I'd ever met. He felt like a supernatural being to me. We had a connection that went beyond gender boundaries. Our*

sex was amazing, probably as a result of our connection, and for a long time, we had the best and the most sex I'd ever had with anyone, especially a man.

Øistein: I'm a cisgender, heterosexual man, born in Kenya to Norwegian expat parents. I'm international in outlook, having spent most of my childhood in East Africa, in South Sudan and Ethiopia, my teens in Norway, most of my twenties in the U.K., thirties and beyond in Brooklyn. I became a naturalized American this year. I grew up in progressive Christian circles. Porn was a patriarchal weapon not to be enjoyed. I didn't drink until I was eighteen, and I didn't have sex until I was twenty. Sex and intimate relationships were never discussed in my family. I didn't see myself as attractive, a catch, or particularly sexual until I met Malena. She showered me with love, filled me with confidence, and it opened the door to a whole new repressed sexual side of me.

Malena: Before coming to the retreat, it was clear that the combination of the pandemic and working too much while raising two kids in the intensity of New York City was really starting to affect us. Working remotely as a psychologist was incredibly draining, and it felt like everywhere I turned—kids, spouse, patients, students—everyone needed something from me. Additionally, our marriage was struggling due to lack of relaxed, intentional moments of connection. I felt annoyed with Øistein a lot. I felt he was just one more person who needed something from me, and him wanting sex when I was so shut down felt like a huge drain. I really saw myself as the problem in our sex lives. In my individual therapy, I worked with parts of me that were completely shut down to the idea of sex and intimacy; a grumpy, old woman holding court in front of a large, unopenable door with no key, or a judgmental nun who saw sex as disgusting and appalling. These parts protected me with a shield of control in a time where I felt little control over so many aspects of our shared lives. For a long time, it felt like the sexual part of me had died. I was convinced that if I wasn't married to Øistein, who wanted so much to have sex, I would have been fine with losing my libido. This is sad to think about considering sexuality and sensuality has always been a huge part of my identity and experience. Sex started to feel like something I had to do because I have such a good husband who does so much for me and our family. I also felt responsible for his mood because it was clear that if we were having sex, he was happy, lighter. If we weren't, he was moody and irritable. It became that sex equaled pressure and responsibility.

Øistein: Coming to the retreat, I experienced our relationship like I would visiting Rome, in awe of its history and what it has achieved, like our kids and our family; impressed by what it has endured, like getting through pandemic life; excited by what it can offer of romance, nightlife and sexiness; tired of the slog of everyday, annoyed about things not working like it used to, and with a sense of melancholy for the many memories of past greatness. There was an underlying tension associated with intimacy—or rather lack of—and whenever it was brought up we would fall into the same track of behaviors and words. I felt our level of togetherness was entirely dependent on Malena's mood. I felt that Malena had explored all she wanted in her young years and was now retiring, just as I was coming out of retirement ready to explore, wanting to experience more sexual adventure.

Malena: During the first ketamine experience, I was sitting with the internal tension and confusion around being a sex object, a mother, and a professional. These parts felt unintegrated; parts within me that cannot and must not coexist. Øistein and I had felt really close that morning. We remembered how much we loved talking together, dancing, being together, just having a lot of fun. That evening, the retreat introduced multiple exercises that dealt very directly with intimacy and sex, and I felt my protectors come up. Øistein and I got into a big argument we could not resolve and went to bed angry, which is very unlike us. But the next morning, I woke up with an important realization. It was about how supportive of my sexuality and sexual exploration Øistein had always been. I felt an immense sense of gratitude towards him, that he'd create no blocks for me to feel what I needed to feel. I came in touch with a feeling of expansiveness, both in my love for him, his support, but also in how much he opens the world up for me. That he creates openness rather than blockages.

Øistein: Ketamine helped me to get in touch with the origin of my deepest insecurity. I came to understand that it's been my insecurity that has perpetuated and helped cause periods of lost physical intimacy in our marriage. I have often blamed this on Malena's lack of desire, or lack of "wanting to want." What makes me feel the smallest and most vulnerable is the fear that I'm only loved because of what I do, not because of who I am. That I am loved for my actions, not my being. As a result I always seek to be helpful, be of service, go the extra mile, volunteer, cook. This dynamic also plays out in our relationship. My father does the same thing. He calls it "love actions." Love for me therefore does not feel unconditional. I have to prove my worth. As I get a lot of positive feedback in return for my actions, it becomes fuel for the cycle to continue. I finally connected this to why I take rejection of intimacy so personally. Intimacy and sex represents who I am, not the things I do. Not actions, just me the being, naked and vulnerable. I realized I had not tried to really understand Malena's perspective. I had shied away from asking why she may be avoiding intimacy for fear of the answer. In my insecurity there was only one answer. She didn't love my being. I made it a vote of confidence about me as a person. Fear of rejection fueled a cycle of hurt people hurting each other.

My most powerful breakthrough was when I started to ask, what was scary about intimacy? What were we avoiding? I voiced my fear of rejection. Malena joined me in tears. When we took the ketamine medicine on the third day of the retreat we held each other tight, both crying. We stayed connected, talking, laughing, crying, cuddling each other. I was able to touch Malena's hair, a point of tension, stress, and anxiety over the last year. I showered her with compliments about her looks, attitude, strength, bravery, and beauty.

In this deep moment of connection, I finally saw another possible reason why Malena had shied away from intimacy. Why she had held on to a deep-seated resentment towards me. Earlier in the retreat we had shared our common memories of "peak intimacy." They took us back to our first moments of meeting. Our throes of passion in the years before children. To bedrooms in Astoria with fig trees in the garden. To youth, sexiness, and gorgeous bodies. It is a truism that becoming parents changes everyone, but I had not appreciated that for Malena it forever physically changed her body. The most beautiful moments between us, our "peak intimacy," ended in a form of sexual violence. Twice over she was cut open in the stomach, as our beautiful babies were delivered through C-sections. She carries the scar and sees it every day on what used to be her favorite part of her body. Her sexuality and youth, cut open and scarred forever. For the first time I understood what she meant when she said "It feels like my wires have been cut," in response to why she didn't feel desire the way she used to. After ten years, I finally understood that she was carrying a sexual trauma, that she had been grieving alone, and naturally holding resentment towards me and avoiding intimacy, because it caused pain.

It was the most humbling, sad, and eventually redemptive and relieving feeling I have ever felt. We held each other, crying, laughing, whispering old jokes, complementing, and apologizing to each other. Surrounded by trees, we both felt a coming together again through common roots, strong trunks intertwined and with long branches and fresh leaves allowed to stretch out in different directions, towards new rays of sun, the blue sky and new opportunities for growth, pleasure, and joy. My hope is that discussing, naming, and understanding my own insecurity will make me more intentional in my actions and choices in my relationship with Malena and my life more broadly. Seeking true happiness and love, not simply a reward for my actions.

Malena: When Øistein shared this epiphany, I received an understanding and compassion from him that I didn't know I needed up until that point. I felt so seen, in a way that I didn't realize I needed to be seen. I felt that I had been carrying a rage inside of me, like unconscious, energetic baggage that could simply relax once Øistein understood how the experience of my C-section births had disempowered me. The anger I'd felt at my body, at the hospital staff, at the whole system which had not taken appropriate care of me. My need to control and resistance to sex went hand in hand. I had been carrying a burden that I didn't know I'd been carrying until Øistein labeled it. It shifted our dynamic also in that suddenly I was not the problem, and now Øistein identified himself as part of the solution. He could see there was lots for him to do in order to help with our intimacy issues, starting with identifying how his own issues around self-worth were impacting us, as well as how he had gone quickly into "protector" mode for me, rather than stopping to understand how these births had impacted me. I felt taken care of for the first time in a long time. Our experience with ketamine helped to expand our understanding of what our dynamic was. It broadened both of our viewpoints into a panorama, rather than our usual used-up peephole. I felt more in love with Øistein than I'd felt in years.

After this kind of work, one feels like you climb a huge, steep mountain, and then get to make space for and enjoy this incredible view from above. It felt majestic. But then you get back to everyday life, and old habits die hard, as they say. Øistein was very supportive, and it is clear, in retrospect, that my protectors were really "on fire" following the retreat. We are in a great place as a couple, but still struggling with sex because we work too much, our kids need a lot from us, and I am too overwhelmed. For the future, I'd like to have more space where we can meet and just enjoy being with each other. But I will say that I am much gentler and more sensitive with Øistein than I was before. The feeling of reconnection that we reached, that feeling lives in our relationship now. It is a "feeling-place" we can connect to if we want to go there together. That gives me a lot of peace and joy.

Øistein: For us, this means walking the path toward regaining our passion and intimacy, free from blame, guilt, and pressure . . . together.

Jake*

Jake is eighty years old, a retired clergy and hospice chaplain, and before that a teacher and college professor. He was born during World War II, just after the United States entered the war against fascism/Nazism on D-Day, June 6, 1944. He shared his story with me of psychedelic revelation and redemption in life's second chapter. Here is his story.

Most of my life I didn't know where I fit. There was no real place—I mean, a geographically real place—a site on the human map. A place where I felt safe and that I could be fully who I was. I didn't even know who that person was or how I was going to find out. I mean, look, it's 1954. I'm in the fourth grade, and I'm on the playground, and some dispute happened, and there I am standing facing the teacher. On one side of me are all the girls, and on the other side looking at me are all the boys, and I knew I didn't belong to either group, and the teacher didn't know what to do with me. I was raised in the military, so this is a school for military kids. If I wasn't moving somewhere else, the other kids are. There one day, and suddenly not there the next. I had no neighborhood. No friends. And it was not a place I wanted to be. I had no fun. So, I started furiously crying, frustrated and lost and with zero guidance or sense of justice. The male teacher just looked down at me. I ran off the playground. Ten years old and already I knew I was a hidden person.

See, I think pleasure, sexuality, place, and justice are so knotted together that if you try to manipulate or control or even undo that knot, you become cruel. Society did that by controlling other people's bodies and punishing them for being different, you know, becoming a capitalist culture—and really I mean any kind of difference—if you're any kind of non-white person you can't hide it in a white-controlled world. But sexuality is different. You can hide it, until you are somehow forced to be honest. Stepping out of the wings, out of the dark, is called coming out. But what it really means is being honest. It really means that I deserve justice, and place, and pleasure, and the gift of my sexuality.

One of the passages in the Bible that sustained me for a long time—and there have really been only two—one of them was, "Thou preparest a table before me in the presence of my enemies." I took that to heart. Whoever that God was in my mind was on my side. I mean, I'm dying here. People were out to annihilate me, and I mean personally, too. And God put a feast in front of me so that the whole friggin' capitalist structure could see that I am well cared for and they didn't provide it. I think that sentence, from Psalm 23, is so radical as to undermine whole social structures. Well, yes, there is one more. It's in Paul's letter to the Galatians, Chapter 5, right at the beginning: "For freedom Christ has set us free. Do not, therefore, submit again to a yoke of slavery." And it was that second one—it was a daily mantra—it got me through a lot of hatred from family and religion, and helped me make sense of psychedelic experience.

I didn't go to psychedelics because I thought it might help me. Really. I was fifty-one years old before I tried it. And I didn't even know what it was. Ayahuasca? I got an invitation from someone I have forgotten. Damn! If I could remember, I'd thank him and kiss his feet. I know what people say about it now, but in 1995 I was new to all this. The whole, entire altered consciousness program in my world was about alcohol. Period. So, I didn't do it to stretch my horizon, nor to expand my consciousness, nor to explore creativity or my sexuality, nor to envelope me within the whispering conversations of the forest, and certainly not to impale myself on the putrid psychotic stake of "ego death," a term to which I have become willfully and increasingly resistant. At the invitation from my unknown benefactor, I didn't yet know that those were things people thought possible and talked about. Curious, but plainly late to the game. These are words from an old man.

I was afraid. Very afraid. Curious and afraid. Fearful to the point of daily thoughts of suicide. I had too many failures. I had a severe lack of self-worth. I was very sure I didn't know what a secure relationship felt like. I mean, did you have a tetherball game on your playground? Remember how you hit it and it spun around a pole, and then someone hit it back? It's a game to teach social skills of serve and receive and sent it back, kind of a teacher of having a social dialogue.

It involved hitting, of course. Maybe I'm too sensitive to violence.

Well, my tether cord was frayed, down to a strand or two, and the ball was about to fly off with the next hit. Eventually, I was diagnosed with multiple personality disorder, but that was before they really understood sexual trauma. Maybe it was the rapes by my uncle and a pastor, in combination with everything else. I heard my father tell his family about putting men's dicks on a chopping block and taking a hatchet to it because of some indiscretion. I took that to heart, too. Death everywhere, and my pleasures were dangerous. I wasn't always so sure about that table of God spread before me.

Psychedelics showed me that I had a neighborhood within. They also helped me not dissociate every time I wanted to have sex, "Danger, Will Robinson, danger." So, I had separate parts that I couldn't get together. Meanwhile, I wanted to have sex with men, not with women to prove that I am a man, and not with men to be an anima to their animus. So, yes, there was a distinct male part and a separate and distinct female part. It was like being on the playground in the fourth grade. I didn't know where I belonged. Once, much later, a leather man I was having sex with pushed me off him and said, "But, you're a woman!" You know, like, who was he talking about? I had lots of moments like that when I was profoundly frightened about my existence.

But here's the heart of the story. Psychedelics helped me heal and find love-justice in my life. Ninety ayahuasca ceremonies in Peru, Brazil, and various sites in the United States. 700 mushroom ceremonies. Bufo. 5-MeO-DMT. San Pedro. 2C-B. 2C-E. MDMA. LSD. And so on. It was a long, long journey. I was resolved to become a unified and healthy soul in defiance of my religious upbringing, in spite of the capitalistic, binary structures of America, despite the rejections of my family. When I came out as gay, my father said, "We assume you will give up all rights to your children and never see them again." Even against the beliefs of therapists who said that I could only hope to manage the damage—because, they said, the damage to my brain was permanent. That was then. That was the world I had to resist in order to heal.

My most loving words to people fighting each other for who has a right to belong to which group: Wake up. Look in the mirror. You have become cruel. At the beginning of my relationship with my current partner, we would take psychedelics every Saturday night when we set aside time to have sex. LSD and MDMA were favorites because I could feel deeply connected and also wide open. I could say the truth and hear it from him, and it was (finally in my life!) very OK. So, he and I consciously used sex to explore our relationships with our fathers. We began role playing daddies and boys. And after four years of this, we realized we were emerging into a new and adult relationship with each other. And after eleven years, he's the best boyfriend I ever had and continue to have. We did it. We did it together. This kind of ripe love grows during the depths of honesty and the manure of struggles. We'll be partners until we die. You know what I want written on my tombstone? "You were the best ever!" Maybe I mean psychedelics, too.

One more note. I was finally able to bring the separate male and female parts of me together in psychedelic ceremonies. In one ceremony I saw the patterns that got me into trouble. I saw how they started. And I gave them up, right there in an ayahuasca ceremony. Two weeks later, during a 5-MeO-DMT ceremony, I externalized both my male and my female parts, in the air over me. My eyes are open. I am looking right at them. The man is naked and is moving down onto my body. The woman is naked, in the air, immediately above him. "What?!" I said. Then I knew I was looking at myself. All that journey from fourth grade to this moment, nearly seventy years later. And the naked woman merged with the naked man and the two of them merged into my body. Then they spun around and together looked out through my eyes, through my flesh, through my sex and my pleasure, and with a visceral feeling, a knowing for justice. I immediately grasped a truth about how, with my body, I nourish other men and also in some way have a very full capacity to nourish anyone, man or woman. "This is my body given for you." My life and my body, a sacrament for others. I feed. I nourish. I support. I help them open to their hidden selves and encourage them to come forward and be seen. I will guard your wounds. On the earth.

I love.

Then words came easily. This is me: Mothering Father. One-to-one, and in intentional ceremonial gathering.

Rabbi Shir Meira

Shir Meira (they/them) is an ordained rabbi, sacred singer and songwriter, student of Jewish mysticism, and spiritual counselor. During our friendship, I watched Shir on a path of personal discovery of gender, sexuality, and self-actualization through spiritual practices and psychedelics. We sat down for a discussion about psychedelics, pleasure, suffering, redemption, and beauty. Here is their story:

Growing up in New York City and in a progressive liberal family, it was okay for me to become whoever I wanted to be. I knew fairly early on that I was not heterosexual. In fact, in high school it was common for people in my grade to identify as bi, although there was always something unsettling for me about the duality of bisexuality. My attractions were about particular people and their particular energies. I felt connected to being outside of a binary before I even had terms for that. I didn't have the language or concepts of nonbinary or genderqueer, but I explored my sexuality quietly, under the radar. I had trouble finding spaces that resonated with me. Gay male spaces often didn't feel right. I would go to Pride parades but those overwhelmed me. I realize now that was probably because of my autistic identity. I do think also that my dad's death was liberatory in a certain way. Not because I think he would have disapproved of me, or would have shamed me for any lifestyle choices, but because I don't think he significantly accomplished an embodied life himself. In fact, the only spiritual message I got from him after his death was, "Go as far as you can into this body, embody yourself as much as possible!" It felt like permission. This message didn't even feel directly from him, but like it was from something from the angelic sphere carrying him off to be recycled into the cosmos. The lesson was, "Take your best shot at living this life." So in the grief there was a liberation and the freedom that came through. Around that time I was also finding folks and friends who were modeling other potentialities and possibilities.

Discussing death leads me to thinking about the Zen Peacemaker Bearing Witness retreats at Auschwitz-Birkenau where I served as a rabbi. Each week—I attended for five consecutive years—we would spend many hours sitting at a place called the Selection Site, a train platform at the arrival spot inside Birkenau. Those who managed to survive the ordeal of being shipped there were "selected" either for internment in the death camp or immediate gassing, with the mere flick of a finger. Left, die immediately; right, die eventually, probably after great suffering. There was something about sitting at that place of selection . . . it was the arbitrary violence that is selection that had already deeply percolated into my being. I would say that psychedelics slowly helped me actually touch and discern the pain of that constant selection, of the myriad ways we are subjected to being selected or separated out. One of the earliest ways we do this is by gender: "Is it a boy?" That is almost to say, "Which team are you playing for?" It happens with religion, nationality, belief systems, and on and on. Psychedelics over time, cumulatively, have given me experiences of great macroscopic and microscopic vision, zooming in deeply or panning out wide, to see the integrity of all the parts of ourselves. The fractal and unitive nature of our being: wild, chaotic, unbridled, and yet whole, seamless, unending.

My general psychedelic history started in my teens with very acute and profound experiences. Then I went dormant for a few decades while I dug deep into Jewish mysticism, practiced meditation, and started a family. But then it reemerged. Later on, after my second Rabbinic ordination, I realized that my public, professional spiritual life and my private psychedelic life were running on parallel tracks. I couldn't bear what felt like duplicity. These two streams were profoundly informing one another, albeit implicitly. But Michael Pollan hadn't been on the front page of the New York Times *fifteen years earlier. Psychedelics weren't part of the general discourse, and I also didn't have a psychedelic community at that time. So the Zen retreats, practicing the tenets of Not Knowing and Bearing Witness, and other meditation and embodiment practices preceded my return to psychedelics. The process of developing the inner witness allowed me to have very deep and strong encounters with psychedelics. It allowed a willingness for psychedelics to thoroughly deconstruct my psyche, tear open and eviscerate, and to explore how I'm making meaning of myriad life experiences. Sitting in a place like Auschwitz is incomprehensible; it's beyond the capacity for the human mind to understand that cruelty, that suffering. Yet the human mind and human body need some sort of containment, need to make some meaning or sense of the experience, and so the place itself—direct experience—becomes the teacher. The raw, sensory encounter of the artifacts that are there, the other people who are on retreat. Practicing and encountering others brings you to this psychedelic expansive state of meaning-making. So then later when I would experience MDMA or mushrooms, I was able to get in touch with the injustice of experiencing being selected, of being labeled. Jew versus non-Jew, or male versus female, or human versus non-human, or human versus nature. How many of us have to live outside of the felt sense, the embodied, birthright experience of belonging to all sides? There is no division, there is no separation, there is no me from them.*

Somehow the work that happens after taking psychedelics, the embodiments that are required to integrate these experiences, have brought me to experience myself beyond the gender binary; to honor the experience of my religious heritage, my genetic and epigenetic Jewish ancestral history as being beyond an ethnic limitation; to experience my humanity, to honor the elemental ancients and our future ancestors. This embodiment also demands an honoring of our connections to the very sexual nature of the entire universe, that everything is inter-penetrating itself. God is a switch and so am I! *This was illuminated by MDMA in particular, and pondering the politics of pleasure. The fear-reduction that comes with Ecstasy, and the meditative grooves I had developed through sitting practice, allowed me to honestly follow sensation; to take somatic, polyvagal healing down into the core of my being. Melting into a soft, undifferentiated awareness helped me realize I never liked picking sides or playing for a team. This wasn't all rainbows and unicorns; there was a very dark burnout period. But it led me to a diagnosis of being on the autism spectrum. This immediately unlocked profound grief and utter relief. My neurodivergence helped me identify my neuroqueerness and to embrace this kaleidoscopic mind. I could stop shaming myself with "Something's wrong with me." My brain doesn't have a bug in the system or a flaw; it's a feature! My social obliviousness or ignorance got me into trouble in certain places, and a pervasive uncomfortable disdain which I have started to dissolve. Some sensory sensitivity that could completely overwhelm me could, in other communities or contexts, connect me to a vast vitality and an incredible aliveness. There was a whole reckoning that started with my autistic diagnosis. Autism, sexuality, gender, and psychedelics and consciousness, they were all about opening and belonging. I've surrendered to something much larger than conceptual frameworks can contain.*

I think pleasure is what we call the body's knowing of its belonging to the universe. It's how we tell we're meant to be here. We're not a mistake. However, pleasure is so narrowly circumscribed, and so are our bodies. It sometimes takes these volcanic, theophanic experiences of high doses of psychedelics for us to get shaken out of our narrow conceptions of what is or isn't pleasurable. As I slowed down and relaxed into my capacity for surrender, I found myself having more sophisticated and subtle relationships with medicines. I have discovered that there's nourishment in the aesthetic. So many of these psychedelics tend to work on our visual cortices. I think that's because the world is beautiful, and we're supposed to be nourished by the exquisite intricacy and diversity of the natural world. Sometimes it feels like a common setting in which we use psychedelics such as, "I'm going to take the time to mindfully be with my friends in nature," would be enough without the mushrooms if we really honored the experience. I'm going to be with someone I care about, we're going to go somewhere beautiful, and we're going to have nothing else to do. Then, if we happen to introduce a mushroom, the mushroom says (they seem to speak in the plural), "Oh, I'm so glad you joined us!" We are all breathing in the infinite chorus of harmony. Look at the ants, how they're on constant parade! Look at the leaves, how they dance! Look at the clouds, how they frolic before the sapphire throne of the Holy One." Once you have that enough times you recognize maybe all it takes is having a relationship with nature, or a good friend, or sitting and taking a deep breath to join that breath of life.

I would also say that pleasure is hidden in plain sight throughout Jewish spiritual practice, in the mystical roots of the Hasidic tradition in particular. Pleasure is the enemy of corporate capitalism, right? I bless this present reality as it is, savor this food, hum this song, sway to this moment. Because if we can just enjoy ourselves as we are—if we don't need anything at all—who will benefit from our sense of scarcity, or from our constant desire for more?

I'm really happy you're writing this book and that there are more sage guides becoming accessible and available to this work. It's not for everyone, but so many people are going for it anyway. I sat with my own psychedelic harm for two decades because I didn't have a community or integration support. So, I'm mostly contributing my story here for the sake of harm reduction. It's not the experiences themselves but the messages we receive and embody that I think are the real medicine. The Talmud teaches that an uninterpreted dream is like an unopened letter. We need each other to reflect the dream of our dreams, to make meaning in relationship. Pleasure and psychedelics can take us to the very edges of our isolated identities, to the voices urging us to grow into a unitive, non-dual, nonbinary consciousness.

Charley and Shelley Wininger

On a warm summer afternoon, I sat down with Charley and Shelley Wininger. Both in their seventies, Charley and Shelley have spent two decades acting as community leaders, mentors, and proselytizers of psychedelic joy. What I love so deeply about them is their apparent and intense love for each other and their dedication to creating community gatherings with psychedelics like MDMA centered on connection, pleasure, and love. Charley is the author of the book *Listening to Ecstasy: The Transformative Power of MDMA*, and Shelley presents at conferences and events on women's sexuality and cannabis. Here's what they had to say.

(This interview has been edited for content and clarity.)

Charley: With MDMA, I would continuously have this uncanny experience of surprise that my body could feel so good, that it was capable of feeling so good. It felt like I was alive, only more so. Like, "I could live like this forever." And the feeling that emanates from my chest on a good MDMA high, that emanates through my whole body and being is one of such expansiveness, where my ego is on vacation for the day, and my body boundaries are dissolving, and I'm feeling that I'm a part of everything. Just the simple pleasure of that, of not being constrained by my ego, my self-concept, or my physical body. Or my age! Not being constrained by my age!

Shelley: I become ageless. I have no age. I don't think about age. My body doesn't hurt. My mind is sharp. On pretty much any psychedelic, I can feel . . . how do I feel? I feel **wonderful!**

Charley: You look like you're in bliss when you're rolling.

Shelley: If we are talking about MDMA, yes. With LSD, I meld with Charley. Once it happened the first time, now it happens on many substances. If I have some cannabis that's a little bit more than usual, I meld with him.

Charley: And there's a pleasure in that. And it's not just a physical pleasure.

Shelley: Oh! Yes, my whole body becomes part of him, and I can't tell where my body begins and where his ends. We're one.

Dee Dee: Charley, you had said Shelley was in bliss when she's on MDMA, and you looked at Shelley, and I could see the love in your eyes. How does it feel to see her in that kind of bliss?

Charley: I'm an empathetic person to begin with, and it's heightened on MDMA. I'm more empathetic with her than I am with anyone else on the planet. So if I see her in bliss, it puts me in bliss. And if she sees me in bliss, it puts her in bliss. It's a cycle. It's ecstatic! And euphoric for me, because she becomes even more beautiful when she's in bliss. So besides that I never thought my body could feel so good, I never thought I could be so in love. I never thought *love could feel so good! Also, with this bliss there is a feeling so profound, it's an easing of the boundaries. For me, that's a relief. Like I said, I'm no longer constrained, but also, I hadn't known I'd been feeling constrained. And my consciousness is wider than what it usually is, and that's a liberating feeling. Ram Dass talked about dying being akin to the experience of taking off an old shoe. So this is like dying being alive. Taking off old clothes that don't fit anymore or old skin that doesn't belong anymore. There's a profound liberation in that. And what could be more pleasurable than that?*

Let's talk about acid. That's even more intense sexually for me. MDMA is not necessarily sexual, depending on how you define sexual. LSD is both hypersensual and hypersexual. Once when I had a guided LSD session, I think it was a disappointment for the guide because he was expecting all kinds of stuff to emerge, but as I was lying there, all I was feeling was my groin. All I really wanted to do was play with myself! I didn't, but the acid was making me feel incredibly alive by having me embody my sexuality.

Dee Dee: *So that's how you interpreted that? That this somatic awakening was a life awakening?*

Charley: *More like an aliveness awakening! I was simply feeling this intensely warm, erotic feeling. Certainly my best orgasms have been on acid or 2C-B. With either of these, once I came, there was a wave of feeling all through me—a wave of release and relief, which had a rippling effect through me over time. Once I'd been turned on to that possibility, I realized I could be sober and have sex of that intensity, and this was a revelation and a liberating one, that my whole body could be sexual, not just the tip of my cock. I didn't know that was possible before acid or psilocybin. It's psychedelics that turned me on to that. It may sound funny, but I didn't know it was allowed! I didn't know God would allow such a thing to happen! It makes me think, who is this God? Not who I thought. God put us here for this too!*

Dee Dee: *Where did the idea come from that that's not why we're* here? I'm curious! Clearly there was an awakening that happened because of psychedelics around how big sexual pleasure could be, how you can connect with your body. What was before that?

Charley: My parents weren't particularly shaming, at least not explicitly. No one said "Don't masturbate." But I had it in my head that I shouldn't. As a fourteen-year-old, I always felt like I should resist the urge. But I couldn't, so I would feel guilty and ashamed. When the counterculture came to town—this was around 1966, when I was sixteen and seventeen—I got in touch with ideas and realizations that there's a more liberated way to look at sex and my body. The revolution, you could say, will not be disembodied! When I was young, I tried to go to high school dances, and I was very awkward and uncoordinated and painfully self-conscious. When I moved into the East Village when I was twenty in 1969, I started smoking cannabis. One day I went to the Fillmore East when the Dead were playing, and people were dancing. And all they were doing was jumping up and down and being in their body. And looking so much happier than me and the kids at the high school dance! They weren't doing a step! They weren't dancing to look good, they were dancing to feel good! I thought, I can do this, and I like it!

Dee Dee: Isn't it amazing what opens up when you think "How does it feel," instead of "How does it look to other people?"

Charley: Yes, getting out of your ego, out of your self consciousness. Cannabis and psychedelics helped me find my own sense of rhythm. With MDMA I feel like I'm being danced. I'm the puppet and it's dancing me across the puppet stage. I feel half my age and half my weight. I can dance and the rhythm is there and I lose myself in it and that's intensely pleasurable. Pleasure is about losing myself. That's what these medicines do. They get me out of my head and into my body. Out of my own way, and I forget myself for a while, the judgements and evaluations relent for a while.

Dee Dee: Somewhere in there is some deeper version of yourself. You're talking about losing yourself, but you're probably connecting to more of what your "Self" actually is.

Charley: *That's right. The real "Self," that was here before I was born and will continue after I'm gone. My essence, that is indestructible. These medicines widen that consciousness.*

Shelley: *I was never told about masturbation. I was eighteen in nursing school, and a book came out about sexual fantasies. I didn't know what a fantasy was for. I was so clueless! I had a lot of one-night stands in the '70s that were never pleasurable. It was just what we did. But I really didn't start getting sexual to the point that it was amazing until I met Charley. I woke up. I woke up to who I am, what my body is capable of. Cannabis was my gateway drug to psychedelics and to sex. We smoked cannabis before we ever did MDMA. And I was like "Wow." When I left my ex-husband, I actually said to myself, "there's got to be more to life than this. I'm just existing." Once I met Charley, I was in a different world. Everything was about being here with him, and learning more about my body, and sex. So, when I started trying LSD and MDMA, it opened up a whole new dimension. It was making me wider and wider. Melding with somebody. And every time we have sex, I do take cannabis.*

Charley: *Because why not?*

Shelley: *Yeah! Especially after menopause—it really helped.*

Charley: *We're proud of our sex life!*

(We all laugh together.)

I'm proud of her. I get a little . . . hmm, what would they call it? Not penis envy, clitoris envy! Shelley will on an average night have twenty orgasms!

Shelley: *Some of them are small. I call them orgs. It comes and goes. Like a little one. But there's more! There's more! I have so many different kinds of orgasms. But I never would have had this, I don't think, unless I had somebody who was sexually awake as he is and using the medicines. Now I can do certain things without the medicines, but the medicines are enhancers. Why not?*

Dee Dee: *You're making an interesting point, both of you. One thing that's emerged from the medical psychedelic model, or it circulates from the idea of how we're supposed to use psychedelics* seriously, which is you use them for a specific goal and then you don't necessarily keep doing them. And what you're talking about is, why not? This is enhancing, and you're obviously conscious about whether it's causing any harm in your life. Keeping that in check.

Charley: Right. We're very careful. And Shelley can now tune into her body without chemical enhancers because once you've been turned on, your mind, your body is opened to what's possible.

Shelley: Most of it is using my brain power. Using fantasy, using music. I use music a lot. Whether it be cannabis, LSD, MDMA, I need music. Can I share one fantasy that would be apropos to the book? I'm ageless. Any medicine makes me ageless. I don't think, "Oh, my God, I'm seventy-two years old and doing this." No! I'm just who I am. So the fantasy is that I'm younger, and being introduced to a medicine for the first time and just lying there. For this particular fantasy the music is rock and roll, and I'm back in the day. I'm fantasizing that this happened to me in my early twenties because I missed it then. I'm making up for lost time. I meet Charley, and I'm telling my body, "Let the medicine work," and I give myself to the medicine. I don't think about orgasms. There's no agenda. I just feel the medicine. So in my mind I'm watching a porn film of myself in the East Village, this whole scenario.

Charley: Hippie porn!

Shelley: Yeah, yeah! And, oh my God. By letting the medicine work, not fighting it, I've had full body orgasms. I do a full body check. Where am I feeling it? My head is buzzing, my arms are buzzing, my toes are buzzing. My whole body is buzzing! Next thing I know I have a whole body orgasm!

Dee Dee: Shelley, you're talking about your fantasy of having this in your twenties, but actually you came to psychedelics as a more mature person. For you, what is the relationship between that emotional maturity and how you experienced psychedelics? Many people do this in their twenties, and they aren't having deep experiences. I don't think recreational is a dirty word at all,

> *but you're coming to this mindfully. Joyfully and mindfully, but mindfully.*
>
> **Shelley:** *If I had really done it back then, I don't think I would have appreciated it. I would have taken it for granted. I wouldn't have used the medicines to learn about myself, especially as I do now, having one partner. I know that when I'm hot, he's hot. And when he's hot, I'm hot. So we're feeding off of each other. It's much more pleasurable, deeper, heart-felt, body-felt. I'm in this intense relationship with this man. I'm him and he's me.*

David Ortmann

David Ortmann is a psychotherapist, sex therapist, minister, and writer. I first encountered David at a sex therapy conference many years ago when he delivered one of the most compassionate and brilliant presentations I've ever seen detailing his work with a highly stigmatized population of therapy clients. He has devoted his career to anti-racist work and supporting sexually marginalized individuals. He is the co-author of *Sexual Outsiders: Understanding BDSM Sexualities and Communities*, and many other professional and popular articles. Here is his story.

Background: 1976–1979

The great Michael Pollan, in his classic game changer How to Change Your Mind, *makes an important point of taking into consideration both one's "set" and "setting" before embarking on any journey involving altered or psychedelic states; I wholeheartedly endorse this. The set and setting that one is born into? That's a different kind of set and setting, not up for choice. My "set" was a small American town, hardly a suburb, influenced by a religious cult of toxic restrictions, terminal neediness, and a pathologically self-absorbed guilt. It was a putrid rot I would later come to call, "spiritual poverty." That set was placed firmly within a larger social "setting" where children were discouraged from saying no, and taught to refrain from asking questions. It was a point in American history where the physical beating of small children by much larger adults wielding objects was common; perversion confused with love. It was a time and a place violently opposed to one boy's unusually open and inquisitive nature. That boy was me.*

Waves: 1976–1978

The riding of waves has been a literal and metaphoric symbol present throughout my life. When not engaged in the endless, repetitive days of grade school, my family spent part of our summer at the beach. From our first meeting, the ocean was both God and Home for me. I practiced body surfing over, under, and through the wild waves of the Atlantic, an elven, blue-eyed, straw-haired child of the 1970s. This was long before sunblock and iPads, before the days when every child got an award, when children were more or less seen and not heard, and before the days when children were taught how to say no. The physical world still held fascination for us, and some of us were misused and damaged in ways subsequent generations cannot understand. At the beach, the difference between my sister and father and my mother and myself became evident. My mother and I ran into the ocean each summer like we were embracing an old friend.

My mother was adventurous, as was her eight-year-old son. Submerged to my waist in the Atlantic Ocean, I learned to ride the waves. Riding a wave involved leaping up to meet it at the precise moment. It was a science and an art, a combination of forces that still thrills me. My mother was an expert at this. We glided over those rollers, and soon I'd feel that anticipatory exhilaration, akin to the tingle in one's stomach when excited, awaiting the huge waves I called "tidal waves," because they looked just like the tidal wave that rolled on, unending, during the opening credits of TV's Hawaii 5-0. *I was too young to understand the show, but I loved watching that wave.*

Those waves "rolled" quite a distance from where we were planted, and we would watch them grow and gain power. Being caught up in those waves was an unavoidable joy for me, better than any rollercoaster. At my size, these majestic crashers completely enveloped me, lifting me off my feet and turning me over and over in submerged summersaults. They pulled me forward in one moment, backward in the next and left me completely uncertain as to which end was up. It was me and the Atlantic Ocean together, as it always felt so natural to be. I was always safe. That inherent knowledge was unshakable. Nature was safe. It took care of me.

People and institutions? They were different.

Waves: 2019

On a Saturday afternoon forty years later, I was no more afraid of the waves from the powerfully strong psychedelic medicine flowing through, under, and over me as those created by the great Atlantic in which I played as a boy.

Never forget to play. If you've forgotten, then remember, relearn, and practice. Play is not only for children. It's a tool that helps us face extraordinary challenges and epiphanies until the day our bodies die. The key lies in not caring about how you appear to others, an inaccurate and limiting thought-trap in us all, and from which we could all benefit from turning the collective volume down.

When journeying through an altered state of consciousness, your best ally is knowing yourself. For example, my body always gets cold at some point on these expeditions and warm bedding and clothing are always at hand. I also get warm and will spend some of that time naked. Water, that magic elixir of life, is never far away either. All journeys require hydration, plus water is super fun to look at when traveling. The journey on which I'd been called that day, was met with conscious intention on my part. I'd been experiencing the emotional equivalent of a splinter working its way toward the surface for months; now it wanted out. Psychedelic states of consciousness have always treated me like a loving, old friend. I, in turn, always maintain a reverential respect for their awesome powers and a childlike affection for their spirited magick.

I knew I must embrace a descent into my own personal hell to do something which needed to be done, so I could evolve into whatever it is I was becoming on the material plane. Transcendence involves letting go. Growth requires change. As the medicine within began to peak, I reassured myself that I was flanked by two powerful traveling partners—the Medicine and the Self—both of which have always had *my back. I knew I was in my sun-drenched bedroom, at the top floor of a Manhattan apartment house, in which I've also always felt safe. I was bundled up in a huge carved oak bed with the kind of quilts and down featherbeds that are common in Europe but not so much in America. The next intake of breath was the breath of a newborn and the breath of the Universe. Slowly, all around me, my bedroom began to fade, growing darker despite the sunlight. I watched it all slowly melt in shadow around me, becoming a place I recognized but had not visited in a long time. I knew what was coming and reminded my body to calm itself, while reminding my mind and spirit that I was safe and everything was going to be okay.*

This, I'd learned, is one of the prices paid by healers and guides, undertaken throughout time, in the interest of later guiding others. My eyelids felt heavy. I let them close and, when I opened them, I found myself in a bathroom. That *bathroom, a cavernous hole carved into the chasmic space beneath the bleachers near a football field in 1982.*

Bill: 1982

I've always known I would see him again.

Bill looked just the same that afternoon during my medicine journey as he did that long, sad summer day back in 1982. I took a deep breath and just went with it, a lesson both instinctual and trained into me after years of meditative and spiritual study. I was still grounded in my New York nest. I was safe. It was 2019, though the medicine was bringing me back to 1982, and here I was, where it all started. The parking lot. I exhaled again, realizing I was meant to remember it all. I was okay with that. Splinters hurt most when being pulled out.

After finishing eighth grade, I was finally free of Iselin Middle School. Next year I'd be a freshman in high school. I joined the John F. Kennedy Memorial High School Cross Country team that summer because I had to belong to something, or someone, somehow. Now, every morning in August 1982, a month before the new school year began, the team gathered to run at 8 a.m. each day in the park. But this was no ordinary practice day. It was special, a charity marathon at neighboring Woodbridge High School. The marathon included both a two- and five-mile run. Our coach decided participation would not only qualify as daily practice, but it would also be a change of scene and allow us to mingle among the greater community of Woodbridge Township.

But why was I alone?

Then, I remembered the two marathons. From the looks of the parking lot, it seemed most people there were running the five, leaving me by myself. I had a lot of downtime after successfully completing the two-mile, finishing my post-run stretching, lingering, and walking it off, while also looking for a place to perch away from the bleachers where it was too windy. Soon I'd found a long cement parking block still close to the track. I've no memory of how long I was sitting there alone before I was no longer alone.

"Hi." I heard a light-spirited, but hearty voice. "Mind if I join you?" I looked up to see a bigger-than-life shadow character backlit by the sun, lending him a glowing God-like aura. He was much older than I, and visibly very fit. And he was addressing me.

"Uh . . . yes. Um, I mean 'no.' I don't mind." He slid down with remarkable speed and eased next to me. Though we were not touching and inches apart, I could feel the heat from his body. Bill, as he introduced himself, had a mane of thick wavy perfectly white hair. He wore a pair of navy blue, polyester coach shorts—a style popular again in 2023—but now referred to as retro. The shorts were very tight and stretchy, ending at his muscular mid-thigh. Tucked into them was a white t-shirt and over that he wore a half-unzipped navy blue track jacket with white piping.

"I can't wait to go home and relax after this." Bill sighed, tilting his head back and looking at the sky. I remember being repulsed by the thick salt and pepper chest hair peeking out from the t-shirt at his throat.

"Yeah, me too." I said, also looking skyward.

What was I supposed to say? I didn't know anything about relaxing. I was always coiled up, preparing for the next onslaught.

When I turned my gaze back to him, Bill's eyes were looking at my legs and his mouth was making words. Relaxing, he expounded, involved his girlfriend (or girlfriends), a fireplace, and low music. It took a while to register that a man was talking to me about girls, and that was a first. I felt noticed and special. I also felt like an actor standing before the all-encompassing, critical eye of the film camera, except someone had given me the wrong script, or perhaps had forgotten to give me a script at all. I was, for several moments, frozen in place.

"You have really nice legs," Bill said, "so muscular for such a young guy." His smile was captivating. I watched his gaze move over my calves and my thighs, just coming into their muscular own. His alpine blue eyes came to rest just a second too long on that mysterious cluster of boyish manhood where my thighs met, an area I'd only recently discovered the pleasures of.

I was confused. Bill was strikingly handsome, like a movie star—and that was confusing too! Sure, I thought some of my male classmates were cute, but guys my dad's age—and Bill was older than them—didn't talk to me like this and I certainly wasn't used to other guys admiring my body or giving me compliments about anything. Before I knew it, the conversation was expertly steered into pretty graphic detail, with Bill describing further his definition of relaxation. Now there was a bed and candles and oil and moisture and slippery slickness culminating in even more wetness and pleasure. I imagined a 1970s bachelor pad, replete with animal skins, candles, and . . . well, that was all. I didn't really know what sex looked like, and that fact made me something of a sitting duck on that parking block. I was still a boy, albeit with muscled legs dusted with downy baby blonde hairs. I don't remember exactly when Bill's talk, which was engaging me just as any secret peek behind the curtains of adult life would, turned dark. Compliments about the outline of my boyish manhood, packed tightly into my cutoff sweat shorts, to my eyes, and to what he was, in about thirty seconds, to call, "The prize—that big cock I can see is already bigger than most other boys your age, am I right?"

I missed that tip of his hand, concealed within a compliment, until just now. Bill had compared the size of the confusing erection in my shorts with those of other boys my age. So, he'd seen the bodies of other boys my age. He'd done this sort of thing before. I thought this whole weird interaction was happening to me only. It never dawned on me that Bill was repeating a pattern. I thought our encounter was by chance. I thought I was special. I didn't have any idea of what another guy's penis looked like, not that I was entirely disinterested in the subject. At that moment, I just liked the idea that mine was, according to a male adult, bigger than most. My total ignorance of comprehending, understanding, creating, and maintaining boundaries with adults had long ago set me up for what was to come. I couldn't draw boundaries any better with my peers, and that bore its own strange fruit. I always admired the confidence of the tough, socially dominant boys in middle school, boys who were developing faster than I was and brimming with a swagger I both wanted and was attracted to.

I was always somehow outside the circles. My stares of unadulterated idolatry toward these boys, though unconscious to me, got me in a lot of trouble at school. Looking back, it was all somehow innocently pre-sexual, or meta-sexual, akin to the realms of being awestruck by art, or a waterfall, or anything beautiful. I stared at those boys the same way I stared at paintings at the Frick in New York City or, years later, at the more-alive-than-life sculpture of Michelangelo's sublime David, forever and always, in Florence.

I was soon getting hit by more than just puberty. At that time and place in history if you were that boy who stared too long at other boys, you'd invariably get beaten, jumped, or targeted, becoming an outlet, a repository for the aggression, and repressed desires of any boy who wanted to use you, especially once you'd been labelled a faggot aloud. After that, the beatings and bullying went epidemic. By then, I noticed teachers and counselors, from the principal to the cleaning staff, turn quietly away, pretending they'd seen nothing . . . leaving me to believe that I was nothing, and that this war against me was just, and deserved. By the third month of seventh grade, I was the school faggot, and that word had the grossly adhesive power to last through high school.

Everything I described above was called "teasing" back then and not taken anywhere nearly as seriously as it is today, and it was reinforced from all fronts. Between church, parenting, ancestral family trauma deeply rooted in generations-long styles of self-medicating, of avoiding—or exploiting—conflict, and my general lack of social sophistication painted a big ol' sparkly pink bullseye on my back, targeting me for men like Bill.

"Wait 'til she takes that big cock in her mouth," Bill was saying now. "That . . . now that *is* pleasure I can hardly describe . . . but I know you'll love it. All guys do."

This conversation was now far out of my control, though it had never been in *my* control, and—even as I write these words from both the safety of my home in 2023 and from the safe distance of four decades—I can still feel the dizzying conflict between the fires of self-preservation, a conflagration in my gut that told me this brief interaction had gone from neutral to friendly, from friendly to curious, from curiosity to sexual, from sexual to borderline unsafe, and from that unsafety to a danger so strong, I was amazed at how still, silent, and undeniably present it was. All that mental, physical and emotional conflict, distorted by the mighty force of a thirteen-year-old boy's arousal. I had no preparation, skill, or choice to do anything to prevent what I knew was, had been, already happening.

By the time Bill was declaring that "A man's gotta get off a lot more than girls do . . . " and something about "helping each other out," I was looking for a way out, but my focus was filled with the static of a lifetime of religious brainwashing, an unconscious, relentless process of being told to reject and disown anything resembling my own needs, the effects of poor parenting, and of a society and a school system that failed to teach me what boundaries were, let alone how to create them, especially with other adults. I was such pathetic easy pickings. Good, obedient, little Catholic boys did what they were told. That's the distillation of all the horrors, lies, and manipulations of being raised without a voice.

Don't fuss.

Don't complain.

Just spread your legs and shut up.

I ventured valiantly with, "Um . . . they're all gonna be done with the five-mile run soon and uh . . . I have to go to the bathroom . . ." I recall now, from the safety and sanity of this moment, that a part of that kid was both coiled to flee and another, well-trained, part of him looked up at Bill, asking his permission. I was not yet a man, but no longer a little boy. I was a freak, just as I was told at school and church and bad things happened to boys who were labeled freaks and faggots and bitches. Even in that moment, looking for an excuse to extract myself from Bill, I was years away from using this kind of language and only barely understood its power or meaning—and I was certainly not aware of its intention, its purpose in keeping me in a line I never consented to queue up in.

My brain, my body, my Self, fought interminably for survival in a world that did not want me in it, kept making that point clear, and didn't look like it was going to change anytime soon. The battle between my instinct for self-preservation and my boyhood conditioning to ask permission was still unfurling inside of me as Bill sprung up after me with, "That's cool. I need to piss, too."

I can remember thinking, "Fuck. Fuck. Fuck," remaining half-aware of my surroundings and half-aware of Bill's movements, looking for other potential avenues of escape. He walked close beside me, on my left, blocking the damn sun again, as I walked slowly to the bathroom at the other end of the parking lot, my heart beating visibly through my brand-new marathon commemoration t-shirt that day, beating out of arousal, fear, and many other words for feelings I didn't understand.

"Maybe I should go in alone?" I ventured. Bill smiled down at me, his head blocking the sun. That smile! It was a powerful weapon that had me in its crosshairs.

"Nah," Bill said dismissively. "We're all men here."

The Bathroom: 1982

In 1982, the bathroom at Woodbridge High School looked like it was pulled right from a horror movie. Any hope I had of escaping *deflated when I saw a long wall of ancient urinals, utterly unprotected by anything like the dividers later, modern public restrooms would come to have. Standing before one of these behemoth sarcophagi, I remember thinking perhaps it was a portal I could escape through, though in the next moment it became a threatening door through which I could not go.*

The stained porcelain alcoves with their rusty hair-clotted drains repelled me. The smell of ammonia, piss, and isolation overcame me. I felt the cold, aching silence of the place. The huge windows were covered with gray paint, shielding any light from the outside, and forbidding any glimmer of sunlight into this space. It was all there. I remember watching some of that paint flake, peel, and fall to the filthy floor. Mostly, it did what it was painted to do—to hide, to cover, to keep the shadow secrets it bore witness to.

Years later I told two trusted loved ones about what Bill did to me in that bathroom, but I was already telling it like it had happened to someone else. Then, I locked it away in a tight, little box, bound with the kind of string once found in old Jersey City bakeries. The red and white twine that doesn't break. I was confident the box containing that day would join the others, filled with their specific horrors, all as well-wrapped and tightly packed as the next. I didn't realize I was building my own closet, or my own coffin. I trusted these woeful secrets would remain contained. And they did. Until they didn't.

The Bathroom: 2019

And now, here deep in my medicine ceremony, we stand together again.

Bill and I have returned to the bathroom.

I can feel it all again, the smell, the sight, the abysmal silence. I see the windows still covered in flaking paint. The urinals stand as tall and ghostly as ever. My awareness of my astral body on this plane is that of a very young—perhaps five-year-old—boy. He's very blonde, and he's got a gentle smile on his face. The other is a glowing idealized form of my current adult body and they meld back and forth with ease because they are, I realize now, the same.

Bill looks exactly as he did that day and I am present enough to recognize his appeal as the extremely attractive and charismatic man he appears as, and still not blame myself for the events of that day. Many things can be true. His form was somewhat cowering and his energy was . . . not dark, but very heavy. His head hung down and I knew he wasn't smiling. I also knew that he had stolen something from me that day, and I made that traumatic encounter even more so by giving into fear, shame, and silence. This is not about blame. It's about exponential conscious awareness.

With each breath I took, this strong, luminous energy coursed through me, a force stronger than electricity or tidal waves. It was both the familiar feeling of immense power and of an acute, profound aliveness. I was now in a position to give Bill something, and I chose to. I don't recall the specifics of how my body went from bundled in bed to standing before him in that metaphysical bathroom, but do remember tucking my hand under his chin and gently bringing his face to meet mine. He was in torment, though that word is too small. There were stains running down his face from the dirty, decades-long tears, fears, regrets and . . . you'll have to excuse me because words fail to capture the psychedelic realm, just as they sometimes do down here in the material realm. Suddenly, I saw him as a boy, but just for the most fleeting of seconds, so brief I couldn't extract any imagery from that moment of sight.

I know this is not really about Bill, or even about me. It is a much bigger part of a vicious earthly cycle of men hurting their fellow men, their brothers. It is but one small example of man's inhumanity to man, in an endless history of our fumbled, all-too-human attempts at connecting and conquering, of bonding and playing. Perhaps we men need to rediscover that basic trust of being close and available to one another . . . and as that thought flies away . . . I'm breathing deeply and expanding with that same simultaneous profound breath of a newborn and the tiny breath of the entire universe. It was my job to end this now. I knew this with an unwavering clarity. I was ending this, on my terms, to free Bill, free a part of me, and for the benefit, somehow, of all of us. The word forgiveness comes to mind and it lingers over us in little sparkly streaks of sunlight that manage to fight their way through the tiny portions of window where the paint has fallen away.

I tell him, aloud, that it is okay. I tell him I forgive him. I hold him in my arms, feeling his body tremble and heave. I hold him close for a long, long time, rocking him like I would rock my own child because, right now, he is. I hold and stroke and console him and my forgiveness pours all over him, covering him in what looks like a blanket of my own powerful light. I know that I get to hold him until it's time to stop. That time comes, and I let him go. He's sort of glowing as he walks off. He stops, turning to wave at me. His lips don't move and he makes no sound, but he is thanking me. Bill disappears and soon the bathroom becomes my bedroom, and 1982 mingles with 2019, and I realize in an ethereal yet embodied way that Bill was worth my forgiveness. The Forgiveness.

And so am I.

And so are we all.

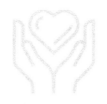

8
BIG LOVE

A Psychedelic Philosophy of the Heart

*Dragonfly out in the sun, you know what I mean, don't
    you know?*
Butterflies all havin' fun, you know what I mean
Sleep in peace when day is done, that's what I mean
And this old world is a new world
And a bold world, for me . . .

"FEELING GOOD" AS SUNG BY NINA SIMONE

WHAT IS LOVE?

What do we mean when we use the word "love?" What do we *really* mean when we say "I love you?" Are we talking about an action, as in the act of loving? Are we describing a feeling, a sensation, an inner knowing? Is it a complex neurochemical reaction that can be inhibited or enhanced? Or is love a calling, a state of grace we must cultivate and work at? When we look in someone's eyes and say "I love you" and hear it in return, often with a mellifluous shifting of emphasis from "I *love* you" to the reciprocal "I love *you*," how can we ever really know that the self-state, the experience of love that is being professed, is actually the same thing at all? Can we ever be too liberal with the words "I love you?" Some family lore about my childhood is that I began to speak in full sentences at nine months old. Of course, no one believed my mother that her nine-month-old kid could do this until she produced a cassette tape recording of my glorious first sentence. On the tape, I just said, "I love you!" over and over. These words, apparently, were my first, and most important mantra, and ones that have served me well even in the worst moments of life.

One of the things I find most thrilling about the expanding discourse on psychedelics is that it pushes the boundaries between what we consider to be the realm of clinical science (symptoms, brain states, neurobiological reactions), and the unconventional marriage that has been forged with the subjective features of the psychedelic experience (the mystical, the noetic quality, and the experience of universal love, or embodying love itself). It seems to be that perhaps the single most pervasive feature of all psychedelic experiences when undertaken with an openness for growth and healing is touching into a quality of transcendent love. Psychedelic science continues to grapple with how exactly to understand, codify, and research these experiences of spiritual connection, deep inner knowing, connection to all things, and psychedelic love. And some wonder whether they need to be codified at all. But one thing that scientists studying these medicines agree on is that these elusive experiences of connection, perspective, and love, though poorly understood by science, seem to change us in fundamentally positive ways and have great utility in our growth process. And yet, the question as to what *love itself* actually is has been woven through the classical philosophy of Plato and Aristotle and recurs through the history of art, literature, and religion with no unifying or concrete answer. Turns out, this universal human experience, and pervasive psychedelic experience, is not easily understood at all.

Thinkers and lovers have always intuitively known that love comes in many unique forms: the familial, the universal, the spiritual, and of course, the erotic. All of these forms of love can be used to soothe, to exhilarate, to heal, to connect. But feelings of love—and the fealty and clannishness that can be an expectation of some socialized expressions of love—can also be used to control, to manipulate, or to inhibit individuation from toxic relationships, community, or family. Perhaps this isn't love at all. Saying "I love you" is at times a milestone, meaning we are somewhere deeply significant in a relationship. Or it can be a spell. A reassurance. Even a tactic. To say "I love you" and then cause harm is a confusing and common occurrence. Can we love and harm at the same time? Or can we love someone who also has harmed us?

It seems, after all, that the way we express love, much like the way we experience psychedelics, takes on the characteristics of our mindset and our setting. Psychedelic visionary Stan Grof once described psychedelics as "non-specific amplifiers,"[1] meaning the medicine illuminates our internal framework that preexists in our psyches that can then be considered, understood, and made meaning of rather than providing a specific or predictable experience from the medicine itself. I believe love, and the way we practice love, may be quite the same. We feel a deep connection or passion for someone. What we choose to do with that love, how we practice love, whether we are willing to surrender to love, is up to us and guided by our ethics, beliefs, and how we are shaped by our life experiences. If this is true, then the most powerful expression of the psychedelic experience might be to baptize us in a boundless ocean of universal love, and the outcome of psychedelic consciousness might be to heal ourselves enough to prepare our hearts to fall deeply and totally in love with the world and with each other.

BIG LOVE

While the forms, flavors, and ways of practicing love are nearly limitless, I will describe a form of love I believe to be enhanced by the psychedelic experience as it relates to sexuality and relationships, and in fact our relationships to ourselves and relationship to the Earth. There are some common threads that can support us in developing a general psychedelic theory of love and understand how psychedelics may help our experience of love to flourish. I will keep my language simple, but my vision wide. Psychedelic love, at its most profound, can be described in two beautiful, bold words: Big Love.

Big Love is an expression of love that is felt directly and practiced in our relationship to ourselves, to others, and to our environment, and is mediated by a perspective that we are not only linked to one another, but also connected to something that is greater than the sum of its parts. Big Love encompasses the expansive universal love for all beings that is nearly ubiquitous in psychedelic experiences, but it is intertwined with a deeply intimate expression of love that creates space for securely attached, personal love between people, and indeed cherishing the individuality and autonomy of those we love. It is the spiritually mature love that allows us to sacrifice our own immediate wants and desires to offer other people the space to be themselves, to be safe, to be free, and to flourish with our love blessing. We are called to step into a giant psychedelic field of love that allows us to actually embrace the state of *being love* itself. Big Love, at its core, dismantles the phrase "*I* love *you*," because it is a state of inner knowing that there is really no "I" or "you," no lover and loved. And yet, the paradox of Big Love means that universal love will never eclipse our very human need for personal love. Psychedelic love also requires that we develop the capacity for true intimacy and connection. That we can, without reservation, allow other people to feel our love in abundance. As it turns out, there is actually no feeling of universal love that is so transcendent that we can bypass the need to give and receive the words "I love *you*," as often as possible.

A PERSONAL NOTE ON LOVE

One of the most profoundly clarifying experiences of my adult life happened a few years ago when my partner and I returned from a strenuous, multi-day hiking trip and, of course, scheduled ourselves to go immediately back to work. We were getting ready in the morning when they started to feel ill. In a few short minutes it became clear something was very, very wrong. Still not understanding the gravity of the situation, I called a cab. A cab. And thank the gods for the kindest cab driver on planet Earth who took us to the nearest emergency room. Let me tell you, if you walk into an emergency room in Brooklyn, New York, no one is rushing to help you like on TV. But after a few preliminary tests, it became clear my partner was experiencing a life-threatening illness.

I was in a state of utter bewilderment and terror. How does a person in their forties who just returned from hiking over a hundred miles, who otherwise lives a very healthy lifestyle, get sick like this? I remember meeting my partner's eyes while they were on a stretcher with doctors circulating around them. Their expression was of fear, but not only that, it was an expression of love. I will never forget that moment for my entire life. Our life together changed completely on that day. You have no idea just how much, and how fully, you love someone until the moment you see with your own eyes that you could lose them. That's the moment when I came to know the space between love and terror, ecstasy and grief. To really love fully is also to accept the greatest risk. The risk of giving yourself fully to love and then having it torn away. The immediate aftermath of the situation was of course shock and trauma. It's a story for a whole other book how that event brought back crippling fear, nightmares, and anxiety. But we got through it.

My partner not only lived, and gained some status as a total medical anomaly ten physicians later, but we decided to live better than ever. We both went to trauma therapy, but more importantly, took everything we ever wanted to change that was in our power to change and did it. Conflict disappeared from our relationship. What's there to fight about when you could die? Hate your job? Change it, because you are going to die. Want to focus more on having the intimate life you want? Do it now. Because death is coming. Strangely, once the initial terror subsided and every day wasn't plagued with the threat of more mystery illness, we started really living. It was that moment in the emergency room when time stopped, where I saw fear in the face of the person I love and was helpless to do anything material to stop what was happening, that I really surrendered. What I *could* do was love completely and embrace vulnerability in that moment, and then the next day, and every day after. My psychedelic experiences prepared me to stand in the face of my greatest fear and embrace it. In facing it, I gained something tremendous. Genuine presence, the ability to identify and live our values as a couple, and opening my heart to the deepest levels of love.

Big Love, psychedelic love, requires that we are willing to be broken open, that we might, for a brief time, lose ourselves entirely for the purpose of connecting to something much, much bigger. It is in this process of losing ourselves that we are found. It is only in the willingness to abandon judgment, to forgive ... to soften, that we can be remolded into something stronger. When we accept and know that we are part of a greater whole, it is only then that we truly realize the harm we do to each other and to the Earth *is harm we inflict on ourselves*. When we apply this psychedelic philosophy of love to our sex life, to our intimate relationships, to our partnerships, we are asked to take a big risk. It is an invitation to go deep. But going deep means that we relinquish our right to protect ourselves from heartbreak. We are fully there, fully invested. Fully present. We surrender to love. We let love annihilate us.

♥

This book is peppered with research, examples, and stories of how psychedelics can occasion certain phenomena like the mystical experience, "ego death," and qualities of inner acceptance and non-judgment. While these are compelling concepts, they are repeated so many times in the literature they have become abstract. The much more important question is *why* are these features of the psychedelic experience important and how do they relate to love? The truth is, if our psychedelic experiences do not lead us to a place that allows us to love more deeply, to accept ourselves and others, to sacrifice our immediate wants and desires for the well-being of ourselves, others, and the Earth, then they are, simply put, a light show. A carnival attraction. An experience we have and brush off unchanged.

Allow me to introduce one psychedelic scientist who has taken the question of entheogenic love quite seriously. Dr. Adele Lafrance is a researcher, clinician, and author. When her name comes up among colleagues, it is generally followed by some form of admiring sigh and the phrase, "I love her." She's a person who is inspiring a field obsessed with scientific legitimacy to think in a new way. In imagining a conclusion for this book, I wanted to feature what to me is perhaps the most important and overlooked research happening in psychedelics today that stands to illuminate a more heart-centered approach to psychedelic science. Adele is one of the architects of The Love Project, a research endeavor aimed at exploring the experience of psychedelic love in all its vastness. The Love Project is not only about documenting the experiences of psychedelic love felt by both medicine guides and journeyers, but to take the findings and use them to influence the way we think about psychedelic—and non-psychedelic—science and therapy. In fact, Adele pointed out, her original impetus to study love was to use the exploration to inform a model that includes love as part of the healing process in conventional health care settings which she believes could be an "instant revolution."

At the time of writing, The Love Project is still very much underway, but preliminary research showed that the most profound experiences of love felt during psychedelic states were love *for* others, the experience of "being love" itself, and experiencing love *from* others. In her research, the experience of love for others, and in fact all beings, was the most common and profound form of love linked to psychedelic experience. Adele shared with me that over eighty percent of her study respondents stated that their psychedelic experiences of love changed their relationship to God, spirituality, and consciousness, and nearly all of the subjects—both psychedelic users as well as guides—believed that the experience of psychedelic love was helpful for healing.

I started my conversation with Adele by asking why she thought that the topic of love is absent from the contemporary psychedelic discourse and why psychedelic therapists are often not talking about love with their clients despite its omnipresence in psychedelic experiences. She laughed,

> I read a research paper recently and I believe the author used the words "positive, strong affective experiences," and I thought, "Oh, I think they're referring to love!" Love has been considered, and continues to be considered by many, as unprofessional, unscientific, and unethical in conventional healing spaces. I also think that clinicians or care providers are afraid that love may be misconstrued if spoken about in clinical settings and therefore could lead to a potential negative impact on either themselves in the form of accusations of professional misconduct, or have a negative impact on the person

that they're supporting due to misunderstanding.* The other piece is that so many of us struggle with using that word with our closest people. Period! So it'd be natural for there to be difficulties with bringing love into clinical work. In our own personal lives we can find all kinds of clever ways to reduce the vulnerability that we experience when expressing love. Instead of saying "I love you," we might say, "I have a lot of love for you," or "love ya." Of course that will be amplified in our professional lives as well. I think we need to be able to talk about love explicitly in our lives, and as therapists with our clients.

How many people have been told by their therapists, doctors, or guides that they are loved? Or asked about love in their lives and how more love can support healing? Adele believes that being able to navigate love with clients in a therapeutic space is just not something therapists are trained to do, but they need to be. She continued, "So many people have been hurt by people they love, and so love ends up being a really scary space that's incredibly vulnerable. In fact," she said, "when it comes to love, we are all in need of a little rehabilitation."

For Adele, and for myself and many other psychedelic clinicians, it seems obvious that training providers to know how to talk about and cultivate love with clients in psychedelic work could change the entire landscape of how we provide care and deepen the impact of psychedelic therapy. But there is a nagging question. What do we do with these psychedelic experiences of all-encompassing universal love when there is still so much suffering in the world? Adele admitted, "Those universal love experiences can be disheartening. We come back to our lives where there are multiple wars going on, active genocide, maltreatment of women and children, racism. It's really hard to have big experiences of psychedelic love and then come back to our current world. It requires a lot of grief work, and the belief that things will get better. I really do believe in an evolution of consciousness towards

---

*It's essential to clarify that Adele is interested in tapping into qualities of universal love in clinical work, not erotic love that would be harmful to a therapeutic relationship.

a more loving reality. But in our lifetimes, it might be limited."

Whether we use psychedelics for our own personal growth and healing, or as part of a family or community ritual, we are called to embrace something beyond just the resolution of our own individual symptoms or traumas, or even to connect with our community for that one experience. Psychedelic work must open us up not only to deeper empathy, but to action. What can we do to actually make the suffering of others better, even if it's small? How can we bear witness to the suffering in the world and keep a tender, loving heart? How do we remain hopeful that, as Adele puts it, a more loving reality is possible? We are called to ask ourselves, on the deepest level, what exactly is our healing for? It's wonderful to feel better, but if that transformation does not extend into more kindness, more love, and more hope, then it is incomplete.

I would like to gently frame that there is indeed a potential shadow side to these big experiences of psychedelic universal love, as profound and transformative as they can be. It is this same shadow that exists in some spiritual disciplines that teach concepts related to the "self" as being illusory, or teach that it is our attachment to our lives, to certain outcomes, or to other people, that is the root cause of suffering. When we have big psychedelic experiences that can give us a glimpse that "all is one," or that the assemblage of personality traits and life experiences we experience as "self" is not exactly who we really are at our core, that can blow open our perception of reality and radically change how we choose to live our lives. But we can also be tempted to assume that this new perception of reality itself is the lesson, and that how we treat ourselves and other people on a very human level is not as important as these spiritual principles. But what if these little glimmers of transcendent reality are actually just playful nudges not to take ourselves so seriously, and not to believe in everything we see or perceive as being how we think it is?

Having a big medicine experience that shows you there is no real "self," isn't very useful to us if we don't first learn to deeply and radically love ourselves in our own humanity and hold that as foundational to how we live our lives. Likewise, and more germane to the topic of this book, universal love is actually pretty hollow if we aren't willing to surrender to the messy, passionate, painful, ecstatic, and transformative power of erotic love with another human being. To me, the practice of psychedelic love is realized when we embrace the suffering, the heartbreak, and welcome the unbearable aching of desire, while still keeping our feet on the ground and our hearts connected to the world. Psychedelic consciousness is the nexus, the singularity, where we feel and witness the big truths about ourselves, the universe, and the interconnection of all things, while simultaneously wrapping ourselves in tender attachment and expressions of personal love in a very human way. The psychedelic spiritual path is not about using our experience of universal Big Love to bypass or transcend the suffering, desire, and heartbreak of our relative existence. But instead, psychedelic consciousness allows us to hang out and revel in the liminal interplay between absolute spiritual truths and the ordinary reality of our beautiful human experience.

THE OCEANIC BOUNDLESSNESS OF PSYCHEDELIC LOVE

What does it mean to enter into the ceremony of the erotic? Who do we become when we shed our chrysalis, unmask ourselves and submit to the wild wanting of the feminine, the soft, the mysterious, and unknowable? What happens to us when we join with our lover, when we take on the very rhythm of one heart beating together, of mouths and tastes, when we become like the wax of a candle dripping, thick and glistening, forming an entirely new shape together born of flame? How does this ritual change when we perform it with the same person for ten years, for twenty, with the nectar of familiarity adding a sweet humor and comfort to our passion? How are we changed when we come back to this erotic prayer over and over again, tracing the same familiar terrain of a body that changes over time, changes so slowly it can barely be noticed? As bodies change, so too do our hearts. We submit to the power that the erotic holds to enliven us, to nourish us to new growth, to take the pieces of our broken and tender hearts and lovingly meld them back together with seams of gold.

It turns out, falling in love is a psychedelic state. We let our beating heart be offered up on the altar of love for sacrifice. The word sacrifice, after all, comes from the roots *sacer*, holy or sacred, and *facere*, to make or do. We make it holy. We participate in the ceremony of erotic love. We offer up our individuality, our fear, our past and future life, to become one being, one mouth, one body, one consciousness, if we are lucky, for a whole lifetime. It's dangerous. And it's awesome. Because we will never be fully free of the specter of grief, the risk of heartbreak. We must pay a steep price to the gods of love for our pleasure. That price is the risk of loss. But it is what must be paid to enter into the deep waters of relationship, fully alive and swimming in the oceanic boundlessness of psychedelic erotic love.

If it's controversial to talk about love when we talk about psychedelics, then psychedelic erotic love is an even riskier endeavor. For the conventional Western psychedelic world, the Psychedelic Erotic sits at the very outskirts. It's like standing at the last outpost on the frontier, and what's left before us is outlaw territory. Fierce and beautiful and expansive. But you better saddle up and be ready for the ride. When we embrace the Psychedelic Erotic, we are going back to our most primal expression of self. We become priests and priestesses and devoted to the ancient gods that rule sensation, desire, joy, and pleasure. We drink from the cup of love. We choose to ride our libidinal energy, rather than be ridden by it. It's a feeling state. A rapturous and feral place that we touch within ourselves, and then we can let it expand out from our hearts to touch others. The Psychedelic Erotic is the practice of edging Eros. We bring ourselves right to the tipping point. Right to the edge where we think we're going to spill out, be consumed, lose our grip. But instead we ride the waves of desire and let it build again and again, with more intensity, more fullness this time, deeper, hotter. Until finally, we release into pleasure.

The Psychedelic Erotic is when we bring all that we are: our lifeforce, our passion, our vulnerability, and our physical bodies in the most naked and honest way to our sexual relationships. But we do it while simultaneously holding the bigger truth that losing ourselves this way with a partner is actually a very deep form of finding ourselves; without pretense, without manipulation, without dysfunctional self-protection. But like all things psychedelic, it first requires that we know we are safe to dissolve and come back together, somehow different than we were before. We have the opportunity to grow, to change, to soften into love. This too is a mystical experience every bit as deep as any plant or molecule can give us. For me, it is deeply beautiful to think of all of the psychedelic plants and molecules as our guides in healing our hearts, but for the very purpose of bringing us to this point. To allow us to stand hand in hand with our lover, looking out over the vast and untamed wildness of erotic love and say yes.

Yes to it all.

The End

Glossary of
Psychedelic Terms

This book refers to key terms and ideas that are used widely in the contemporary discourse on psychedelics. If you are new to psychedelics, understanding these concepts will help to support your reading of the book. This list is not exhaustive, but rather a good primer to accompany your reading. These are not academic definitions, but rather explanations situated within the context of this book drawn from research, cultural discourse, and my own personal experience.

Animism: The belief that all things contain spirit and are animate. In modern psychedelic culture, this term is related to not only the healing "spirits" experienced with sacred plant medicines (such as Grandfather Huachuma or Mother Ayahuasca), but is evolving to include the spirits of even synthetic psychedelics such as ketamine, thought to possess a feminine healing spirit. It is believed that these spirits can be reached and conspire to enhance psychedelic experience and healing, and, more importantly, offer valuable information about what is needed for life alignment and health.

Cast: A late addition to the psychedelic encyclopedia, *cast* is perhaps the most overlooked and most important aspect to consider in a psychedelic journey. Cast refers to the "who," as in who is with you when you are embarking on a medicine journey. As previously stated, safety trumps all. Are there unpredictable, unknown, or unsafe people in the environment? Not good for a safe trip. More difficult to quantify, but no less important, is the "vibe." Are you journeying with someone that expects talking and interaction all night when you want quiet and introspection? If you are in a group context, are all participants able to handle a group dynamic? Conversely, what makes a good guide or tripping partner, or even more important, a good facilitator? Research into the efficacy of traditional psychotherapy finds that there is very little difference between modalities in terms of which one is better (for example, cognitive behavioral, somatic, or psychodynamic). But what did predict therapeutic success? How positively the client felt toward their therapist and the alliance between them.[1] I venture that this is even more true in psychedelic contexts meaning choosing the right guide, journeying partner, or friend to trip with is as important as the medicine itself.

Ceremonial/Ritual Contexts: Ceremonial contexts for psychedelic healing encompass a wide range of settings, including ceremonies within Indigenous healing traditions and neo-shamanic ritual settings. These ceremonies may be facilitated by a shaman or medicine person with robust training who may also belong to family or community lineage of healers rooted in identity and place, neo-shamanic rituals that incorporate live music and other elements often held in a group, or individual work by a facilitator either trained in a shamanic lineage or inspired by (or appropriating) shamanic approaches to healing. Advantages to this approach are that it validates a wide variety of reasons for psychedelic use, including community building, healing spiritual/physical health issues, personal development, and ancestral healing normally excluded from the medical approach. While few critiques exist for this form of psychedelic healing, cautions include problematic participation by people disrespectful of Indigenous healing practices, spaces that heavily emphasize traditional gender roles and may be unsafe or unwelcoming for gender non-conforming people, limited recourse in the event of sexual abuse, and limited medical oversight in cases of destabilized psychological states or health issues.

Empathogen/Entactogen: is another modern descriptor most related to MDMA. *Empathogen* means to generate a state of empathy, and

Entactogen means to "touch within." These terms relate to a quality of openness, increased empathy, and particularly connection with yourself and others.

Entheogen: What a gorgeous word! Entheogen is a term that means "god within," or loosely "taking the divine within." The term leans more toward the spiritual and visionary aspects of psychedelics and implies a heightened experience of sacredness, connection with the divine, and higher truth. Throughout this book, I occasionally use this word synonymously with the term "psychedelic" for style or alliteration. Strictly speaking, they are different as "entheogen" generally refers only to classic psychedelics such as psilocybin and mescaline that reliably offer mystical experiences.

Medical/Clinical Model: The medical model for psychedelic healing is rapidly becoming the dominant mode in the United States and Europe. This term generally refers to both clinical research and psychedelic for-profit ventures targeted to treat specific mental health disorders. If MDMA and psilocybin are rescheduled for medical use, this venue for psychedelic work will likely flourish in the United States. Advantages to the medical model are that psychedelic work can be monitored and guided by trained therapists, physical health can be monitored carefully, substances are ensured to be of pure quality limiting risk from adulterants, and there are (hopefully) means of recourse should there be an ethical breach of conduct on the part of the therapist. Some critiques of the medical model are as follows; it hinges on a pathology-centered perspective requiring a diagnosis and measurable results when in fact psychedelics have far broader spiritual and psychological benefits; the medical model is situated within a for-profit health care system that is not equipped to serve many of those who could benefit from psychedelic work; it gatekeeps ancestral medicines and initiates barriers to access; and it medicalizes experiences that have traditionally been held in community settings by elders.

Naturalistic Contexts: simply refer to using psychedelics in nature, at home with a friend or partner, or even at transformational festivals.

With proper education and precaution, millions of people have safely used psychedelics in this way. The movement most closely connected to naturalistic contexts is the decriminalization movement, which strives to end criminal prosecution for the cultivation, possession, and use of psychedelics, particularly those that are naturally-occurring. The championing of naturalistic psychedelic use is also linked to the critique of the medical model which some believe seeks to medicalize and control psychedelic access for profit within a corrupt health care system. Naturalistic psychedelic use is also associated with most social movements including peace and ecological movements that have been bolstered by psychedelic consciousness.

Plant Medicine: A term that refers to naturally occurring psychedelics all of which have roots in Indigenous traditions. Some medicines are ingested as the whole plant and some processed as an admixture of plants or an extraction. Plant medicines include psilocybin mushrooms, ayahuasca, peyote, huachuma, and iboga.

Psychedelic: The term "psychedelic" was first coined by British psychiatrist Humphry Osmond, and is derived from the Greek roots *psyche* and *delos* which combined mean "mind manifesting."[2] Psychedelic refers broadly to a variety of substances. Originally, the term referred to what is now known as the classic psychedelics, LSD, psilocybin, mescaline, and DMT (and DMT-containing medicines like ayahuasca) that induce strong affective states and visual distortions. Now most people use it broadly to refer to all medicines that alter perception and have healing properties, including ketamine and MDMA. For the purpose of this book, "psychedelic" can also be thought of as an aspirational state or philosophy meaning expansive, erotic, rooted in humanistic values, and consciousness-oriented.

Recreational Contexts: I don't imagine I have to spell out the definition of recreational. This means to use psychedelics for enjoyment and pleasure. It is worth pointing out that in many years of therapeutic practice and after conducting hundreds of psychedelic integration sessions, what can masquerade behind the veneer of recreation is quite often deeply therapeutic because social connection, peak experiences, and embodied joy do heal us.

Set: *Set* broadly refers to the mindset of a person about to have a psychedelic experience and can be thought to consist of the personality, preparation, expectations, and intentions of the journeyer. Readiness for a psychedelic experience is related to emotional and physical preparedness. Clear intentions, physical wellness, and preparation (including *la dieta*, or shamanic diet for medicines like ayahuasca), as well as approaching the experience with manageable levels of anticipatory anxiety all contribute to a psychedelic experience being meaningful and positive.

Mindset is a powerful indicator of what may happen in a psychedelic experience as well as a predictor of treatment efficacy in clinical work. A recent study of people who microdose psychedelics showed that expecting to benefit from microdosing predicted a positive outcome.[3]

Another concept rarely uttered in the same sentence as *set* but intrinsically linked nonetheless is *placebo*. The link between placebo response and set (as well as setting) is beautifully articulated by Ido Hartogsohn, who states that understanding set and setting in psychedelic work could benefit our understanding of placebo, but more importantly, describes that since psychedelics amplify the perception of meaning, this heightened sense of meaning in a meaningful setting—whether it be clinical or ritual—could magnify the benefits of psychedelic work.[4] Clinical research has been focused on trying to separate the discrete effects of psychedelic medicines (the "real" effect) from the psychological impact of *believing* you will be helped by it. With my clients, I frame it this way: Placebo is a concept maligned by Western science. But considered in a different way, placebo can be thought of as the power of your mind to heal you when supported by ritual and intention, and in the case of psychedelics, with the introduction of a non-human sentience there to assist your healing. In other words, magic.

Setting: *Setting* commonly refers to the context or environment in which a psychedelic experience takes place. Setting is actually a more complex concept than it might seem. Once basics are established, such as whether the environment is fundamentally safe (from legal risk, predation, etc.), an enduring psychedelic truth is that one type of setting is not good for all people. People traumatized in medical environments might feel very unsafe within a medical setting, while a person worried about health risks might find that same environment absolutely the safest for them. Transformative festivals might be a context for peak psychedelic experiences for some while for others chaotic and overwhelming for others. Moreover, advocates for decriminalization and community-based healing believe that safely held, nonhierarchical community healing spaces are excellent settings, preferable for many over clinical ones. Setting is also important to traditional or "shamanic" healing rituals that can be rooted to specific geographic places, nature, or with elaborate altars and implements for ceremony.

Shamanic/Shaman: Here is what a *shaman* is not; white guys with dreads sleeping with younger women and calling themselves a shaman, drug dealers with lots of beads, people appropriating cultural traditions they are unauthorized to practice and lording it over others. It is far beyond this book to present a robust exploration of what shamanism is, but it does feel important to have some understanding of the roots of *shamanic* practices and understand how that word is used (sometimes problematically), in the contemporary "underground" use of psychedelics.

Roger Walsh quotes French anthropologist Roberte Hayamon: "For more than a century the question of shamanism really is in the final analysis has hindered all attempts to define it."[5] Shamanism is a pancultural practice that is unified by one core experience, that the shaman is a person who enters into an altered state of consciousness, often traveling out of the corporal body, to access the spirit world and use that access in service to their community for healing, sorcery, finding lost objects, or other practices. In present day psychedelic ritual, shamanic healing ceremonies may be held by actual shamans from traditions such as the Shipibo, Q'ero, Native

American, or Bwiti that nearly all contain healing songs, implements, and other rituals.

There is also a proliferation of practices we might call "neo-shamanic" that may include elements of these practices. Some of these facilitators are appropriating wisdom traditions without proper training. However, I feel personally very enthusiastic about people creating new ritual forms inspired by shamanic ritual practices without appropriating traditions to which they do not belong that are rooted in their own cultural music, places of origin, and healing traditions. A vibrant Jewish psychedelic resurgence is currently happening, in fact! Remember, all people of this planet are children of Earth-based spiritual practices before the advent of Christian colonization and violent oppression. For those of us from European ancestry, we may have lost our original Earth-based practices, but there are ways of connecting back to your own traditions, or the place you live right now, and integrating new forms of psychedelic healing rituals into your practice without engaging in harmful appropriation.

Notes

INTRODUCTION

1. Fotiou, "The Role of Indigenous Knowledges in Psychedelic Science."

CHAPTER 1. HEALING IN BLISS

1. Corbyn, "The Firms Hoping to Take Psychedelics Mainstream."
2. Muttoni, Ardissino, and John, "Classical Psychedelics for the Treatment of Depression and Anxiety: A Systematic Review," 11–24.
3. Krediet, Bostoen, Breeksema, Van Schagen, Passie, and Vermetten, "Reviewing the Potential of Psychedelics for the Treatment of PTSD," 385–400.
4. Sessa, "Is It Time to Revisit the Role of Psychedelic Drugs in Enhancing Human Creativity?" 821–27.
5. Gandy, "Psychedelics and Potential Benefits in 'Healthy Normals': A Review of the Literature," 280–87.
6. Qiu and Minda, "Psychedelic Experiences and Mindfulness Are Associated with Improved Wellbeing," 1–11.
7. Schultes, Hoffman, and Rätsch, *Plants of the Gods*, 9.
8. Hofmann, *LSD, My Problem Child*, 35.
9. Nichols and Walter, "The History of Psychedelics in Psychiatry," 151–66.
10. Prince, at al., "Examination of Recreational and Spiritual Peyote Use Among American Indian Youth," 366–70.
11. Fotiou, "The Role of Indigenous Knowledges in Psychedelic Science," 1–8.
12. Stolaroff, *Secret Chief Revealed*, xi.
13. Bøhling, "Psychedelic Pleasures: An Affective Understanding of the Joys of Tripping," 133–43.

14. Lozada, "Men Have Lost Their Way. Josh Hawley Has Thoughts about How to Save Them."
15. van der Kolk, *The Body Keeps the Score: Brain, Mind, and Body in the Transformation of Trauma*, 51–64.
16. Fisher, *Healing the Fragmented Selves of Trauma Survivors: Overcoming Internal Self-Alienation*, 31.
17. Resnick, *The Pleasure Zone*, 18.
18. Resnick, *The Pleasure Zone*, 18.
19. "Public Enemy Number One: A Pragmatic Appraoach to America's Drug Problem."
20. Smith, "Modeling the Flesh of God: Semantic Hyperpriming and the Teonancátl Cults of Mexico," 297–308.
21. Carod-Artal, "Hallucinogenic Drugs in Pre-Columbian Mesoamerican Cultures," 42–49.
22. Letcher, *Shroom: A Cultural History of the Magic Mushroom*, 21.
23. White, "Race and Class in Early Anti-Drug Legislation in the United States."
24. Hart, *Drug Use for Grown-Ups: Chasing Liberty in the Land of Fear*, 33.
25. Trickey, "Inside the Story of America's 19th-Century Opiate Addiction."
26. Dawson, *The Peyote Effect: From the Inquisition to the War on Drugs*, 45–47.
27. Wing, "Marijuana Prohibition Was Racist from the Start. Not Much Has Changed."
28. Miller, *The Hippies and American Values*, XV.
29. Siegel Watkins, "How the Pill Became a Lifestyle Drug, The Phamaceutical Industry and Birth Control in the United States Since 1960," 1464.
30. Flannagan, "The Wild History of the Summer of Love Explained."
31. Dyck, "Flashback: Psychiatric Experimentation with LSD in Historical Perspective," 381–88.
32. DiPaolo, "LSD and the Hippies: A Focused Analysis of Criminalization and Persecution In the Sixties."
33. Stanger, "'Moral Panic' in the Sixties: The Rise and Rapid Declination of LSD in American Society," 3–4.
34. Nuwer, *I Feel Love*, 49–54.
35. Nuwer, *I Feel Love*, 34.
36. Shulgin, *PIKHAL: A Chemical Love Story*, 504, 736.
37. Holland, *Ecstasy: The Complete Guide, A Comprehensive Look at the Risks and Benefits of MDMA*, 14–16.

38. SAMHA, "Highlights by Race/Ethnicity for the 2022 For the National Survey on Drug Use and Health."
39. Fisher, *Healing the Fragmented Selves of Trauma Survivors: Overcoming Internal Self-Alienation*, 21.
40. Heaven, *Cactus of Mystery: The Shamanic Powers of the Peruvian San Pedro Cactus. Vermont*, 6.
41. Jay, *Mescaline: A Global History of the First Psychedelic*, 15.
42. Anderson, *Transcending Trauma: Healing Complex PTSD with Internal Family Systems*, xvii.

CHAPTER 2. PSYCHEDELIC SEXUALITY

1. Bouso, Dos Santos, Alcázar-Córcoles, and Hallak, "Serotonergic Psychedelics and Personality: A Systematic Review of Contemporary Research," 118–32.
2. MacLean, Johnson, and Griffiths, "Mystical Experiences Occasioned by the Hallucinogen Psilocybin Lead to Increases in the Personality Domain of Openness," 1453–61.
3. Morin, *The Erotic Mind: Unlocking the Inner Sources of Sexual Passion and Fulfillment*, 306.
4. Blatchford, Bright, and Engel, "Tripping over the Other: Could Psychedelics Increase Empathy?" 163–70.
5. Weiss, Miller, Carter, and Campbell, "Examining Changes in Personality Following Shamanic Ceremonial Use of Ayahuasca."
6. Agin-Liebes, Ekman, Anderson, Malloy, Haas, and Woolley, "Participant Reports of Mindfulness, Posttraumatic Growth, and Social Connectedness in Psilocybin-Assisted Group Therapy: An Interpretive Phenomenological Analysis."
7. Kane, "The 9 Attitudes of Mindfulness according to Jon Kabat-Zinn."
8. Chowdhury, "The Five Facet Mindfulness Questionnaire (FFMQ)."
9. Weiner, Cannon, and Avery-Clark, "Reclaiming the Lost Art of Sensate Focus: A Clinician's Guide."
10. Brotto, *Better Sex Through Mindfulness: How Women Can Cultivate Desire*, 33.
11. Radakovic, et al., "Psychedelics and Mindfulness: A Systematic Review and Meta-Analysis," 137–53.
12. Ueda, et al., "Trends in Frequency of Sexual Activity and Number of Sexual Partners among Adults Aged 18 to 44 Years in the US, 2000–2018."

13. Williams, "Psychedelics Are Queer, Just Saying."
14. Yurcaba, "Nearly Half of Trans People Have Been Mistreated by Medical Providers, Report Finds."
15. Montero, "LGBT Adults' Experiences with Discrimination and Health Care Disparities: Findings from the KFF Survey of Racism, Discrimination, and Health."
16. Belser and Keating, "A Queer Vision for Psychedelic Research," 4.
17. Ens, "LSD and Mescaline Psychedelic Conversion Therapies in Postwar North America," 49.
18. Jay. "Why is psychedelic culture dominated by privileged white men?"
19. Davidson, "Psyched Straight: The Early Life of LSD as a Conversion Therapy Drug," 54
20. Dubus, "High Dose Psychedelic Shock Therapy with LSD and Mescaline: The Conversion Treatment of a French Doctor on Two Adolescents in the 1960s," 59–64.
21. Ens, "LSD and Mescaline Psychedelic Conversion Therapies in Postwar North America," 45.
22. Alempijevic, et al., "Statement on Conversion Therapy."
23. Ens, "LSD and Mescaline Psychedelic Conversion Therapies in Postwar North America," 51.
24. McClure, "Psychedelic Studies Have Marginalized LGBTQI+ Communities for Years—These Researchers Are Changing That."
25. Belser and Keating, "A Queer Vision for Psychedelic Research," 7.
26. Goldpaugh, "Reclaiming Ecstasy: A Radical Queer Perspective on the Power of Pleasure in Psychedelic Healing," 231–237.
27. Margolin, "The Inherent Queerness of Psychedelics."
28. Veaux, et al., *More Than Two: A Practical Guide to Ethical Polyamory*, 8.
29. Levine and Heller, *Attached: The New Science of Adult Attachment and How It Can Help You Find—and Keep—Love*, 9.
30. Katz and Katz, "Reconceptualizing Attachment Theory through the Lens of Polyamory," 792–809.
31. Stauffer, et al., "Psilocybin-Assisted Group Therapy and Attachment: Observed Reduction in Attachment Anxiety and Influences of Attachment Insecurity on the Psilocybin Experience," 526–32.
32. Levine, "What Is 'Radical Monogamy'?"
33. Hammers, "Reworking Trauma Through BDSM," 491–512.
34. Hammers, "Reworking Trauma Through BDSM," 491–512.

35. Ogden, *Expanding the Practice of Sex Therapy*, 60.
36. Pollan, *How to Change Your Mind: The New Science of Psychedelics*, 95.
37. Timmermann, et al., "Psychedelics Alter Metaphysical Beliefs."
38. Ko, et al., "Psychedelics, Mystical Experience, and Therapeutic Efficacy: A Systematic Review."
39. Garcia-Romeu, Griffiths, and Johnson, "Psilocybin-Occasioned Mystical Experiences in the Treatment of Tobacco Addiction," 157–164.
40. Goldpaugh, "Finding the Divine Within: Exploring the Role of the Sacred in Psychedelic Integration Therapy for Sexual Trauma and Dysfunction," 314–23.
41. Ogden, *Expanding the Practice of Sex Therapy*, 60.
42. Illing, "The Psychedelic Roots of Christianity."
43. Brown, "The Immortality Key: The Secret History of the Religion with No Name," 5–8.
44. Muraresku, *The Immortality Key*, 27–31.
45. Crowley, *Secret Drugs of Buddhism: Psychedelic Sacraments and the Origins of the Vajrayana*, 116.

CHAPTER 3. SEXUAL HEALING

1. Haagen, at al., "The Efficacy of Recommended Treatments for Veterans with PTSD: A Metaregression Analysis," 184–94.
2. Krediet, et al., "Reviewing the Potential of Psychedelics for the Treatment of PTSD," 385–400.
3. Lawlor, "Psychedelic Bypassing: When Avoidance Is Mistaken for Healing."
4. Krayer, et al., "The Influence of Child Sexual Abuse on the Self from Adult Narrative Perspectives," 135–51.
5. Haines, *Healing Sex: A Mind-Body Approach to Healing Sexual Trauma*, xvii.
6. Crocq and Crocq, "From Shell Shock and War Neurosis to Posttraumatic Stress Disorder: A History of Psychotraumatology," 48.
7. Sutterlin, "History of Trauma Theory," 11–13.
8. Crocq and Crocq, "From Shell Shock and War Neurosis to Posttraumatic Stress Disorder: A History of Psychotraumatology," 47–55.
9. van der Kolk, *The Body Keeps the Score: Brain, Mind, and Body in the Transformation of Trauma*, 19.
10. Herman, *Trauma and Recovery: The Aftermath of Violence from Domestic Abuse to Political Terror*, 13–15.

11. Herman, "Complex PTSD: A Syndrome in Survivors of Prolonged and Repeated Trauma," 377–91.
12. Fisher, *Healing the Fragmented Selves of Trauma Survivors: Overcoming Internal Self-Alienation*, 34–38.
13. Carpenter, *Life, Reinvented: A Guide to Healing from Sexual Trauma for Survivors and Loved Ones*, 67–74.
14. Basile, at al., "The National Intimate Partner and Sexual Violence Survey: 2016/2017 Report on Sexual Violence."
15. National Sexual Violence Resource Center, "Sexual Violence and Transgender and Non-Binary Communities."
16. Liebschutz, et al., "The Relationship between Sexual and Physical Abuse and Substance Abuse Consequences," 121–28.
17. RAINN, "Perpetrators of Sexual Violence: Statistics."
18. Yehuda, Lehrner, and Rosenbaum, "PTSD and Sexual Dysfunction in Men and Women," 1107–19.
19. Haines, *Healing Sex: A Mind-Body Approach to Healing Sexual Trauma*, 13.
20. Maté and Maté, *The Myth of Normal: Trauma, Illness, and Healing in a Toxic Culture*, 20.
21. Visser, "Decolonizing Trauma Theory: Retrospect and Prospects," 250–26.
22. Linklater, *Decolonizing Trauma Work: Indigenous Stories and Strategies*, 22.
23. Richter-Levin and Sandi, "Labels Matter: Is It Stress or Is It Trauma?"
24. National Council on Family Relations, *Inclusion and Diversity Committee Report: What's Your Social Location*?
25. Shifren, et al.,"Sexual Problems and Distress in United States Women," 970–78.
26. Kleinplatz and Ménard, *Magnificent Sex*, 54.
27. Laan, et al., "In Pursuit of Pleasure: A Biopsychosocial Perspective on Sexual Pleasure and Gender," 1–21.
28. Informed Health, "How effective are antidepressants?"
29. Atmaca, "Selective Serotonin Reuptake Inhibitor-Induced Sexual Dysfunction: Current Management Perspectives," 1043–1050.
30. Earp and Savulescu, *Love Drugs: The Chemical Future of Relationships*, 59–60.
31. Kleinplatz and Ménard, *Magnificent Sex*, 20.
32. Blatchford, Bright, and Engel, "Tripping over the Other: Could Psychedelics Increase Empathy?"

33. MacLean, Johnson, and Griffiths, "Mystical Experiences Occasioned by the Hallucinogen Psilocybin Lead to Increases in the Personality Domain of Openness," 1453–61.
34. Weiss, et al., "Examining Changes in Personality Following Shamanic Ceremonial Use of Ayahuasca."
35. Wagner, et al., "Relational and Growth Outcomes Following Couples Therapy with MDMA for PTSD."

CHAPTER 4. PSYCHEDELIC PREPARATION AND INTEGRATION FOR SEXUAL HEALING AND EXPANDED PLEASURE

1. Earleywine, et al., "Integration in Psychedelic-Assisted Treatments: Recurring Themes in Current Providers' Definitions, Challenges, and Concerns."
2. Bathje, Majeski, and Kudowor, "Psychedelic Integration: An Analysis of the Concept and Its Practice."
3. Nardou, et al., "Oxytocin-Dependent Reopening of a Social Reward Learning Critical Period with MDMA," 116–20.
4. Nardou, et al., "Psychedelics Reopen the Social Reward Learning Critical Period," 1–9.
5. hooks, *All About Love: New Visions*, 10.
6. Cornell Law School, Legal Information Institute, "Decriminalization."
7. Erowid, "25I-NBOMe (2C-I-NBOMe) Vault: Fatalities / Deaths."
8. Anderson, "Toé: The Witchcraft Plant That's Spoiling Ayahuasca Tourism."
9. Gorman, et al., "Psychedelic Harm Reduction and Integration: A Transtheoretical Model for Clinical Practice."
10. Haijen, et al., "Predicting Responses to Psychedelics: A Prospective Study."
11. Nuwer, *I Feel Love*, 41–43.

CHAPTER 5. HIGH IMPACT

1. Timmermann, Watts, and Dupuis, "Towards Psychedelic Apprenticeship: Developing a Gentle Touch for the Mediation and Validation of Psychedelic-Induced Insights and Revelations," 691–704.
2. Otgaar, et al., "Oversimplifications and Misrepresentations in the Repressed Memory Debate: A Reply to Ross," 1–11.
3. Patihis, et al., "Are the 'Memory Wars' Over? A Scientist-Practitioner Gap in Beliefs about Repressed Memory," 519–30.

4. Jay, Mescaline: A Global History of the First Psychedelic, 86.
5. Otgaar, Howe, and Patihis, "What Science Tells Us about False and Repressed Memories," 1–6.
6. Patihis, et al., "Are the 'Memory Wars' Over? A Scientist-Practitioner Gap in Beliefs about Repressed Memory," 519–30.
7. Otgaar, Howe, and Patihism, "What Science Tells Us about False and Repressed Memories," 1–6.
8. Weiss, et al., "Prevalence and Therapeutic Impact of Adverse Life Event Reexperiencing under Ceremonial Ayahuasca."
9. Carbonaro, et al., "Survey Study of Challenging Experiences after Ingesting Psilocybin Mushrooms: Acute and Enduring Positive and Negative Consequences," 1268–78.
10. Pilgrim and Guinan, "From Mitigation to Culpability: Rethinking the Evidence about Therapist Sexual Abuse," 153–68.
11. Celenza and Gabbard, "Analysts Who Commit Sexual Boundary Violations: A Lost Cause?" 617–36.
12. Celenza and Gabbard, "Analysts Who Commit Sexual Boundary Violations: A Lost Cause?" 617–36.
13. Celenza and Gabbard, "Analysts Who Commit Sexual Boundary Violations: A Lost Cause?" 617–36.
14. Hamilton and Spruill, "Identifying and Reducing Risk Factors Related to Trainee–Client Sexual Misconduct," 318–27.
15. Norris, Gutheil, and Strasburger, "This Couldn't Happen to Me: Boundary Problems and Sexual Misconduct in the Psychotherapy Relationship," 476–82.
16. Shulgin, "The New Psychotherapy: MDMA and the Shadow," 197–204.
17. Hamilton and Spruill, "Identifying and Reducing Risk Factors Related to Trainee–Client Sexual Misconduct," 318–27.
18. Romero, "In Brazil, Some Inmates Get Therapy with Hallucinogenic Tea."
19. Brennan, et al., "A Qualitative Exploration of Relational Ethical Challenges and Practices in Psychedelic Healing."
20. Peluso, et al. "Reflections on Crafting an Ayahuasca Community Guide for the Awareness of Sexual Abuse," 24–33.

CHAPTER 6. IN THE GARDEN OF EARTHLY DELIGHTS

1. Barba, et. al., "Psychedelics and sexual functioning: a mixed-methods study, 1–16.

2. Jacobs, Banbury, and Lusher, "Micro-Dosing Psychedelics as a Plausible Adjunct to Psychosexual and Couple's Therapy: A Qualitative Insight," 1–14.
3. Maxwell, "Chemsex behaviors among men who have sex with men: A systematic review of the literature," 74–89
4. Moyle, et al., "Pharmacosex: Reimagining Sex, Drugs and Enhancement."
5. Gateway Foundation, "Molly vs. Ecstasy: What's the Difference?"
6. Buffum and Moser, "MDMA and Human Sexual Function," 355–59.
7. Buffum and Moser, "MDMA and Human Sexual Function," 355–59.
8. Zemishlany, Aizenberg, and Weizman, "Subjective Effects of MDMA ('Ecstasy') on Human Sexual Function," 127–30.
9. Passie, et al., "Ecstasy (MDMA) Mimics the Post-Orgasmic State: Impairment of Sexual Drive and Function during Acute MDMA-Effects May Be due to Increased Prolactin Secretion," 899–903.
10. Sessa, et al., "Debunking the Myth of 'Blue Mondays.' No Evidence of Affect Drop after Taking Clinical MDMA," 360–67.
11. Tukano, "A Medicine Heritage of 160 Indigenous Peoples: The Origins of Ayahuasca before Globalization."
12. Holyanova, "Ayahuasca May Have Aided in the Rescue of Children Lost in the Amazon Forest."
13. Domínguez-Clavé, et al., "Ayahuasca: Pharmacology, Neuroscience and Therapeutic Potential," 89–101.
14. Peluso, "Ayahuasca's Attractions and Distractions: Examining Sexual Seduction in Shaman-Participant Interactions."
15. Espinoza, "Sexual Healing with Amazonian Plant Teachers: A Heuristic Inquiry of Women's Spiritual-Erotic Awakenings," 109–20.
16. Cavnar, "The Effects of Ayahuasca Ritual Participation on Gay and Lesbian Identity," 252–60.
17. Harner, *The Way of the Shaman*, 7–9.
18. Letcher, *Shroom: A Cultural History of the Magic Mushroom*, 21.
19. Froese, Guzman and Davalos, "On the Origin of the Genus Psilocybe and Its Potential Ritual Use in Ancient Africa and Europel," 103–14.
20. Stamets, *Psilocybin Mushrooms of the World: An Identification Guide*, 12.
21. Smith, "Modeling the Flesh of God: Semantic Hyperpriming and the Teonancatál Cults of Mexico," 297–308.
22. Pollan, *How to Change Your Mind: The New Science of Psychedelics*, 109.
23. Beyer, "The Tragedy of Maria Sabina."

24. Lechtner, *Shroom: A Cultural History of the Magic Mushroom*, 100.
25. Pollan, *How to Change Your Mind: The New Science of Psychedelics*, 114.
26. Lechtner, *Shroom: A Cultural History of the Magic Mushroom*, 108.
27. Woodruff and Hatsis, "Memeing Maria Sabina: How Social Media Whitewashes Culture."
28. *High Times*, "High Times Greats: R. Gordon Wasson, the Magical Mushroom Quest of R. Gordon Wasson (1898–1986)."
29. Pollan, *How to Change Your Mind: The New Science of Psychedelics*, 110.
30. Pollan, *How to Change Your Mind: The New Science of Psychedelics*, 114.
31. Weinberger, "When the C.I.A. Was into Mind Control (Published 2019)."
32. Peplow and Nature Biotechnology, "Should Next-Generation Psychedelics Skip the Trip?"
33. The New York Times, "Taking the Magic out of Magic Mushrooms."
34. Stone. "Microdosing and tripping on mushrooms is on the rise in the U.S."
35. Busby. "Psychedelic Mushrooms Are Getting Much, Much Stronger."
36. Glover, "How to Take a Heroic Dose of Mushrooms."
37. Rucker and Young, "Psilocybin: From Serendipity to Credibility?"
38. Kiraga, et al., "Decreases in State and Trait Anxiety Post-Psilocybin: A Naturalistic, Observational Study Among Retreat Attendees."
39. Mason, et al., "Sub-Acute Effects of Psilocybin on Empathy, Creative Thinking, and Subjective Well-Being," 123–34.
40. Gwynne, *Empire of the Summer Moon: Quanah Parker and the Rise and Fall of the Comanches, the Most Powerful Indian Tribe in American History*, 314.
41. Bruhn, et al., "Mescaline Use for 5700 Years."
42. Jay, *Mescaline: A Global History of the First Psychedelic*, 79.
43. Huxley, *The Doors of Perception*, 6.
44. Jay, *Psychonauts: Drugs and the Making of the Modern Mind*, 293–294.
45. Fetty, "Origins of the Term 'Psychedelic.'"
46. Jay "What Happened to Mescaline?"
47. Lorde, "The Uses of the Erotic: The Erotic As Power," 29.
48. Lawrence, et al., "Phenomenology and Content of the Inhaled N, N-Dimethyltryptamine (N, N-DMT) Experience."
49. Barker, "Administration of N,N-dimethyltryptamine (DMT) in psychedelic therapeutics and research and the study of endogenous DMT," 1749–63.
50. Psymposia, "After a Year of Controversy, MAPS Canada Executive Director Mark Haden Announces Resignation."

51. De Greef, "The Pied Piper of Psychedelic Toads."
52. Ermakova, et al., "A Narrative Synthesis of Research with 5-MeO-DMT," 273–94.
53. Oroc, *Tryptamine Palace: 5-MeO-DMT and the Sonoran Desert Toad*, 27.
54. Jay, *Psychonauts: Drugs and the Making of the Modern Mind*, 2.
55. Jay, *Psychonauts: Drugs and the Making of the Modern Mind*, 1–3.
56. Bernal, et al., "Reactivations after 5-Methoxy-N,N-Dimethyltryptamine Use in Naturalistic Settings: An Initial Exploratory Analysis of the Phenomenon's Predictors and Its Emotional Valence."
57. Dymock, Mechen, and Moyle, "Acid and the Sexual Psychonauts."
58. L.A. Times Archive, "Thelma Schnee Moss; Writer, UCLA Psychology Professor."
59. Newland, *My Self and I*, 5.
60. Ling and Buckman, "The Treatment of Frigidity With LSD and Ritalin," 231–39.
61. Ling and Buckman, "The Treatment of Frigidity With LSD and Ritalin," 231–39.
62. Margolin, "Sexual Frigidity: The Social Construction of Masculine Privilege and Feminine Pathology."
63. Castleman, "The Truth About Vaginal Orgasms."
64. Prause, et al., "Clitorally Stimulated Orgasms Are Associated With Better Control of Sexual Desire, and Not Associated With Depression or Anxiety, Compared With Vaginally Stimulated Orgasms."
65. Shulgin and Shulgin, *Pihkal: A Chemical Love Story*, 218.
66. Fischer, *Therapy with Substance: Psycholytic Psychotherapy in the Twenty First Century*, 86.
67. Kim, et al., "Ketamine: Mechanisms and Relevance to Treatment of Depression." 129–43.
68. Li and Vlisides, "Ketamine: 50 Years of Modulating the Mind."
69. Cornfield, et al., "Exploring the effects and experiences of ketamine in group couples therapy."
70. Neubert, Anderson, and Mason, "Psychedelic Intimacy: Altered States of Consciousness in Romantic Relationships."
71. Neubert, Anderson, and Mason, "Psychedelic Intimacy: Altered States of Consciousness in Romantic Relationships."

CHAPTER 8. BIG LOVE

1. Shreck, "Stanislav and Christina Grof: Cartographers of the Psyche."

GLOSSARY

1. Flückiger, Del Re, Wampold, and Horvath, "The Alliance in Adult Psychotherapy: A Meta-Analytic Synthesis," 316–40.
2. Bauer, "Humphry Osmond."
3. Kaertner, et al., "Positive Expectations Predict Improved Mental-Health Outcomes Linked to Psychedelic Microdosing."
4. Hartogsohn, "Set and Setting, Psychedelics and the Placebo Response: An Extra-Pharmacological Perspective on Psychopharmacology," 1259–67.
5. Walsh, *The World of Shamanism, New Views of an Ancient Tradition*, 11.

BIBLIOGRAPHY

Agin-Liebes, Gabrielle, Eve Ekman, B. Anderson, Maxx Malloy, Alexandra Haas, and Josh Woolley. "Participant Reports of Mindfulness, Posttraumatic Growth, and Social Connectedness in Psilocybin-Assisted Group Therapy: An Interpretive Phenomenological Analysis." *Journal of Humanistic Psychology*, June 12, 2021, 002216782110229.

Alempijevic, Djordje, Rusudan Beriashvili, Jonathan Beynon, Bettina Birmanns, Marie Brasholt, Juliet Cohen, Maximo Duque, et al. "Statement on Conversion Therapy." *Journal of Forensic and Legal Medicine*. 2020. 72 (1): 101930.

Anderson, Brian. "Toé: The 'Witchcraft Plant' That's Spoiling Ayahuasca Tourism." *Vice*. February 13, 2013. Accessed October 31, 2024.

Anderson, Frank. *Transcending Trauma: Healing Complex PTSD with Internal Family Systems*. Eau Claire, WI: PESI Publishing, 2021.

Ardissino, Maddalena, Christopher John, and Silvia Muttoni. "Classical Psychedelics for the Treatment of Depression and Anxiety: A Systematic Review." *Journal of Affective Disorders* 258 (November 2019): 11–24.

Atmaca, M. "Selective Serotonin Reuptake Inhibitor-Induced Sexual Dysfunction: Current Management Perspectives." *Neuropsychiatric Disease and Treatment* 16 (2020): 1043–50.

Barba, T., H. Kettner, C. Radu, et al. "Psychedelics and sexual functioning: a mixed-methods study." *Nature Scientific Reports* 14, 2181 (2024).

Barker, Stephen A. "Administration of N,N-dimethyltryptamine (DMT) in psychedelic therapeutics and research and the study of endogenous DMT." *Psychopharmacology*, 239(6) (2023): 1749–63.

Basile, K.C., S.G. Smith, M. Kresnow, S. Khatiwada, and R.W. Leemis. *The National Intimate Partner and Sexual Violence Survey: 2016/2017 Report on Sexual Violence*. Atlanta, GA: National Center for Injury Prevention and Control, Centers for Disease Control and Prevention, 2022.

Bathje, Geoff J., Eric Majeski, and Mesphina Kudowor. "Psychedelic Integration: An Analysis of the Concept and Its Practice." *Frontiers in Psychology* 13 (August 4, 2022).

Bauer, Barbara E. "Humphry Osmond." Psychedelic Science Review. December 19, 2018. Accessed January 6, 2024.

Belser, Alex and Ava Keating. "A Queer Vision for Psychedelic Research: Past Reckonings, Current Reforms, and Future Transformations." *Queering Psychedelics: From Oppression to Liberation in Psychedelic Medicine*, edited by Alex Belser, Clancy Cavnar, and Beatriz Labate, 3–11. Santa Fe and London: Synergetic Press, 2022.

Beyer, Steve. "The Tragedy of Maria Sabina." Singing to the Plants (Steve Beyer's Blog on Ayahuasca and The Amazon). February 17, 2008. Accessed December 28, 2023.

Blatchford, Emily, Stephen Bright, and Liam Engel. "Tripping over the Other: Could Psychedelics Increase Empathy?" *Journal of Psychedelic Studies* 4, no. 3 (September 2020): 163–70.

Bøhling, Frederik. "Psychedelic Pleasures: An Affective Understanding of the Joys of Tripping." *The International Journal on Drug Policy* 49 (November 2017): 133–43.

Bouso, José Carlos, Rafael G. dos Santos, Miguel Ángel Alcázar-Córcoles, and Jaime E.C. Hallak. "Serotonergic Psychedelics and Personality: A Systematic Review of Contemporary Research." *Neuroscience & Biobehavioral Reviews* 87 (April 2018): 118–32.

Brennan, William, Margo A. Jackson, Katherine MacLean, and Joseph G. Ponterotto. "A Qualitative Exploration of Relational Ethical Challenges and Practices in Psychedelic Healing." *Journal of Humanistic Psychology*, September 2021: 1–31.

Brotto, Lori A. *Better Sex through Mindfulness: How Women Can Cultivate Desire*. Vancouver: Greystone Books, 2018.

Brown, Jerry. "The Immortality Key: The Secret History of the Religion with No Name." *Journal of Psychedelic Studies*, 5, no. 1 (2021): 5–8.

Bruhn, Jan, Peter A. G. M. De Smet, Hesham El-Seedi, and Olof Beck. "Mescaline Use for 5700 Years." *The Lancet* 359 (May 2002): 1866.

Buffum, John, and Charles A. Moser. "MDMA and Human Sexual Function." *Journal of Psychoactive Drugs* 18, no. 4 (October 1, 1986): 355–59.

Busby, Mattha. "Psychedelic Mushrooms Are Getting Much, Much Stronger." *Wired*, October 18, 2024. Accessed October 31, 2024.

Carbonaro, Theresa M., Matthew P. Bradstreet, Frederick S. Barrett, Katherine A. MacLean, Robert Jesse, Matthew W. Johnson, and Roland R. Griffiths. "Survey Study of Challenging Experiences after Ingesting Psilocybin Mushrooms: Acute and Enduring Positive and Negative Consequences." *Journal of Psychopharmacology* 30, no. 12 (2016): 1268–78.

Castleman, Michael. "The Truth About Vaginal Orgasms." *Psychology Today*, May 2, 2021. Accessed October 30, 2024.

Carod-Artal, F.J. "Hallucinogenic Drugs in Pre-Columbian Mesoamerican Cultures." *Neurología* (English Edition) 30, no. 1 (January-February, 2015): 42–49.

Carpenter, Erin. *Life, Reinvented: A Guide to Healing from Sexual Trauma for Survivors and Loved Ones*. Denver, CO: Quantum Publishing Group, 2014.

Cavnar, Clancy. "The Effects of Ayahuasca Ritual Participation on Gay and Lesbian Identity." *Journal of Psychoactive Drugs* 46, no. 3 (2014): 252–60.

Celenza, Andrea, and Glen O. Gabbard. "Analysts Who Commit Sexual Boundary Violations: A Lost Cause?" *Journal of the American Psychoanalytic Association* 51, no. 2 (2003): 61736.

Chowdhury, Madhuleena Roy. "The Five Facet Mindfulness Questionnaire (FFMQ)." *Positive Psychology*. August 27, 2019. Accessed December 1, 2023.

Corbyn, Zoe. "The Firms Hoping to Take Psychedelics Mainstream." BBC website. Last modified September 14, 2023.

Cornell Law School, Legal Information Institute. "Decriminalization." Last modified September, 2022.

Cornfield, Mark, Susan McBride, Joseph LaTorre, Daniel Zalewa, Jade Gallo, Mehdi Mahammadki, and Monnica Williams. "Exploring the effects and experiences of ketamine in group couples therapy." *Journal of Psychedelic Studies* (May 2024).

Crocq, Marc-Antoine, and Louis Crocq. "From Shell Shock and War Neurosis to Posttraumatic Stress Disorder: A History of Psychotraumatology." *Dialogues in Clinical Neuroscience* 2, no. 1 (March 2000): 47–55.

Crowley, Mike. *Secret Drugs of Buddhism: Psychedelic Sacraments and the Origins of the Vajrayana*. Santa Fe: Synergetic Press, 2019.

Davidson, Tal. "Psyched Straight: The Early Life of LSD as a Conversion Therapy Drug." In *Queering Psychedelics: From Oppression to Liberation in Psychedelic Medicine*, edited by Alex Belser, Clancy Cavnar, and Beatriz Labate, 53–54. Santa Fe and London: Synergetic Press, 2022.

Dawson, Alexander S. *The Peyote Effect: From the Inquisition to the War on Drugs*. Oakland, California: University of California Press, 2018.

De Greef, Kimon. "The Pied Piper of Psychedelic Toads." *The New Yorker*. Condé Nast. March 21, 2022. Accessed December 11, 2023.

DiPaolo, Miranda. LSD and the Hippies: A Focused Analysis of Criminalization and Persecution In the Sixties. The PIT Journal, Social Sciences, Cycle 9, 2018. Accessed October 28, 2024.

Domínguez-Clavé, Elisabet, Joaquim Soler, Matilde Elices, Juan C Pascual, Enrique Álvarez, Mario de la Fuente Revenga, Pablo Friedlander, Amanda Feilding, and Jordi Riba. "Ayahuasca: Pharmacology, Neuroscience and Therapeutic Potential." *Brain Research Bulletin* 126 (Pt 1) (2016): 89–101.

Dubus, Zoe. "High Dose Psychedelic Shock Therapy with LSD and Mescaline: The Conversion Treatment of a French Doctor on Two Adolescents in the 1960s." *Queering Psychedelics: From Oppression to Liberation in Psychedelic Medicine*, edited by Alex Belser, Clancy Cavnar, and Beatriz Labate, 59–64. London, England: Synergetic Press, 2022.

Dyck, Erika. "Flashback: Psychiatric Experimentation with LSD in Historical Perspective." *The Canadian Journal of Psychiatry* vol. 50, no. 7, (2005) 381–388.

Dymock, Alex, Ben Mechen, and Leah Moyle. "Acid and the Sexual Psychonauts." Wellcome Collection. January 16, 2019. Accessed December 22, 2023.

Earleywine, M., Low, F., Lau, C., & De Leo, J. "Integration in Psychedelic-Assisted Treatments: Recurring Themes in Current Providers' Definitions, Challenges, and Concerns." *Journal of Humanistic Psychology* (2022).

Earp, Brian D., and Julian Savulescu. *Love Drugs: The Chemical Future of Relationships*. Stanford, California: Redwood Press, 2020.

Ens, Andrea. "LSD and Mescaline Psychedelic Conversion Therapies in Postwar North America." *Queering Psychedelics: From Oppression to Liberation in Psychedelic Medicine*, edited by Alex Belser, Clancy Cavnar, and Beatriz Labate, 45–52. Santa Fe and London: Synergetic Press, 2022.

Ermakova, Anna O., Fiona Dunbar, James Rucker, and Matthew W. Johnson. "A Narrative Synthesis of Research with 5-MeO-DMT." *Journal of Psychopharmacology* 36, 3: (2021) 273–94.

Erowid. "25I-NBOMe (2C-I-NBOMe) Fatalities/Deaths." *The Vaults of Erowid* (website). Accessed December 8, 2023.

Espinoza, Yalila. "Sexual Healing with Amazonian Plant Teachers: A Heuristic Inquiry of Women's Spiritual–Erotic Awakenings." *Sexual and Relationship Therapy* 29, no. 1 (2014): 109–20.

Fetty, Nick. "Origin of the Term "Psychedelic," *New York Academy of Science Blog.* August 2024. Accessed October 30, 2024.

Fisher, Janina. *Healing the Fragmented Selves of Trauma Survivors: Overcoming Internal Self-Alienation.* London: Taylor & Francis, 2017.

Flannagan, S. "The Wild History of the Summer of Love Explained," *Grunge.* Jan 13, 2021. Accessed October 27, 2024.

Flückiger, Christoph, A. C. Del Re, Bruce E. Wampold, and Adam O. Horvath. "The Alliance in Adult Psychotherapy: A Meta-Analytic Synthesis." *Psychotherapy* 55, no. 4 (December 1, 2018): 316–40.

Fotiou, Evgenia. "The Role of Indigenous Knowledges in Psychedelic Science." *Journal of Psychedelic Studies* 4, no. 1 (2019): 16–23.

Froese, Tom, Gaston Guzman, and Laura Guzman Davalos. "On the Origin of the Genus Psilocybe and Its Potential Ritual Use in Ancient Africa and Europe." *Economic Botany* 70, no. 2 (2016):103–14.

Gandy, Sam. "Psychedelics and Potential Benefits in 'Healthy Normals': A Review of the Literature." *Journal of Psychedelic Studies* 3, no. 3 (September 2019): 280–87.

Garcia-Romeu, Albert, Roland R. Griffiths, and Matthew W. Johnson. "Psilocybin-Occasioned Mystical Experiences in the Treatment of Tobacco Addiction." *Current Drug Abuse Reviews* 7, no. 3 (February 20, 2015): 157–64.

Gateway Foundation. "Molly vs. Ecstasy: What's the Difference?" Gateway Foundation. Accessed October 7, 2024.

Glover, Ella. "How to Take a Heroic Dose of Mushrooms." *Dazed.* Last modified October 13, 2023.

Goldpaugh, Dee Dee. "Finding the Divine Within: Exploring the Role of the Sacred in Psychedelic Integration Therapy for Sexual Trauma and Dysfunction." *Sexual and Relationship Therapy,* (October 2022): 314–323.

Goldpaugh, Dee Dee. "Reclaiming Ecstasy: A Radical Queer Perspective on the Power of Pleasure in Psychedelic Healing." *Queering Psychedelics: From Oppression to Liberation in Psychedelic Medicine,* edited by Alex Belser,

Clancy Cavnar and Beatriz Labate, 231237. London, England: Synergetic Press, 2022.

Gorman, Ingmar, Elizabeth M. Nielson, Aja Molinar, Ksenia Cassidy, and Jonathan Sabbagh. "Psychedelic Harm Reduction and Integration: A Transtheoretical Model for Clinical Practice." *Frontiers in Psychology* 12 (March 2021).

Gwynne, S. C. *Empire of the Summer Moon: Quanah Parker and the Rise and Fall of the Comanches, the Most Powerful Indian Tribe in American History.* London: Constable, 2011.

Haagen, Joris F.G., Geert E. Smid, Jeroen W. Knipscheer, and Rolf J. Kleber. "The Efficacy of Recommended Treatments for Veterans with PTSD: A Metaregression Analysis." *Clinical Psychology Review* 40 (August 2015): 184–194.

Haagen, Joris F.G., Geert E. Smid, Jeroen W. Knipscheer, and Rolf J. Kleber. "The Efficacy of Recommended Treatments for Veterans with PTSD: A Metaregression Analysis." *Clinical Psychology Review* 40 (August 2015): 184–194.

Haijen, Eline C. H. M., Mendel Kaelen, Leor Roseman, Christopher Timmermann, Hannes Kettner, Suzanne Russ, David Nutt, et al. "Predicting Responses to Psychedelics: A Prospective Study." *Frontiers in Pharmacology* 9 (November 2018).

Haines, Staci. *Healing Sex: A Mind-Body Approach to Healing Sexual Trauma.* San Francisco, CA: Cleis Press, 2010.

Hamilton, James C., and Jean Spruill. "Identifying and Reducing Risk Factors Related to Trainee–Client Sexual Misconduct." *Professional Psychology: Research and Practice* 30, no. 3 (1999): 318–27.

Hammers, Corie. "Reworking Trauma Through BDSM." *Signs: Journal of Women in Culture and Society* 44, no. 2 (2019): 491–512.

Harner, Michael. *The Way of the Shaman.* New York: Harper & Row, 1980.

Hart, Carl L. *Drug Use for Grown-Ups: Chasing Liberty in the Land of Fear.* New York: Penguin Books, 2022.

Hartogsohn, Ido. "Set and Setting, Psychedelics and the Placebo Response: An Extra-Pharmacological Perspective on Psychopharmacology." *Journal of Psychopharmacology* 30, no. 12 (2016): 1259–67.

Heaven, Ross. *Cactus of Mystery: The Shamanic Powers of the Peruvian San Pedro Cactus.* Rochester, VT:, Park Street Press, 2012.

Herman, Judith. "Complex PTSD: A Syndrome in Survivors of Prolonged and Repeated Trauma." *Journal of Traumatic Stress* 5, no. 3 (July 1992): 377–391.

Herman, Judith. *Trauma and Recovery: The Aftermath of Violence from Domestic Abuse to Political Terror*. New York: Basic Books, 1992.

High Times. "R. Gordon Wasson, the Magical Mushroom Quest of R. Gordon Wasson (1898–1986)." *High Times*. September 22, 2020. Accessed December 1, 2023.

Hofmann, Albert. *LSD, My Problem Child*. Oxford: Beckley Foundation, 2019.

Holland, Julie. *Ecstasy: The Complete Guide: A Comprehensive Look at the Risks and Benefits of MDMA*. Rochester, VT: Park Street Press, 2001.

Holyanova, Maria. "Ayahuasca May Have Aided in the Rescue of Children Lost in the Amazon Forest." Psychedelic Spotlight. June 19, 2023. Accessed December 20, 2023.

hooks, bell. *All About Love: New Visions*. New York: Harper Perennial, 1999.

Huxley, Aldous. *The Doors of Perception*. New York: Harper Perennial, (1954) 2009.

Illing, Sean. "The Psychedelic Roots of Christianity." *Vox*. March 4, 2021. November 12, 2023.

InformedHealth. "Depression: How effective are antidepressants?" Cologne, Germany: Institute for Quality and Efficiency in Health Care (IQWiG); 2006. Updated Jun 18, 2020.

Jacobs, Lucy, Samantha Banbury, and Joanne Lusher. "Micro-Dosing Psychedelics as a Plausible Adjunct to Psychosexual and Couple's Therapy: A Qualitative Insight." *Sexual and Relationship Therapy*, February 2022: 1–14.

Jay, Mike. *Mescaline: A Global History of the First Psychedelic*. New Haven: Yale University Press, 2019.

Jay, Mike. *Psychonauts: Drugs and the Making of the Modern Mind*. New Haven; London: Yale University Press, 2023.

Jay, Mike. "What Happened to Mescaline?" Yale University Press. August 6, 2019. Accessed November 4, 2023.

Jay, Mike. "Why is psychedelic culture dominated by privileged white men?" June 26, 2019. Accessed October 31st, 2024.

Kaertner, L. S., M. B. Steinborn, H. Kettner, M. J. Spriggs, L. Roseman, T. Buchborn, M. Balaet, C. Timmermann, D. Erritzoe, and R. L. Carhart-

Harris. "Positive Expectations Predict Improved Mental-Health Outcomes Linked to Psychedelic Microdosing." *Scientific Reports* 11 (2021): 1.

Kane, Ryan. "The 9 Attitudes of Mindfulness according to Jon Kabat-Zinn." Mindfulnessbox. February 3, 2022. Accessed October 21, 2023.

Kim, Ji-Woon, Kanzo Suzuki, Ege T. Kavalali, and Lisa Monteggia. "Ketamine: Mechanisms and Relevance to Treatment of Depression." *Annual Review of Medicine* 75. (2024): 129–43.

Kiraga, Maggie Kamila, Kim P. C. Kuypers, Malin Vedoy Uthaug, Johannes G. Ramaekers, and Natasha Leigh Mason. "Decreases in State and Trait Anxiety Post-Psilocybin: A Naturalistic, Observational Study Among Retreat Attendees." *Frontiers in Psychiatry* 13 (July 2022).

Kleinplatz, Peggy J., and A. Dana Ménard. *Magnificent Sex*. London: Routledge, 2020.

Ko, Kwonmok, Gemma Knight, James J. Rucker, and Anthony J. Cleare. "Psychedelics, Mystical Experience, and Therapeutic Efficacy: A Systematic Review." *Frontiers in Psychiatry* 13 (July 2022).

Krayer, Anne, Diane Seddon, Catherine A. Robinson, and Hefin Gwilym. "The Influence of Child Sexual Abuse on the Self from Adult Narrative Perspectives." *Journal of Child Sexual Abuse* 24, no. 2 (March 2015): 135–151.

Krediet, Erwin, Tijmen Bostoen, Joost Breeksema, Annette van Schagen, Torsten Passie, and Eric Vermetten. "Reviewing the Potential of Psychedelics for the Treatment of PTSD." *International Journal of Neuropsychopharmacology* 23, no. 6 (June 2020).

L.A. Times Archives. "Thelma Schnee Moss: Writer, UCLA College Professor." Feb 5th, 1997. Accessed October 28th, 2024.

Laan, Ellen T. M., Verena Klein, Marlene A. Werner, Rik H. W. van Lunsen, and Erick Janssen. 2021. "In Pursuit of Pleasure: A Biopsychosocial Perspective on Sexual Pleasure and Gender." *International Journal of Sexual Health* 33 (4): 1–21.

Lawlor, Sean. "Psychedelic Bypassing: When Avoidance Is Mistaken for Healing." Psychedelics Today. November 18, 2021. Accessed December 1, 2023.

Lawrence, David Wyndham, Robin Carhart-Harris, Roland Griffiths, and Christopher Timmermann. "Phenomenology and Content of the Inhaled N, N-Dimethyltryptamine (N, N-DMT) Experience." *Scientific Reports* 12

(May, 2022): 8562. *Shroom: A Cultural History of the Magic Mushroom.* New York: Harper Perennial, 2008.

Levine, Nick. "What Is 'Radical Monogamy'?" *Vice.* March 8, 2022. Accessed December 2, 2023.

Li, Linda, and Phillip E. Vlisides. "Ketamine: 50 Years of Modulating the Mind." *Frontiers in Human Neuroscience* 10, no 612. (November 2016).

Liebschutz, Jane, Jacqueline B. Savetsky, Richard Saitz, Nicholas J. Horton, Christine Lloyd-Travaglini, and Jeffrey H. Samet. "The Relationship between Sexual and Physical Abuse and Substance Abuse Consequences." *Journal of Substance Abuse Treatment* 22, no. 3 (April 2002): 121–28.

Ling, Thomas and John Buckman. "The Treatment of Frigidity with LSD and Ritalin." *The Psychedelic Reader,* edited by Gunter M. Weill, Ralph Metzner, and Timothy Leary. New Hyde Park, NY: University Books, 1965.

Linklater, Renee. *Decolonizing Trauma Work: Indigenous Stories and Strategies.* Halifax and Winnipeg: Fernwood Publishing, 2014.

Lorde, Audrey, "Uses of the Erotic." in *Pleasure Activism*, ed. adrienne marie brown. Chico, Edinburgh: AK Press. 2019.

Lozada, Carlos. "Review of Men Have Lost Their Way. Josh Hawley Has Thoughts about How to Save Them." *New York Times*, June 1, 2023.

Lyons, Richard D. "Psychiatrists, in a Shift, Declare Homosexuality No Mental Illness." *The New York Times.* December 16, 1973.

MacLean, Katherine A., Matthew W. Johnson, and Roland R. Griffiths. "Mystical Experiences Occasioned by the Hallucinogen Psilocybin Lead to Increases in the Personality Domain of Openness." *Journal of Psychopharmacology* 25, no. 11 (September 2011): 1453–61.

Margolin, Leslie. "Sexual Frigidity: The Social Construction of Masculine Privilege and Feminine Pathology." *Journal of Gender Studies*, 2016, 26 (5): 583–94.

Margolin, Madison. "The Inherent Queerness of Psychedelics." *DoubleBlind Magazine.* Updated August 19th, 2020. Accessed October 30, 2024.

Mason, Natasha L., Elisabeth Mischler, Malin V. Uthaug, and Kim P. C. Kuypers. "Sub-Acute Effects of Psilocybin on Empathy, Creative Thinking, and Subjective Well-Being." *Journal of Psychoactive Drugs* 51 (2, 2019): 123–34.

Maté, Gabor, and Daniel Maté. *The Myth of Normal: Trauma, Illness, and Healing In a Toxic Culture.* New York: Avery/Penguin Random House, 2022.

Maxwell, Steven, Maryam Shahmanesh, Mitzy Gafos. "Chemsex behaviors among men who have sex with men: A systematic review of the literature." *International Journal of Drug Policy*. Vol 63, January 2019, 74–89.

McClure, James. "Psychedelic Studies Have Marginalized LGBTQI+ Communities for Years—These Researchers Are Changing That." *DoubleBlind Magazine*. June 1, 2020. Accessed October 31, 2024.

Meckel Fischer, Friederike. *Therapy with Substance: Psycholytic Psychotherapy in the Twenty-First Century*. London: Muswell Hill Press, 2015.

Miller, Timothy. *The Hippies and American Values*. Knoxville, TN: University of Tennessee Press, 1992.

Montero, Alex, Liz Hamel, Samanthan Artiga, Lindsay Dawson. "LGBT Adults' Experiences with Discrimination and Health Care Disparities: Findings from the KFF Survey of Racism, Discrimination, and Health," KFF, April 2, 2024. Accessed October 30, 2024.

Morin, Jack. *The Erotic Mind: Unlocking the Inner Sources of Sexual Passion and Fulfillment*. New York: Harper Perennial, 1996.

Moyle, Leah, Alex Dymock, Alexandra Aldridge, and Ben Mechen. "Pharmacosex: Reimagining Sex, Drugs and Enhancement." *International Journal of Drug Policy* 86 (December 2020): 102943.

Muraresku, Brian C. *The Immortality Key*. New York, NY: St, Martin's Press, 2020.

Nardou, Romain, Edward Sawyer, Young Jun Song, Makenzie Wilkinson, Yasmin Padovan-Hernandez, Júnia Lara de Deus, Noelle Wright, et al. "Psychedelics Reopen the Social Reward Learning Critical Period." *Nature* (2023): 1–9.

Nardou, Romain, Eastman M. Lewis, Rebecca Rothhaas, Ran Xu, Aimei Yang, Edward S. Boyden, and Gül Dölen. "Oxytocin-Dependent Reopening of a Social Reward Learning Critical Period with MDMA." *Nature* 569, no. 7754 (April 3, 2019): 116–20.

National Council on Family Relations. *Inclusion and Diversity Committee Report: What's Your Social Location?* 2019 NCFR Report. Accessed October 3, 2024.

National Sexual Violence Resource Center. "Sexual Violence and Transgender and Non-Binary Communities." 2019. [PDF: Transgender Infrographic] National Sexual Violence Resource Center.

Neubert, Jonas J., Katie Anderson, and Natasha Mason. "Psychedelic Intimacy:

Altered States of Consciousness in Romantic Relationships." PsyArXiv. (August 25, 2023).

Newland, Constance. *My Self and I*. New York: Cowar-McCann. 1962.

The New York Times. "Taking the Magic out of Magic Mushrooms." *The New York Times*. Accessed October 3, 2024.

Nichols, David E., and Hannes Walter. "The History of Psychedelics in Psychiatry." *Pharmacopsychiatry* 54, no. 4 (2020).

Norris, Donna M., Thomas G. Gutheil, and Larry H. Strasburger. "This Couldn't Happen to Me: Boundary Problems and Sexual Misconduct in the Psychotherapy Relationship." *Focus* 5, no. 4 (January 1, 2007): 476–82.

Nuwer, Rachel. *I Feel Love: MDMA and the Quest for Connection in a Fractured World*. Bloomsbury Publishing USA, 2023.

Ogden, Gina. *Expanding the Practice of Sex Therapy*. New York and London: Routledge, 2018.

Oroc, James. *Tryptamine Palace: 5-MeO-DMT and the Sonoran Desert Toad*. Rochester, VT: Park Street Press. 2009.

Ortiz Bernal, Ana María, Charles L. Raison, Rafael L. Lancelotta, and Alan K. Davis. "Reactivations after 5-Methoxy-N,N-Dimethyltryptamine Use in Naturalistic Settings: An Initial Exploratory Analysis of the Phenomenon's Predictors and Its Emotional Valence." *Frontiers in Psychiatry* 13 (November, 2022).

Otgaar, Henry, Olivier Dodier, Maryanne Garry, Mark L. Howe, Elizabeth F. Loftus, Steven Jay Lynn, Ivan Mangiulli, Richard J. McNally, and Lawrence Patihis. "Oversimplifications and Misrepresentations in the Repressed Memory Debate: A Reply to Ross." *Journal of Child Sexual Abuse* 32, no. 1 (October 13, 2022): 116–26.

Otgaar, Henry, Mark L. Howe, and Lawrence Patihis. "What Science Tells Us about False and Repressed Memories." *Memory* 30, no. 1 (2021): 1–6.

Pai, Anushka, Alina M. Suris, and Carol S. North. "Posttraumatic Stress Disorder in the DSM-5: Controversy, Change, and Conceptual Considerations." *Behavioral Sciences* 7, no. 1 (February 2017): 7.

Passie, Torsten, Uwe Hartmann, Udo Schneider, Hinderk M. Emrich, and Tillmann H.C. Krüger. "Ecstasy (MDMA) Mimics the Post-Orgasmic State: Impairment of Sexual Drive and Function during Acute MDMA-Effects May Be Due to Increased Prolactin Secretion." *Medical Hypotheses* 64, no. 5 (2005): 899–903.

Patihis, Lawrence, Lavina Y. Ho, Ian W. Tingen, Scott O. Lilienfeld, and Elizabeth F. Loftus. "Are the 'Memory Wars' Over? A Scientist-Practitioner Gap in Beliefs about Repressed Memory." *Psychological Science* 25, no. 2 (2013): 519–30.

Peluso, Daniela. "Ayahuasca's Attractions and Distractions: Examining Sexual Seduction in Shaman-Participant Interactions." In *Ayahuasca Shamanism in the Amazon and Beyond,* edited by Beatriz Labate and Clancy Cavnar, 231-55. Oxford, United Kingdom: Oxford University Press, 2014.

Peluso, Daniela, Emily Sinclair, Beatriz Labate, and Clancy Cavnar. "Reflections on Crafting an Ayahuasca Community Guide for the Awareness of Sexual Abuse." *Journal of Psychedelic Studies* 4, no. 1 (2020): 24–33.

Peplow and Nature Biotechnology. "Should Next-Generation Psychedelics Skip the Trip?" *Scientific American*. June 22, 2024.

Petry, Luke G., Monica Sharma, Aaron Wolfgang, David A. Ross, and Joseph J. Cooper. "Any Questions? A Sober Look at MDMA." *Biological Psychiatry* 90, no. 3 (August 1, 2021): e7–e8.

Pilgrim, David, and Pat Guinan. "From Mitigation to Culpability: Rethinking the Evidence about Therapist Sexual Abuse." *European Journal of Psychotherapy & Counselling* 2, no. 2 (1999): 153–68.

Pollan, Michael. *How to Change Your Mind: The New Science of Psychedelics.* London: Penguin Books, 2018.

Prause N, Kuang L, Lee P, Miller G. "Clitorally Stimulated Orgasms Are Associated With Better Control of Sexual Desire, and Not Associated With Depression or Anxiety, Compared With Vaginally Stimulated Orgasms." *Journal of Sexual Medicine*. Vol. 13, No. 11. (November 2016) 1676–1685.

Prince, Mark A., Maeve B. O'Donnell, Linda R. Stanley, and Randall C. Swaim. "Examination of Recreational and Spiritual Peyote Use Among American Indian Youth." *Journal of Studies on Alcohol and Drugs*, 80(3) (2019): 366–70.

Psymposia. "After a Year of Controversy, MAPS Canada Executive Director Mark Haden Announces Resignation." *Psymposia*. February 19, 2021. Accessed December 9, 2023.

Qiu, Tianhong Tim, and John Paul Minda. "Psychedelic Experiences and Mindfulness Are Associated with Improved Wellbeing." *Journal of Psychoactive Drugs* 55, no. 2 (April 2022): 1–11.

Radakovic, Chelsea, Ratko Radakovic, Guy Peryer, and Jo-Anne Geere.

"Psychedelics and Mindfulness: A Systematic Review and Meta-Analysis." *Journal of Psychedelic Studies* 6, no. 2 (2022): 137–53.

RAINN. "Perpetrators of Sexual Violence: Statistics." Accessed October 28, 2024.

Resnick, Stella. *The Pleasure Zone*. Berkeley, CA: Publishers Group West, 1997.

Richter-Levin, Gal, and Carmen Sandi. "Labels Matter: Is It Stress or Is It Trauma?" *Translational Psychiatry* 11 (385), June, 2021.

Romero, Simon. "Review of In Brazil, Some Inmates Get Therapy with Hallucinogenic Tea." *New York Times*, March 28, 2015.

Rucker, James J., and Allan H. Young. "Psilocybin: From Serendipity to Credibility?" *Frontiers in Psychiatry* 12 (April 2021).

SAMHA. "Highlights by Race/Ethnicity for the 2022 For the National Survey on Drug Use and Health." Accessed October 30, 2024.

Schultes, Richard Evans, Albert Hoffman, and Christian Rätsch. *Plants of the Gods*. Rochester, VT: Healing Arts Press, 2001.

Sessa, Ben. "Is It Time to Revisit the Role of Psychedelic Drugs in Enhancing Human Creativity?" *Journal of Psychopharmacology* 22, no. 8 (February 2008): 821-27.

Sessa, Ben, Jacob S. Aday, Steve O'Brien, H. Valerie Curran, Fiona Measham, Laurie Higbed, and David J. Nutt. "Debunking the Myth of 'Blue Mondays': No Evidence of Affect Drop after Taking Clinical MDMA." *Journal of Psychopharmacology* 36, no. 3 (2021): 360-67.

Shifren, Jan L., Brigitta U. Monz, Patricia A. Russo, Anthony Segreti, and Catherine B. Johannes. 2008. "Sexual Problems and Distress in United States Women." *Obstetrics & Gynecology* 112 (5): 970–78.

Shreck, Mason. "Stanislav and Christina Grof: Cartographers of the Psyche." MAPS Bulletin, Volume XXI, Number 3. 2021.

Shulgin, Alexander T., and Ann Shulgin. *Pihkal: A Chemical Love Story*. Berkeley, CA: Transform Press, 2019.

Shulgin, Ann. "The New Psychotherapy: MDMA and the Shadow." *Psychoactive Sacramentals: Essays on Entheogens and Religion*, edited by Thomas Roberts and Francis Vaughn, 197–204. Council on Spiritual Practices, 2001.

Siegel Watkins, Elizabeth. "How the Pill Became a Lifestyle Drug, The Pharmaceutical Industry and Birth Control in the United States Since 1960." *American Journal of Public Health*, Vol 102 No 8 (2012): 1462–1472.

Smith, Kaleb R. "Modeling the Flesh of God: Semantic Hyperpriming and the Teonancátl Cults of Mexico." *NeuroQuantology* 14, no. 2 (2016): 298.

Stanger, Abigail M. "'Moral Panic' in the Sixties: The Rise and Rapid Declination of LSD in American Society," *The Cardinal Edge*: Vol. 1, Article 16 (2021).

Stamets, Paul. *Psilocybin Mushrooms of the World: An Identification Guide.* Berkeley, Calif.: Ten Speed Press, 1996.

Stolaroff, Myron J. *Secret Chief Revealed*, Revised 2nd Edition. Multidisciplinary Association for Psychedelic Studies, 2022.

Stone, Will. "Microdosing and tripping on mushrooms is on the rise in the U.S." NPR website. June 28th, 2024. Accessed October 31, 2024.

Sutterlin, Nicole. "History of Trauma Theory." In *The Routledge Companion to Literature and Trauma*, edited by Colin Davis and Hanna Meretoja, 11–13. London and New York: Routledge, 2020.

Timmermann, Christopher, Hannes Kettner, Chris Letheby, Leor Roseman, Fernando E. Rosas, and Robin L. Carhart-Harris. "Psychedelics Alter Metaphysical Beliefs." *Scientific Reports* 11, no. 1 (November 2021).

Timmermann, Christopher, Rosalind Watts, and David Dupuis. "Towards Psychedelic Apprenticeship: Developing a Gentle Touch for the Mediation and Validation of Psychedelic-Induced Insights and Revelations." *Transcultural Psychiatry* 59, no. 5 (March 2022): 691–704.

Trickey, Erick. "Review of Inside the Story of America's 19th-Century Opiate Addiction." *Smithsonian Magazine*, January 4, 2018.

Tukano, Daiara. "A Medicine Heritage of 160 Indigenous Peoples: The Origins of Ayahuasca before Globalization." Chacruna. April 6, 2022. Accessed December 9, 2023.

Ueda, Peter, Catherine H. Mercer, Cyrus Ghaznavi, and Debby Herbenick. "Trends in Frequency of Sexual Activity and Number of Sexual Partners among Adults Aged 18 to 44 Years in the US, 2000–2018." *JAMA Network Open* 3, no. 6 (June 12, 2020): e203833.

van der Kolk, Bessel. *The Body Keeps the Score: Mind, Brain and Body in the Transformation of Trauma.* London: Penguin Books, 2014.

Veaux, Franklin, Eve Rickert, Janet W. Hardy, and Tatiana Gill. *More than Two: A Practical Guide to Ethical Polyamory.* Portland, OR: Thorntree Press, 2014.

Visser, Irene. "Decolonizing Trauma Theory: Retrospect and Prospects." *Humanities* 4 (2015): 250–65.

Wagner, Anne C., Rachel E. Liebman, Ann T. Mithoefer, Michael C. Mithoefer, and Candice M. Monson. "Relational and Growth Outcomes Following Couples Therapy with MDMA for PTSD." *Frontiers in Psychiatry* 12 (June 2021).

Walsh, Roger. *The World of Shamanism: New Views of an Ancient Tradition.* Woodbury, MI: Llewellyn Worldwide, 2014.

Weinberger, Sharon. "When the C.I.A. Was into Mind Control." *The New York Times,* September 10, 2019.

Weiner, Linda, Neil Cannon, and Constance Avery-Clark. "Review of Reclaiming the Lost Art of Sensate Focus: A Clinician's Guide." *Family Therapy Magazine,* September 2014.

Weiss, Brandon, Aleksandra Wingert, David Erritzoe, and W. Keith Campbell. "Prevalence and Therapeutic Impact of Adverse Life Event Reexperiencing under Ceremonial Ayahuasca." *Scientific Reports* 13, no. 1 (2023).

Weiss, Brandon, Joshua D. Miller, Nathan T. Carter, and W. Keith Campbell. "Examining Changes in Personality Following Shamanic Ceremonial Use of Ayahuasca." *Scientific Reports* 11, no. 1 (March 2021).

White, William. "Race and Class in Early Anti-Drug Legislation in the United States." Chestnut Health Systems, 2014. Accessed September 2, 2023.

Williams, Bett. "Psychedelics Are Queer, Just Saying." Chacruna. September 27, 2018. Accessed October 28, 2024.

Wing, Nick. "Marijuana Prohibition Was Racist from the Start. Not Much Has Changed." HuffPost. Accessed January 14, 2014.

Woodruff, Eden, and Tom Hatsis. "Memeing Maria Sabina: How Social Media Whitewashes Culture." Psanctum, March 21, 2022. Accessed November 11, 2023.

Yehuda, Rachel, Amy Lehrner, and Talli Y. Rosenbaum. "PTSD and Sexual Dysfunction in Men and Women." *The Journal of Sexual Medicine* 12, no. 5 (May 2015): 1107–19.

Yurcaba, Jo. "Review of Nearly Half of Trans People Have Been Mistreated by Medical Providers, Report Finds." NBC News. Last updated August 19, 2021.

Zemishlany, Z., D. Aizenberg, and A. Weizman. "Subjective Effects of MDMA ('Ecstasy') on Human Sexual Function." *European Psychiatry* 16, no. 2 (2001): 127–30.

INDEX

2C-B, 238, 241
5-MeO-DMT, 95, 134
   integration theme of, 236–38
   overview of, 230–36
25I-NBOMe, 140

Aaliyah (case example), 115–17
acceptance, 41
accepting, 93–94
achievement, 16
agreeableness, 42
Aldridge, Alexandra, 200
amrita, 81
ancestors, 173, 210
Anderson, Frank, 38
Anderson, Katie, 245
Anslinger, Harry, 21
anti-narcotics ordinance, 20–21
anxiety, 10, 48
Aristotle, 286
arousal, 110–11
arousing experience, 114
art, 236–37
attachment theory, 67–68
attention, 46–47
attunement, 17
authoritarian guidelines, 44

autonomy, 189
awareness, 17, 47
ayahuasca, 44, 79, 92
   integration theme of, 212–14
   overview of, 207–12
Aztecs, 19–20, 215–16

bad trips, 173
Banisteriopsis caapi vine, 209–10
Barba, Tommaso, 195–99
Bathje, Geoff, 124
BDSM, 16, 70–73
Belser, Alex, 60–61, 182
Ben (case example), 49–50
Big Five personality domains, 42
Big Love, 287–88
biotech companies, 9
BIPOC people, 2. *See also* Black and Brown people; People of Color
birth control pill, 22
Black and Brown people, 2, 18, 21, 25, 60, 109, 114
bladder cystitis, 242
bliss. *See* pleasure
body, 55–56, 71, 78, 128–30, 135–36
body bliss, 121–22
Bøhling, Frederik, 13

borderline personality disorder, 111–13
boundaries, 44–45, 54–55, 66–67, 72, 180, 187–93
Bouso, José Carlos, 42
breathing, 129
Brennan, Bill, 182–84, 186, 188–89
Breuer, Josef, 106
Brotto, Lori, 46–47
Buddhism, 76, 177
Buffum, John, 203
Bufo Alvarius, 233–34

cannabis, 19, 21
capitalism, 16, 106
Carpenter, Erin, 107
Catholic Church, 19, 177, 216, 245
Cavnar, Clancy, 212
Celenza, Andrea, 178, 179
ceremony, 73
chacruna, 209–10
channeling, 36
Charcot, Jean-Martin, 165
Chavín de Huantar, 34
chemsex, 200
Chinese, 21
Christianity, 13–14, 80–81
client-driven service, 186
climate change, 4–5
clothing, 71–72
cocaine, 110
coffee, 13
Cognitive Behavioral Therapy, 86, 184
colonization, 19
community-oriented psychedelic spaces, 64–65
compassion, 55

complex post-traumatic stress disorder (C-PTSD), 105, 107–8, 111
confrontation, 171–72
connection, 42, 64–65, 68, 90, 96, 146–47, 229–30
connective emotional experiences, 93–94
conscientiousness, 42
conscious non-monogamy (CNM), 66
consent, 16, 54–55, 70, 71
containers, 16–17, 29, 81
controlled releases, 99
Controlled Substances Act of 1970, 11, 12
conversion therapy, 61–63
Cortez, Hernando, 216
countertransference, 180–84
couples, 10–11
  central themes of psychedelic use, 245–47
  ketamine and, 243–44
  psychedelic preparation for, 141–47
  psychedelic integration, 148–49
Coyote, Peter, 22
creativity, 8, 10, 221
Crowley, Aleister, 227
Crowley, Mike, 81
crystals, 137–38
curiosity, 8, 41

Dance Safe, 140
Davis, Wade, 234
Dawson, Alexander, 21
death, 210, 289
decision making, psychedelics and, 55
decommodified healing, 192
decriminalization, 10

Default Mode Network (DMN), 88–89
depression, 10, 48, 196–97
diet, 210
dignity, 41
DiPaolo, Miranda, 23
discernment, 212–14
discrimination, 15
distraction, 46–47
divergent thinking, 221
divination, 209
Divine, 7–8, 74, 136–38, 214
DMT, 209–10, 220, 231
Dolan, Gul, 134
dosage, 53
dual relationships, 189
Dubus, Zoë, 61
Durán, Diego, 19
Dymock, Alex, 200

Earp, Brian, 120
ego dissolution, 221–22, 289
EMBARK model, 182–83
embodiment, 18, 90, 114, 205–7
EMDR, 102, 166, 170–71
emotional connections, 67–68, 203–4
emotional first aid, 56
empathy, 43–45
Encountering Bliss, 246
Ens, Andrea, 62
entheogens, 80, 93
erotica, 17
erotic countertransference, 180–84
erotic identity, 43
erotic parts, 129–30
erotic play, 43
erotic shadows, 43
erotic transference, 180–84

erotic unwinding, 129
Espinoza, Yalila, 210, 214
ethical non-monogamy (ENM), 66
ethics, 18, 43–44
Eucharist, 80–81
Eve (personal narrative), 249–53
expansion, 236–38
extraversion, 42

false memories, 166
fantasy, 43
fatphobia, 30
fear, 69, 86–87, 213
Federal Bureau of Narcotics, 21
feeling, 91–92
felt sense, 79
Female Sexual Arousal Disorder, 240–41
fentanyl, 204
Fischer, Friederike Mickel, 241
Fisher, Janina, 29
flashbacks, 47, 236
Fotiou, Evgenia, 4
Free Love movement, 11, 19, 22–23, 65
Freud, Sigmund, 106, 165, 234, 240–41
frigidity, 239–40
fun, 13, 146–47

Gabbard, Glen, 178, 179
gender, 11, 18, 30, 41, 58, 135–36, 139, 188, 235–36
genderless God, 235
God, 75–76, 137, 235
Goldpaugh, Dee Dee, 1–5
  connecting with present moment, 32–38
  connection with grandmother, 30–31
  journey of healing trauma, 26–30

on modern Buddhism, 76–77
note on love, 288–90
personal experiences of, 169–70, 224–25, 228
sexual trauma and, 51
grief, 4–5
Grof, Stanislov, 61, 287
guides
boundaries and, 189
as perpetrators, 178–79
gurus, 76
Guss, Jeffrey, 87–89

Haines, Staci, 105
Hammers, Corie, 70–71
happiness, 16
harm reduction, 51, 72, 139–41, 220
Harner, Michael, 213
Hatsis, Tom, 217
healing. *See* sexual healing
healing in bliss, 6–8
Heffter, Arthur, 226
Herman, Judith, 106
heroic doses, 220
heroin, 110
Higher Power, 75–76, 173
hippies, 22
HIV, 44–45
Hofmann, Albert, 10, 234, 238
Holliday, Billie, 21
hooks, bell, 135–36
huachuma medicine, 32–38, 79, 224–29
Huxley, Aldous, 226–27
hysteria, 106

imagery, 236–37
Indigenous healers, 190, 208–9

Indigenous peoples, 4, 9–10, 11
inner children, 8
insecurity, 69
integration. *See* psychedelic integration
intentions, 127–28, 144, 145
Internal Family Systems (IFS), 103, 130, 171, 222
interracial sex, 11
intimacy, psychedelic, 246

Jake (personal narrative), 259–63
Jay, Mike, 226, 234
jealousy, 66–67
journaling, 97
joy, 7–8, 14, 33, 90, 96–97

Kabat-Zinn, Jon, 45–46
Keating, Ava, 60–61
ketamine, 87, 95, 238, 241–44
kindness, 45
kink, 16
Kleinplatz, Peggy, 48, 119, 121
Kolk, Bessel van der, 15
Kudowor, Mesphina, 124
kykeon, 80

Lafrance, Adele, 290–92
Leary, Timothy, 42, 61
Lee, Martin, 23
Letcher, Andy, 19
Levine, Nick, 70
Lewin, Louis, 226
LGBTQIA+, 108–9, 212
chemsex and, 200–201
defining, 57–58
queer identities, 57–65

life force, 8
life satisfaction, 10
life worth living, 146–47
living ritual, 125–27, 149
loneliness, 92–93, 170–71
Lorde, Audre, 230
love, 7–8, 45, 52, 66, 82–83
   author's note on, 288–90
   Big Love, 287–88
   boundlessness of psychedelic love, 294–96
   meaning of, 285–87
   universal love, 45, 290–94
Love Project, The, 290–92
low desire, 117, 118
LSD, 10–11, 19, 22, 87, 140
   erotic significance of, 238–41
   vilification of, 23–24

MacLean, Katherine, 42
magnificent sex, 119
Majeski, Eric, 124
Malena (personal narrative), 249–53
Manson Family, 23
MAOI, 209–10
Margolin, Leslie, 240
masculinity, 14
Mason, Natasha, 245
Masters, Robert Augustus, 101
Masters and Johnson, 46
masturbation, 111
Maté, Gabor, 113
Maya, 215–16
MDMA, 10–11, 24–25, 54, 87, 91, 134, 142
   integration theme of, 205–7
   overview of, 201–5

meaning making, 100–104
Mechen, Ben, 200
medical model, 182–83, 216–17, 228, 245
Meira, Shir (personal narrative), 263–67
memory, 161–73
memory reconsolidation, 162–63
Memory Wars, 165–66
Men of Color, 20
mescaline, 10, 34
   integration theme of, 229–30
   overview of, 224–29
microdosing, 9, 219
Miller, Timothy, 22
mindfulness, 10, 45–47, 221
MK-ULTRA, 218
Molly (case example), 161–64
monogamy, 54
moral decay, 19
morality, 14, 44
moral panic, 21
Morin, Jack, 44
Moser, Charles, 203
Moss, Thelma, 239
Most, Albert, 234
Moyle, Leah, 200
Muraresku, Brian C., 80
mushrooms, 6–7
mystical experiences, 77–78

narcissism, 178–79
narratives
   Charley and Shelley Wininger, 267–73
   David Ortmann, 273–84
   deconstructing, 100–104
   Eve, 249–53

Jake, 259–63
Malena and Øistein, 253–58
questioning, 133–35
Shir Meira, 263–67
Native American Church, 225
Native Americans, 21, 225
Natoli, Justin, 59–60, 64–65
Navigating Anxiety, 245–46
negative beliefs, 78–79, 102–3
Neubert, Jonas, 245
neurodiversity, 58
neuroplasticity, 87
neuroticism, 42, 220
Newland, Constance, 239
new relationship energy, 67
New World, 19–20, 216
Nixon, Richard Milhous, 18
noetic quality, 163
non-judgement, 220, 289
non-monogamy, 54, 65–70, 66
non-specific amplifiers, 287
Northrup, Laura Mae, 93–94, 107–8
North Star, 127–28
not knowing, 170
Nuwer, Rachel, 24

oceanic boundlessness, 78
Ogden, Gina, 73–74, 79
Øistein (personal narrative), 253–58
openness, 42, 220, 221
opium dens, 20–21
Oppenheim, Hermann, 105
Oppenheimer, Robert, 238–39
orgasm, 119, 240–41
Original Lover, 201–7
Ortmann, David, 273–84
Osmond, Humphry, 227

Palo Santo, 34
Parker, Quanah, 225
partner choice, 56–57
parts of self, 45, 103–4, 130, 138–39
Peluso, Daniela, 210
pelvic pain, 118
People of Color, 60, 109, 114
perpetrators, 56–57, 178–84
personality change, 41–49
perspective, 30–31, 94
peyote cactus, 10, 225–26
pharmacosex, 201
plant spirits, 79–80
Plato, 286
pleasure, 11
    as birthright, 45
    healing power of, 7–9, 104
    making space for, 132–33
    principle of, 13–18
    psychedelic research and, 12–13
    restoration of, 95–96
    returning to, 138–39
    war on, 18–26
political revolution, 11
Pollan, Michael, 216, 273
polyamory, psychedelics and, 65–70
polycules
    psychedelic integration, 148–49
    psychedelic preparation, 141–47
post-traumatic stress disorder
    (PTSD), 104–7
poverty, 14
power dynamics, 160–61, 187–93
predators, in psychedelic spaces,
    185–87
Predictive Processing, 88–89
presence, 14

projections, 190
prolactin, 204
Prolonged Exposure, 86
protective parts, 130
psilocybin mushrooms, 10–11,
    44–45, 79, 87, 92
  integration theme of, 222–24
  overview of, 215–22
Psychedelic Erotic, 295–96
psychedelic integration, 77–78, 123–25
  5-MeO-DMT and, 236–38
  case study of Valeria, 150–59
  for couples and polycules, 148–49
  for erotic enhancement, 132–41
  memories and, 170–72
  mescaline and, 229–30
  strategies for sexual trauma, 96–104
  themes of, 205–7, 212–14, 222–24, 229–30
psychedelic integration psychotherapy, 27–29
psychedelic intimacy, 246
psychedelic medicines. *See also specific substances*
  as helpers, 8
  overview of for sexual healing, 194–201
psychedelic preparation, 123–25
  case study of Valeria, 150–59
  for couples and polycules, 141–47
  for erotic enhancement, 127–32
Psychedelic Renaissance, 7
psychedelic research, 7, 11–12, 196–99
Psychedelic Sexuality
  boundlessness of psychedelic love, 294–96
  personality change, 41–49

polyamory and, 65–70
power of psychedelic love, 82–83
role of BDSM, 70–73
sex on psychedelics? 50–57
spirituality and, 73–81
vision of, 39–41
psychedelic spaces
  predators in, 185–87
  sexual harm in, 174–77
psychedelic world, end of, 8–13
psychonauts, 11–12
psychopathy, 178–79
PTSD, 172, 201–2
"public safety," 11
purging, 98–99
purification practice, 214
Puritanism, 13–14, 16
purity culture, 74

queer identities, psychedelics and, 57–65

radical monogamy, 70
Raul (case example), 162–63
reactivation, 236
recovered memories, 160–61
  example of Molly, 161–64
  example of Raul, 162–63
reenactments, 70–71
rejection, 43
relational violence, 8, 14, 29–30
releasing, 94–95
Reshaping Practices, 245–46
resilience, 108–13
Resnick, Stella, 16
responsibility, 45
restorative justice, 186–87
retreat centers, 220

Richter-Levin, Gal, 114
right sexual conduct, 44
Rinpoche, Chogyam Trungpa, 81
risk, 72
ritual, 73, 147
Rucker, James, 220

Sabina, Maria, 217–18
sacred sexuality, 74
Sacred Valley, Peru, 32–38
safety, 14, 16–17, 29
Sahagún, Bernardino de, 215–16
Sandi, Carmen, 114
San Pedro. *See* huachuma medicine
savoring, 14
Savulescu, Julian, 120
secure attachment, 67–69
self, 293–94
self-acceptance, 133, 212, 289
self as unknown, 102
self-blame, 102–3
self-control, 16
self-energy, 49
self-esteem, 114
self-knowledge, 145–46
self-perception, 114
self-rejection, 61
self-touch, 17
Sensate Focus, 46
sensation, 14
sensorimotor psychotherapy, 171
sensual pleasure, 17–18
sex. *See also* Psychedelic Sexuality
　optimal components of, 121–22
　research on frequency, 48
　sexual dysfunction, 117–20
sex positivity, 74–75

sex therapy, 46
sexual abandon, 19, 21
sexual abuse, 160–73, 178–84
sexual desires, 43
sexual dysfunction, 117–20, 198–99
sexual enhancement, 11
sexual ethics, 43–44, 49
sexual harm, 56–57, 174–77
sexual healing
　overview of psychedelics for, 194–201
　psychedelics and healing trauma, 86–91
　violence and, 84–86
sexuality. *See* Psychedelic Sexuality
sexual pleasure, 16–18
sexual satisfaction, 196–99
sexual trauma, 15, 86–87
　BDSM and, 70–73
　considerations for survivors, 131–32
　developing an expanded definition, 113–15
　history of, 106–8
　integration strategies, 96–104
　psychedelics and, 86–91, 172–73
　resilience of survivors, 108–13
　stages of healing, 91–96
sexual violence, 8, 84–86
shaking out, 99
shame, 18, 43, 61, 103, 109, 139
shapeshifting, 57
Shiva, 81
Shlain, Bruce, 23
Shulgin, Alexander "Sasha," 24–25, 201–2, 227, 241
Shulgin, Ann, 180
sober sitters, 220
Somatic Experiencing, 170–71

somatic work, 98–100
South America, 81
spiritual bypassing, 101, 136
spiritual growth, 11
spirituality, 73–81, 136–38
SSRIs, 86, 87, 119–20, 196–97
Stamets, Paul, 215–16
Stevens, Jay, 23
storyboards, 214
stress, 14, 48, 114
submission, 71
substance abuse, 109–10
suffering, 292
suffering pleasures, 72–73
Summer of Love, 22
surrender, 71, 222–24

tenderness, 45
therapy and therapists, 26–27, 178–79
toad, Sonoran, 233–34
transference, 180–84
transgender people, 59, 60, 109
trauma, 8, 10. *See also* sexual trauma
   author's journey with, 26–30
   brief history of, 104–8
   capacity for goodness, 33–34
   impact of everyday traumas, 115–17
   parts of self and, 103–4
   pleasure and, 15–16
   reprocessing, 100–104
   sexual abuse, 160–73
traumatic memories
   making sense of, 97–98
   reexperiencing of, 172–73
truffles, 220
Tukano, Daiara, 208–9

underground work, 11–12, 170, 190–92
Universal Consciousness, 75–76
universal love, 45, 290–94
untamed sexuality, 18

vaginal orgasm, 240–41
Valeria (case example), 150–59
veterans, 105–6
Vietnam War, 22–23
vocalization, 99
vulnerability, 145–46

Wagner, Anne, 142–43, 147
warm blanket, 92
War on Drugs, 12, 18–26
Wasson, R. Gordon, 217, 218
Weil, Andrew, 234
white women, 20
Wider Power, 75–76
Williams, Bert, 58–59, 65
Wininger, Charley, 267–73
Wininger, Shelley, 267–73
wisdom, 55, 67, 189
witches and witchcraft, 58
witnessing, 92–93
women, sexual autonomy and, 23
Woodruff, Eden, 217
World War II, 22

Yahuda, Rachel, 110–11
Yeats, W. B., 227
Young, Allan, 220

Zeff, Leo, 142

BOOKS OF RELATED INTEREST

Tantric Sex for Lovers
by Diana Richardson and Michael Richardson

In this boxed set, renowned tantric sex teachers Diana and Michael Richardson present practices to help couples enrich their sex life and relationship with the spiritual, healing power of sex. Includes three books: *Tantric Orgasm for Women*, *Tantric Sex for Men*, and *Slow Sex*.

Psychedelic Medicine
The Healing Powers of LSD, MDMA, Psilocybin, and Ayahuasca
by Dr. Richard Louis Miller

Embracing the revival of psychedelic research and the discovery of new therapeutic uses, Dr. Richard Louis Miller discusses what is happening today in psychedelic medicine—and what will happen in the future—with top researchers in this field, including Rick Doblin, Stanislav Grof, James Fadiman, Julie Holland, and Dennis McKenna.

The Neuroscience of Psychedelics
The Pharmacology of What Makes Us Human
by Genís Ona, PhD
Foreword by José Carlos Bouso, PhD

Longtime pharmacological researcher Genís Ona examines the main pharmacological properties of psychedelic substances, including LSD, DMT, psilocybin, ayahuasca, mescaline, ketamine, ibogaine, salvia, tropane alkaloids, and MDMA. Exploring how psychedelics work within the brain, Ona shares results from his extensive research to reveal the physiological mechanisms that allow these molecules to have their visionary effects.

 Scan the QR code and save 25% at InnerTraditions.com. Browse over 2,000 titles on spirituality, the occult, ancient mysteries, new science, holistic health, and natural medicine.

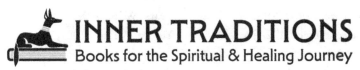

INNER TRADITIONS
Books for the Spiritual & Healing Journey

— SINCE 1975 • ROCHESTER, VERMONT —

InnerTraditions.com • (800) 246-8648